Contents

Preface to the second edition

It is hoped that this book will be of practical help to doctors and nurses confronted by typical management problems in the cardiac patient. As a practical guide it is necessarily dogmatic and much information is given in list format or in tables, especially in sections dealing with drug therapy.

Some subjects in cardiology are often not well covered in clinical training and it is intended that some sections will help fill any gaps in the doctors' or nurses' clinical course, e.g. sections on congenital heart disease, pacing, and cardiac investigations.

Practical procedures such as cardiac catheterisation cannot be learnt from a book and technical aspects of catheterisation are not covered here. However, interpretation of catheter laboratory data is discussed and it is hoped that the book will be of value to the doctor learning invasive cardiology. A practical subject like echocardiography cannot be covered in depth in a book of this size, but the fundamentals and common cardiac conditions are discussed.

Since the publication of the first edition there have been enormous advances in many aspects of cardiology, particularly in the management of ischaemic heart disease. New sections include thrombolysis, percutaneous transluminal coronary angioplasty, management of hyperlipidaemias, Doppler echocardiography, plus advances in pacing and electrophysiology. The sections dealing with drug therapy have been up-dated and the discussion of calcium antagonists and ACE inhibitors extensively revised. The chapter on congenital heart disease now includes a section on management problems of cyanotic congenital heart disease in the adult.

Nuclear cardiology has not been included. It is a vital and growing branch of cardiology but the subject cannot be covered without including many colour diagrams and pictures. This would greatly increase the expense of the book, and I have reluctantly decided to exclude it.

POCKET CONSULTANT

Cardiology

R.H. Swanton
MA, MD, FRCP
Consultant Cardiologist
The Middlesex Hospital
Mortimer Street
London W1N 8AA

SECOND EDITION

Blackwell Scientific Publications
OXFORD LONDON EDINBURGH
BOSTON MELBOURNE

Editorial offices:
Osney Mead, Oxford OX2 0EL
(*Orders:* Tel: 0865 240201)
25 John Street, London WC1N 2BL
23 Ainslie Place, Edinburgh EH3 6AJ
3 Cambridge Center, Suite 208
Cambridge, Massachusetts 02142, USA
107 Barry Street, Carlton
Victoria 3053, Australia

First published 1984
Italian edition 1986
Reprinted 1986
Second edition 1989
Italian edition in preparation
Reprinted 1990

Set by Times Graphics, Singapore
Printed and bound in Great Britain by
The Alden Press, Oxford

DISTRIBUTORS

Marston Book Services Ltd
PO Box 87
Oxford OX2 0DT
(*orders*: Tel. 0865 791155
Fax: 0865 791927
Telex: 837515)

USA
Year Book Medical Publishers
200 North LaSalle Street
Chicago, Illinois 60601
(*Orders:* Tel: (312) 726-9733)

Canada
The C.V. Mosby Company
5240 Finch Avenue East
Scarborough, Ontario
(*Orders:* Tel: (416) 298-1588)

Australia
Blackwell Scientific Publications (Australia) Pty Ltd
107 Barry Street
Carlton, Victoria 3053
(*Orders:* Tel: (03) 347-0300)

British Library
Cataloguing in Publication Data

Swanton, Robert Howard
Cardiology—2nd ed.
(Pocket consultant)
1. Man. Heart. Diseases
I. Title
616.1′2

ISBN 0-632-02044-X

Acknowledgements

I would like to thank my wife Lindsay and my secretaries Mrs Evelyn Beinart and Mrs Jane West for their enormous help in typing the manuscript.

The work of a large number of authors has contributed to the body of knowledge in this book and it would be impossible to thank them individually or to provide detailed references to their work in a pocket book. The list of further reading incorporates references and my thanks to them all. My thanks also to my many colleagues who have helped with suggestions and alterations. I am also indebted to Dr R. Sutton and Medtronic Ltd for permission to modify their pacing code diagrams and to Dr P.E. Gower for permission to include the nomogram for body surface area.

Acknowledgements

1 Cardiac symptoms and physical signs

1.1 Common cardiac symptoms

Angina

Typical angina presents as a chest tightness or heaviness brought on by effort and relieved by rest. The sensation starts in the retrosternal region and radiates across the chest. Frequently it is associated with a leaden feeling in the arms. Occasionally it may present in more unusual sites, e.g. pain in the jaws or teeth on effort, without pain in the chest. It may be confused with oesophageal pain, or may present as epigastric or even hypochondrial pain. The most important feature is its relation to effort. Unilateral chest pain (submammary) is not usually cardiac pain, which is generally symmetrical in distribution.

Angina is typically exacerbated by heavy meals, cold weather (just breathing in cold air is enough) and emotional disturbances. Arguments with colleagues or family and watching exciting television are typical precipitating factors.

Stable angina

Angina induced by effort and relieved by rest. Not increasing in frequency or severity, and predictable in nature. Associated with ST segment depression on ECG.

Decubitus angina

Angina induced by lying down at night or during sleep. It may be due to an increase in LVEDV (and hence wall stress) on lying flat, associated with dreaming, or getting into cold in sheets. Coronary spasm may occur in REM sleep. It may respond to a diuretic or calcium antagonist taken in the evening.

Unstable (crescendo) angina

Angina of increasing frequency and severity. Not only induced by effort but coming on unpredictably at rest. It may progress to myocardial infarction.

Variant angina (Prinzmetal angina)
Angina occurring unpredictably at rest associated with transient ST segment elevation on the ECG. It is not common. It is associated with coronary spasm often in the presence of additional arteriosclerotic lesions.

Other types of retrosternal pain

- *pericardial pain* is described in **7.1**. It is usually retrosternal or epigastric, lasts much longer than angina and is often stabbing in quality. It Is related to respiration and posture (relieved by sitting forward). Diaphragmatic pericardial pain may be referred to the left shoulder.
- *aortic pain* (p. 369). Acute dissection produces a sudden tearing intense pain retrosternally radiating to the back. Its radiation depends on the vessels involved. Aortic aneurysms produce chronic pain especially if rib or vertebral column erosion occurs.
- *non-cardiac pain*. May be oesophageal or mediastinal with similar distribution to cardiac pain but not provoked by effort. Oesophageal pain may be provoked by ergonovine, making it a useless test for coronary spasm. Chest wall pain is usually unilateral. Stomach and gall bladder pain may be epigastric and lower sternal and be confused with cardiac pain.

Dyspnoea
An abnormal sensation of breathlessness on effort or at rest. With increasing disability orthopnoea and paroxysmal nocturnal dyspnoea (PND) occur. Pulmonary oedema is not the only cause of waking breathless at night: it may occur in non-cardiac asthma. A dry nocturnal cough is often a sign of impending PND. With acute pulmonary oedema pink frothy sputum and streaky haemoptysis occur. With poor LV function Cheyne – Stokes ventilation makes the patient feel dyspnoeic in the fast cycle phase.

1 Cardiac symptoms and physical signs

1.1 Common cardiac symptoms

Effort tolerance is graded by New York Heart Association criteria as follows:

Class 1
Patients with cardiac disease but without resulting limitations of physical activity. Ordinary physical activity does not cause undue fatigue, palpitation or angina.

Class 2
Patients with cardiac disease resulting in slight limitation of physical activity. They are comfortable at rest. Ordinary physical activity results in fatigue, palpitation, dyspnoea or angina (e.g. walking up two flights stairs, carrying shopping basket, making beds, etc.). By limiting physical activity patients can still lead a normal social life.

Class 3
Patients with cardiac disease resulting in marked limitation of physical activity. They are comfortable at rest, but even mild physical activity causes fatigue, palpitation, dyspnoea or angina (e.g. walking slowly on the flat). Cannot do any shopping or housework.

Class 4
Patients with cardiac disease who are unable to do any physical activity without symptoms. Angina or heart failure may be present at rest. They are virtually confined to bed or a chair and are totally incapacitated.

Syncope
Syncope may be due to several causes.
• *vasovagal* (vasomotor, simple faint) is the commonest cause. Sudden dilation of venous capacitance vessels associated with vagal-induced bradycardia. Induced by pain, fear, emotion.

1.1 Common cardiac symptoms

• *postural hypotension*. Usually drug induced (by vasodilators). May occur in true salt depletion (by diuretics) or hypovolaemia.
• *carotid sinus syncope*. A rare condition with hypersensitive carotid sinus stimulation (e.g. by tight collars) inducing severe bradycardia.
• *cardiac dysrhythmias*. Commonest causes are sinus arrest, complete AV block, ventricular tachycardia. 24-hour ECG monitoring is necessary.
• *obstructing lesions*. Aortic or pulmonary stenosis, left atrial myxoma or ball valve thrombus, HOCM, massive pulmonary embolism. Effort syncope is commonly secondary to aortic valve or subvalve stenosis in adults and Fallot's tetralogy in children.
• *cerebral causes*. Sudden hypoxia, transient cerebral arterial obstruction, spasm or embolism.
• *cough syncope*. This may be due to temporarily obstructed cerebral venous return.
• *micturition syncope*. This often occurs at night, and sometimes in men with prostatic symptoms. It may be in part due to vagal overactivity and partly due to postural hypotension.

The commonest differential diagnosis needed is sudden syncope In the adult with no apparent cause. Stokes–Adams attacks and epilepsy are the main contenders.

Stokes–Adams attacks	**Epilepsy**
No aura or warning	Aura often present
Transient unconsciousness (often only a few seconds)	More prolonged unconsciousness
Very pale during attack	Tonic/clonic phases
Rapid recovery	Prolonged recovery. Very drowsy
Hot flush on recovery	Absent

A prolonged Stokes–Adams episode may produce an epileptiform attack from cerebral hypoxia. It is not always possible to distinguish the two clinically.

1 Cardiac symptoms and physical signs

1.1 Common cardiac symptoms

Cyanosis

Central cyanosis should be detectable when arterial saturation is less than 85% and when there is more than 5g reduced haemoglobin present. It is more difficult to detect if the patient is also anaemic. Cardiac cyanosis may be caused by poor pulmonary blood flow (e.g. Pulmonary atresia), by right-to-left shunting (e.g. Fallot's tetralogy) or common mixing situations with high pulmonary blood flow (e.g. TAPVD).

Cyanosis from pulmonary causes should be improved by increasing the FiO_2. This will not affect cyanosis from cardiac causes and is a useful test in the cyanosed neonate.

Peripheral cyanosis in the absence of central cyanosis may be due to peripheral vasoconstriction, poor cardiac output or peripheral sludging of red cells (e.g. polycythaemia).

Embolism

Both systemic and pulmonary embolism are common in cardiac disease. Predisposing factors in cardiology are:

Pulmonary emboli	Systemic emboli
Prolonged bed rest	Aortic stenosis (calcium)
High venous pressure	HOCM
Central lines	Mitral stenosis in AF
Femoral vein catheterisation	Infective endocarditis
Pelvic disease (tumour, inflammation)	LA myxoma
Tricuspid endocarditis	Prosthetic aortic or mitral valves
Deep vein thrombosis	Closed mitral valvotomy with a calcified valve (calcium)

Either or both

Myocardial infarction
Dilated cardiomyopathy
CCF
Polycythaemia
Diuretics
Pro-coagulable state
Eosinophilic heart disease

1 Cardiac symptoms and physical signs

1.1 Common cardiac symptoms

Oedema

Factors important in cardiac disease are: elevated venous pressure (CCF, pericardial constriction), increased extracellular volume (salt and water retention), secondary hyperaldosteronism, hypoalbuminaemia (liver congestion, anorexia and poor diet), venous disease and secondary renal failure.

Acute oedema and ascites may develop in pericardial constriction. Protein losing enteropathy can occur with a prolonged high venous pressure exacerbating the oedema.

Other symptoms

These are discussed under relevant chapters:
Palpitation: Principles of paroxysmal tachycardia diagnosis **6.10**.
Haemoptysis: Mitral stenosis **3.1**.
Cyanotic attack: Catheter complications **10.3**.

1.2 Physical examination

Hands

It is important to check for:

- dilated hand veins with CO_2 retention
- temperature (? cool periphery with poor flows, hyperdynamic circulation)
- peripheral cyanosis
- clubbing: cyanotic congenital heart disease, infective endocarditis
- capillary pulsation; aortic regurgitation, PDA
- Osler's nodes, Janeway lesions, splinter haemorrhages: infective endocarditis
- nail fold telangiectases: collagen vascular disease
- arachnodactyly: Marfan syndrome
- polydactyly, syndactyly, triphalangeal thumbs: ASD
- tendon xanthomata

Facial and general appearance

Down's syndrome (AV canal), elf-like facies (supravalvar aortic stenosis), Turner's (coarction, AS), moon-like plump facies (pulmonary stenosis), Noonan's syndrome (pulmonary stenosis, peripheral pulmonary artery stenosis)
Mitral facies with pulmonary hypertension
Central cyanosis.
Differential cyanosis in PDA + Pulmonary hypertension or interrupted aortic arch
Xanthelasma
Teeth: must be checked as part of general CVS examination
Dysphoea at rest. ? Accessory muscles of respiration

Jugular venous pulse (JVP)

Waveform examples are shown in Fig. 1.1. It should fall on inspiration. Inspiratory filling of the neck veins occurs in pericardial constriction (Kussmaul's sign). The waves produced are as follows:

'a' wave. Atrial systole. It occurs just before the carotid pulse. It is lost in AF. Large 'a' waves indicate a raised RVEDP (e.g. PS. PHT). Cannon 'a' waves occur in: junctional tachycardia, complete AV block, ventricular ectopics (atrial systole against a closed tricuspid valve).

'c' wave. Not visible with the naked eye. Effect of tricuspid valve closure on atrial pressure.

'x' descent. Fall in atrial pressure during ventricular systole due to downward movement of base of heart.

'v' wave. Atrial filling against a closed tricuspid valve.

'y' descent. Diastolic collapse following tricuspid valve opening.

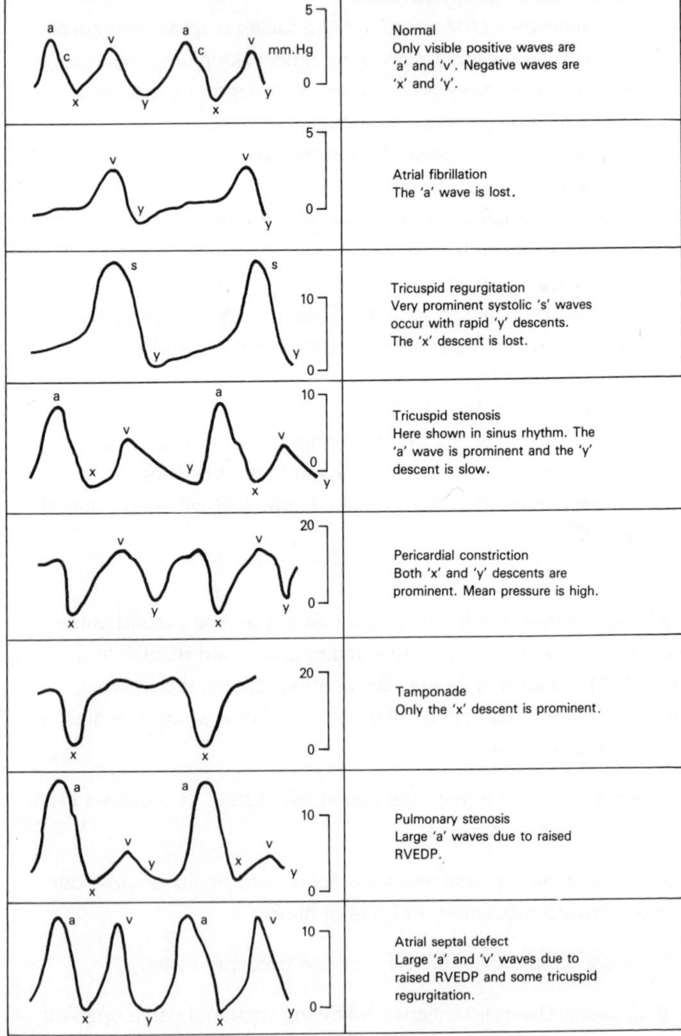

Normal
Only visible positive waves are 'a' and 'v'. Negative waves are 'x' and 'y'.
Atrial fibrillation
The 'a' wave is lost.
Tricuspid regurgitation
Very prominent systolic 's' waves occur with rapid 'y' descents. The 'x' descent is lost.
Tricuspid stenosis
Here shown in sinus rhythm. The 'a' wave is prominent and the 'y' descent is slow.
Pericardial constriction
Both 'x' and 'y' descents are prominent. Mean pressure is high.
Tamponade
Only the 'x' descent is prominent.
Pulmonary stenosis
Large 'a' waves due to raised RVEDP.
Atrial septal defect
Large 'a' and 'v' waves due to raised RVEDP and some tricuspid regurgitation.

Fig. 1.1 Examples of waveforms seen on jugular venous pulse.

's' wave occurs in tricuspid regurgitation. Fusion of 'x' descent and 'v' wave into a large systolic pulsation with rapid 'y' descent.

The normal range of jugular venous pressure is −7 to +3 mmHg. The patient sits at 45° and sternal angle is used as a reference point. Distinction of the JVP from the carotid pulse involves the following 5 features: timing, the ability to compress and obliterate the JVP, the demonstration of hepatojugular reflux, the alteration of the JVP with position and the site of the pulsation itself.

The carotid pulse

Waveform examples are shown in Fig. 1.2. There are three components to the carotid pulse: percussion wave, tidal wave and dicrotic notch.

Percussion wave: a shock wave transmitted up the elastic walls of the arteries. *Tidal wave*: reflection of the percussion wave with forward moving column of blood. It follows the percussion wave and is not usually palpable separately. *Dicrotic notch* times with aortic valve closure.

All the pulses are felt: radials and femorals simultaneously (coarctation). Any pulse may disappear with dissection of the aorta. Right arm and carotid pulses area stronger than left in supra-valve aortic stenosis p. 94).

Palpation

This checks for: thrills, apex beat, abnormal pulsation, and palpable sounds. Systolic thrill in the aortic area suggests aortic stenosis. Feel for thrills in other sites:

Left sternal edge: VSD or HOCM.

Apex: ruptured mitral chordae.

Pulmonary area: Pulmonary stenosis.

Subclavicular area: subclavian artery stenosis.

Diastolic thrills are less common: Feel for apical diastolic thrill in mitral stenosis with patient lying on left side and breath held

1.2 Physical examination

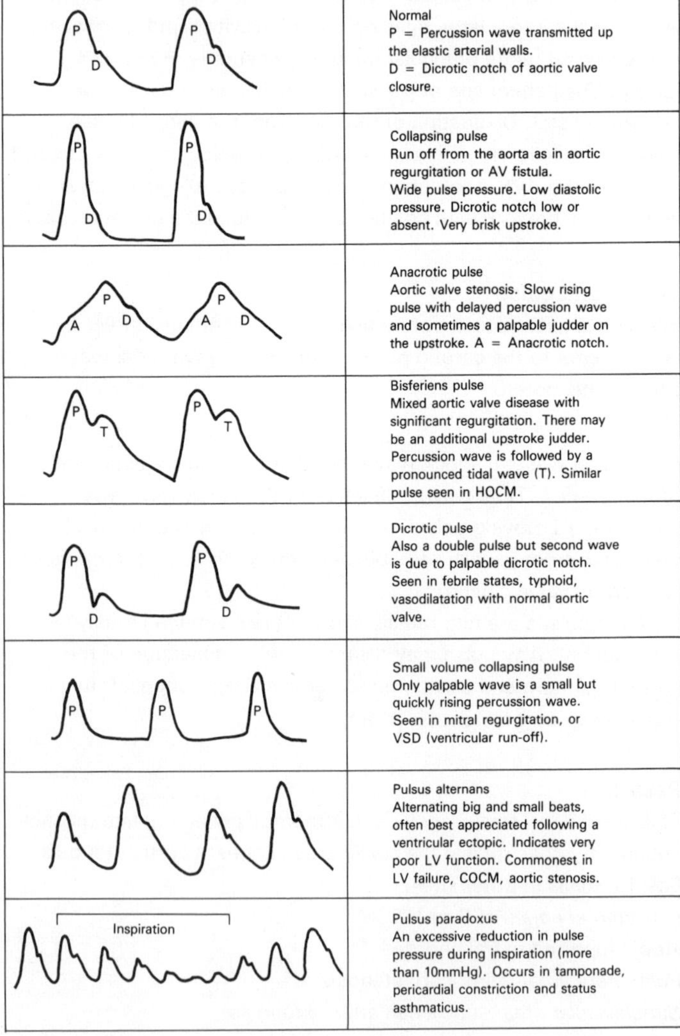

P
D
Normal
P = Percussion wave transmitted up the elastic arterial walls.
D = Dicrotic notch of aortic valve closure.
Collapsing pulse
Run off from the aorta as in aortic regurgitation or AV fistula.
Wide pulse pressure. Low diastolic pressure. Dicrotic notch low or absent. Very brisk upstroke.
A
Anacrotic pulse
Aortic valve stenosis. Slow rising pulse with delayed percussion wave and sometimes a palpable judder on the upstroke. A = Anacrotic notch.
T
Bisferiens pulse
Mixed aortic valve disease with significant regurgitation. There may be an additional upstroke judder. Percussion wave is followed by a pronounced tidal wave (T). Similar pulse seen in HOCM.
Dicrotic pulse
Also a double pulse but second wave is due to palpable dicrotic notch. Seen in febrile states, typhoid, vasodilatation with normal aortic valve.
Small volume collapsing pulse
Only palpable wave is a small but quickly rising percussion wave. Seen in mitral regurgitation, or VSD (ventricular run-off).
Pulsus alternans
Alternating big and small beats, often best appreciated following a ventricular ectopic. Indicates very poor LV function. Commonest in LV failure, COCM, aortic stenosis.
Inspiration
Pulsus paradoxus
An excessive reduction in pulse pressure during inspiration (more than 10mmHg). Occurs in tamponade, pericardial constriction and status asthmaticus.

Fig. 1.2 Examples of carotid pulse waveforms.

in expiration. Left sternal edge diastolic thrill occasionally in aortic regurgitation .

Apex beat and cardiac pulsations
Heart is displaced, not enlarged (e.g. scoliosis, pectus excavatum)?

Normal apex beat is in the 5th left intercostal space in the mid-clavicular line. It is palpable but does not lift the finger off the chest. In abnormal states distinguish between:

- Normal site but thrusting, e.g. HOCM, pure aortic stenosis, hypertension, all with good LV.
- Laterally displaced and hyperdynamic, e.g. mitral and/or aortic regurgitation, VSD.
- Laterally displaced but diffuse, e.g. COCM, LV failure.
- High dyskinetic apex, e.g. LV aneurysm.
- Double apex (enhanced by 'a' wave), in HOCM, hypertension.
- Left parasternal heave: RV hypertrophy, e.g. pulmonary stenosis, cor pulmonale, ASD.
- Dextrocardia with apex in 5th right intercostal space.

Abnormal pulsations are very variable, e.g. ascending aortic aneurysm pulsating in aortic area, RVOT aneurysm in pulmonary area, collateral pulsation round the back in coarctation. Pulsatile RVOT in ASD.

Palpable heart sounds represent forceful valve closure, or valve situated close to the chest wall, e.g. palpable S_1 (mitral closure) in mitral stenosis; P_2 in pulmonary hypertension; A_2 in transposition; both S_1 and S_2 in thin patients with tachycardia.

1.3 Auscultation

Heart sounds

First and second heart sounds are produced by valve closure. Mitral (M_1) and aortic (A_2) are louder than and precede tricuspid (T_1) and pulmonary (P_2). Inspiration widens the split.
Widely split second sound in mitral regurgitation and VSD is due

1.3 Auscultation

First sound (S_1) = $M_1 + T_1$

Loud	Soft	Variable	Widely split
Short PR interval	Long PR interval	3° AV block	RBBB
Tachycardia	Heart block	AF	LBBB
Mitral stenosis	Delayed ventricular contraction (e.g. AS, infarction)	Nodal tachycardia or VT	VPBs VT

Second sound (S_2) = $A_2 + P_2$

Loud A_2	Widely split	Reversed split	Single
Tachycardia	RBBB	LBBB	Fallot
Hypertension	PS (soft P_2)	Aortic stenosis	Severe PS Severe AS
Transposition	Deep inspiration Mitral regurgitation VSD	PDA	Pulmonary atresia Eisenmenger Large VSD Hypertension
Loud P_2	**Fixed split**		
PHT	ASD		

to early ventricular emptying and consequent early aortic valve closure. However the widely split sound is rarely heard as the loud pan-systolic murmur usually obscures it.

Third sound (S_3)

This is pathological over the age of 30 years. It is thought to be produced by rapid LV filling, but the exact source is still debated. Loud S_3 occurs in a dilated LV with rapid early filling (mitral regurgitation, VSD) and is followed by a flow murmur. It also occurs in a dilated LV with high LVEDP and poor function (post infarction, COCM). A higher pitched early S_3 occurs in restrictive cardiomyopathy and pericardial constriction.

Fourth sound (S_4)

The atrial sound not normally audible but is produced at end diastole (just before S_1) with a high end-diastolic pressure or with a long PR interval. It disappears in AF. It is commonest in systemic hypertension, aortic stenosis, HOCM (LV.S_4) or pulmonary stenosis (RV.S_4).

Triple rhythm

A triple/gallop rhythm is normal in children and young adults but is usually pathological over the age of 30 years. S_3 and S_4 are summated in SR with a tachycardia.

S_3 and S_4 are low pitched sounds. Use the bell of the stethoscope and touch the chest lightly.

Added sounds

Ejection sound. In bicuspid aortic or pulmonary valve (not calcified) i.e. young patients.

Mid systolic click. Mitral leaflet prolapse.

Opening snap, mitral. Rarely tricuspid (TS, ASD, Ebstein).

Pericardial clicks (related to posture).

Innocent murmurs

Very common in children and young adults. Usually a pulmonary flow murmur heard at left sternal edge radiating into pulmonary area.

Characteristics of innocent murmur

- ejection systolic. Diastolic or pan systolic murmurs are pathological. The only exceptions are a venous hum or mammary souffle
- no palpable thrill

- no added sounds (e.g. ejection click)
- no signs of cardiac enlargement
- left sternal edge to pulmonary area. May be heard at apex
- normal ECG. CXR or echocardiogram may be necessary for confirmation

The venous hum is a continuous murmur, common in children, reduced by neck vein compression, turning the head laterally, bending the elbows back or lying down. They are loudest in the neck and around the clavicles. They may reappear in pregnancy.

Pathological murmurs

These are organic (valve or subvalve lesion) or functional (increased flow, dilated valve rings, etc.). They are discussed under individual conditions in subsequent chapters.

They should be graded as just audible, soft, moderate or loud. Grading on a 1–6 basis is unnecessary and unhelpful. The murmur should also be classified as to site, radiation, timing (systolic or diastolic, and which part of each), and behaviour with respiration and position. Many murmurs can be accentuated with effort. Alteration of the murmur with position (e.g. squatting) is important in HOCM, mitral prolapse and Fallot's tetralogy. The quality of the murmur itself should also be described, e.g. low or high pitched, rasping, musical, or honking in quality.

Some systolic murmurs can be accentuated by particular manoeuvres. Pansystolic murmur of VSD and mitral regurgitation are increased by hand grip, and decreased by amyl nitrate inhalation. The systolic murmur of hypertrophic obstructive cardiomyopathy is typically accentuated during the valsalva manoeuvre and by standing suddenly from a squatting position. The murmur in HOCM is reduced by passive leg elevation, hand grip, and by squatting from a standing position. (See **4.2**, p. 117.)

2 Congenital heart disease

2 Congenital heart disease

Congenital heart disease occurs in approximately 8 per 1000 live births. Although divided into cyanotic and acyanotic, there are several conditions which start acyanotic and become cyanotic with time, e.g. Fallot's tetralogy, Ebstein's anomaly, and left-to-right shunts developing the Eisenmenger syndrome.

The table below shows the commonest lesions presenting as a neonate and those presenting in the infant and older child.

Most congenital heart disease should be detected by a good neonatal examination or at a 6 week check-up.

	Neonate	**Infant and older child**
Cyanotic	TGA	TGA
	Tricuspid atresia	Fallot's tetralogy
	Obstructed TAPVD	
	Severe PS	
	Pulmonary atresia	
	Severe Ebstein with ASD	
	Hypoplastic left heart	
Acyanotic	Congenital aortic stenosis	VSD
	Coarctation + VSD/PDA	ASD
		PDA
		Congenital aortic stenosis
		Coarctation
		Pulmonary stenosis
		Partial APVD + ASD

Cyanotic congenital heart disease

The table overleaf shows the cyanotic group divided into those conditions with pulmonary plethora or oligaemia, and those with LV or RV hypertrophy.

The addition of pulmonary stenosis to a lesion causes oligaemic lung fields and RV hypertrophy.

Pulmonary plethora	Pulmonary oligaemia
TGA	Fallot's tetralogy
Single atrium	DORV + PS
AV canal	Single ventricle + PS
Truncus arteriosus	Ebstein + PS + ASD
TAPVD	Pulmonary atresia with poor collaterals
DORV	
Primitive ventricle	
Tricuspid atresia with no PS	

With RV hypertrophy	With LV hypertrophy
Fallot's tetralogy	Tricuspid atresia
DORV + PS	Pulmonary atresia with no VSD
Single ventricle + PS/ Sub PS	Single ventricle
TGA + PS (LVOT obstruction)	
Pulmonary atresia + VSD	
TAPVD	
Severe pulmonary stenosis	

2.1 Ventricular septal defect (VSD)

The most common congenital heart lesion is an isolated VSD (2 per 1000 births). It also occurs as part of more complex lesions, e.g.

Fallot's tetralogy DORV Truncus arteriosus	VSD an integral part of the syndrome
Tricuspid atresia Pulmonary atresia TGA Coarctation	often associated with a VSD

2 Congenital heart disease

2.1 Ventricular septal defect

Pathophysiology and symptoms

The immediate effects of a VSD in the neonate depend on its size and the pulmonary vascular resistance (PVR). The site of the VSD becomes important later.

As the PVR falls in the first few days of life, and RV pressure falls below systemic LV pressure, the VSD results in a gradually increasing left-to-right shunt. If the defect is large (> 1 cm^2/m^2 body surface area) the PVR does not fall with the large L → R shunt. The neonatal LV cannot cope with the large volume load and pulmonary oedema develops. There are the typical features of heart failure in infancy:

- tachypnoea
- failure to thrive. Feeding difficulties. Failure to suck adequately
- sweating on feeding
- intercostal recession (increased respiratory work with stiff lungs)
- hepatomegaly

Persisting high pulmonary blood flow results in frequent chest infections, retarded growth and chronic ill health in the untreated case.

Irreversible pulmonary changes start from about the age of 1 year with initial hypertrophy and secondary thrombotic obstruction of pulmonary arterioles.

Physical signs

These are summarised in the next table. Cases in which the VSD murmur is not pansystolic are either very small or very large. With increasing defect size biventricular hypertrophy is evident both clinically and on the ECG. With shunt reversal and pulmonary hypertension at systemic levels, right sided signs are prominent and the murmurs are softer or disappear.

Cardiomegaly and enlargement of the PA conus are not as great as in ASD, except in infants with big shunts.

The second sound in very small VSDs is normal. A_2 is

Grades of ventricular septal defect

Size	Very small	Small	Moderate	Large	Eisenmenger
Thrill	No	Yes	Yes	Yes	No
Murmur and site	Early ejection systolic LSE only	Loud pansystolic LSE→Apex and PA	As in small, but additional mitral diastolic at apex	Pansystolic decrescendo to S_2. Pulmonary ejection systolic + click Possible pulmonary regurgitation	None at LSE. Ejection systolic. PA (soft) + pulmonary regurgitation
Apex	Normal	Normal or LV + slight	LV + RV + slight	LV + RV +	RV + + PA palpable
S_2	Normal. A_2 easily heard	A_2 obscured by murmur, but S_2 split on inspiration	Obscured by murmur	A_2 obscured. P_2 may be loud	Loud single palpable S_2

ECG	Normal	Normal	LV + LA + LAD	LV + LA + RV +	RV + RA + RAD
CxR	Normal	Normal heart size Mild pulmonary plethora	Slight cardiomegaly PA +. Pulmonary plethora	Cardiomegaly (both ventricles). Large PAs. Pulmonary plethora	Large PAs. No plethora. Peripheral pruning
Differential diagnosis	Mild AS or sub-AS. Mild PS or infundibular PS	MR. TR. HOCM. Pulmonary stenosis	MR. TR. Pulmonary stenosis	Severe MR. Mixed AVD	Eisenmenger ASD. PDA, etc.
Prognosis or treatment	Spontaneous closure	Probable spontaneous closure. Observe	Surgery	Surgery	Medical treatment

Antibiotic prophylaxis (dental procedures, etc.) for all grades

obscured by the pansystolic murmur of larger defects, and with equal ventricular pressures S_2 is single.

Spontaneous closure
This occurs in 30–30% of VSDs. It is common in muscular defects, or defects of the membranous septum. It does not occur in defects adjacent to valves, in infundibular (supra-cristal) defects, in AV canal type defects, or in malalignment defects.

Sites of VSD

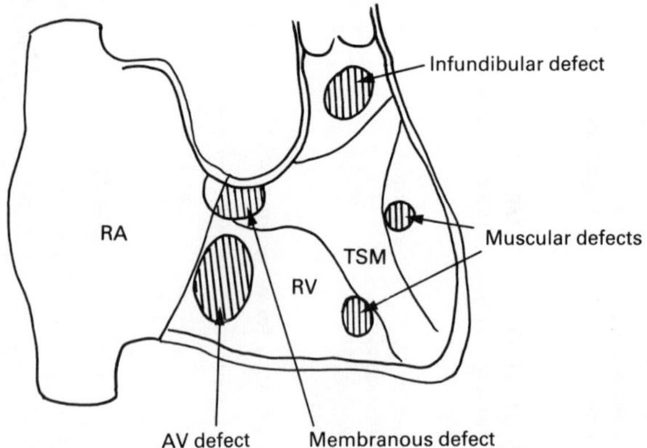

Ventricular septal defects and left ventricular angiography

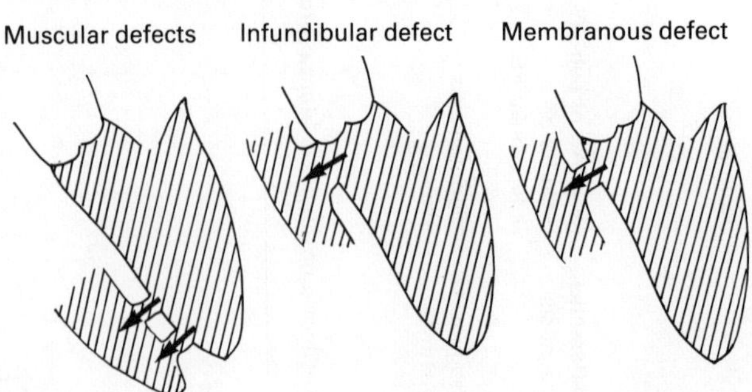

2 Congenital heart disease

2.1 Ventricular septal defect

Fig. 2.1 shows the four common sites simplified.

- Membranous (infracristal). The commonest, just behind the medial papillary muscle of the tricuspid valve which may oppose it and help to close it spontaneously. On closure an aneurysm of the membranous septum may occur.
- Muscular. Variable in site and may be multiple. Acquired muscular VSD after septal infarction is usually of the Swiss-cheese-type.
- Posterior (AV defect). Paratricuspid defect similar to the site of a VSD in AV canal defect, but this VSD may be present with normal AV valves: 'inlet' VSD.
- Infundibular ('supracristal'). A high VSD just beneath the pulmonary valve and below the right coronary cusp of the aortic valve. This may be inadequately supported and prolapse causing aortic regurgitation. This VSD does not close spontaneously.

The infundibular VSD may be associated with malalignment of the infundibular septum, e.g.

VSD + shift of septum to right: Fallot's tetralogy

VSD + shift of septum to left: Double outlet LV with subaortic stenosis

Cardiac catheterisation

Confirms a step up in O_2 saturation in the RV and can quantitate the L → R shunt. LV cines in the 45° and 60° LAO views visualise the interventricular septum with head up tilt. Aortography checks aortic valve competence and excludes PDA or coarctation. RV angiography checks the RVOT. The site of

---

◀ **Fig. 2.1** (opposite) Ventricular septal defect. The sites of the four common VSDs are shown. TSM = trabecula septomarginalis. The bottom panel shows an LV cineangiogram diagrammatically in the 45° LAO projection with 30° craniocaudal tilt. Muscular VSDs tend to be low in the septum and are often multiple. The infundibular defect is immediately subaortic. The membranous defect tends to be a more discrete jet with a small gap between the jet and the aortic valve.

the VSD can be diagnosed at catheter. Muscular VSDs are usually lower in the septum and may be multiple. The infundibular VSD is high, immediately subaortic and there is no gap between the aortic valve and the VSD jet (Fig.2.1). The membranous VSD is usually a discrete jet with a slight gap between the jet and the aortic valve (Fig. 2.1).

Complications of VSD

• Aortic regurgitation. Occurs in about 5% of VSDs. It may occur with membranous (infra-cristal) or infundibular (supra-cristal) defects. The right coronary cusp is unsupported in the infundibular defect and often prolapses into or through the VSD obscuring it on angiography. With membranous defects the non-coronary cusp may also be involved.

• *Infundibular stenosis*. Muscular infundibular obstruction develops in about 5% of VSDs and is progressive—commoner in older patients, and those who have had pulmonary artery banding. Infundibular stenosis improves flooded lungs, but causes shunt reversal and cyanosis.

• *Infective endocarditis*. Possible with any VSD. All should have antibiotic prophylaxis for dental procedures, etc.

• *Pulmonary hypertension*. VSD is the commonest cause of hyperkinetic pulmonary hypertension (large PAs on the CxR and pulmonary plethora). Calculation of pulmonary vascular resistance at catheter is important as this gradually rises as irreversible intimal hypertrophy develops without causing much change on the chest x-ray.

Associated lesions

• AV canal or simple secundum ASD (see ASDs)

• aortic regurgitation (see above)

• PDA. A common association (10% of VSDs). The early diastolic murmur heard in the left upper chest may be confused with aortic or pulmonary regurgitation. Aortography is mandatory in VSDs

• pulmonary stenosis: Valvar (congenital), infundibular (congenital or acquired). The effects depend on the size of the VSD, the severity of the pulmonary stenosis and the systemic vascular resistance. With mild PS a left-to-right shunt persists. If PS is severe and the VSD small the condition mimics severe PS alone. If PS is severe and the VSD large right-to-left shunting occurs (effects similar to Fallot's tetralogy)
• coarctation
• TGA, or corrected transposition
• more complex lesions: DORV, DOLV, truncus arteriosus, tricuspid atresia
• Gerbode defect. Left ventricular to right atrial shunt. Either direct or through the membranous septum first to RV, then to RA via tricuspid regurgitation

Management

In infancy medical management is with digoxin and diuretics in an attempt to hold the situation. With large defects the baby is catheterised early with a view to surgery at about 3 months if the baby is failing to thrive on medical treatment. The VSD is closed, or if multiple, PA banding is performed to reduce pulmonary flow.

If medical treatment is successful, and with only moderate size defects, the VSD is closed in preschool years (e.g. age approx. 3 yr).

Closure of small defects may be justified on the grounds of infective endocarditis risk, but minute defects are usually left.

The high incidence of spontaneous closure in the first year of life (approx. 50%) must encourage medical management at this age where possible.

Management of the child with elevated pulmonary vascular resistance (PVR) is more difficult. If the PVR is <8 units the VSD is usually closed. If the PVR is > 8 units a lung biopsy may be indicated to assess the severity of intimal proliferation before deciding on surgery. (See Table on p. 460 for calculation.)

2.2 Atrial septal defect (ASD)

From the fifth week of intrauterine life the fetal common atrium starts to be divided by the septum primum. This crescentic ridge grows down from the cranial and dorsal part of the atrium towards the endocardial cushions. The foramen primum develops at the junction of the septum with the endocardial cushions. The foramen secundum develops at the top of the septum primum as the foramen primum closes. The septum secundum develops as a second crescentic ridge to the right of the septum primum which fuses with the endocardial cushions. The limbic ledge forms the lower part of the septum secundum and the foramen ovale maintains right-to-left atrial flow in fetal life.

Types of ASD (Fig. 2.2)

- patent foramen ovale
- primum
- secundum
- sinus venosus defect
- IVC defect
- coronary sinus anomalies

Patent foreman ovale (PFO)

Not strictly an ASD. May occur in up to 25% of young children. There is no physiological inter-atrial shunting unless an additional cardiac lesion is present (e.g. pulmonary stenosis when a high RA pressure may cause right-to-left shunting). A PFO does not require closure unless this situation arises. It is useful in catheterisation allowing left atrial catheterisation easily. On withdrawal from LA to RA however there is a difference in mean pressures. This differentiates a PFO from an ASD, where the mean pressures are the same or virtually so. A PFO does not need prophylactic antibiotics for dental procedures etc. Rarely it may allow the passage of a paradoxical embolus.

2.2 Atrial septal defect

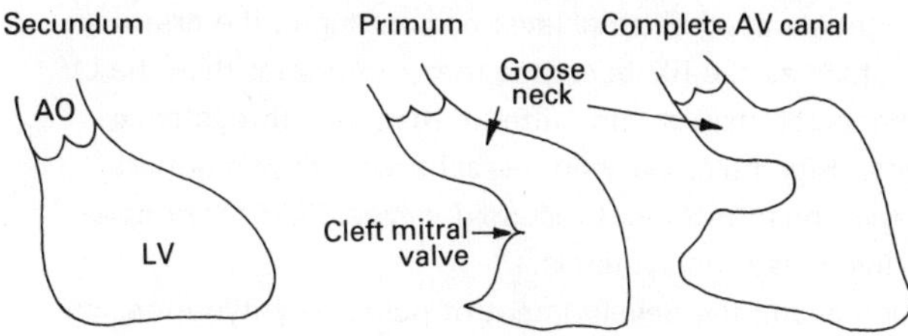

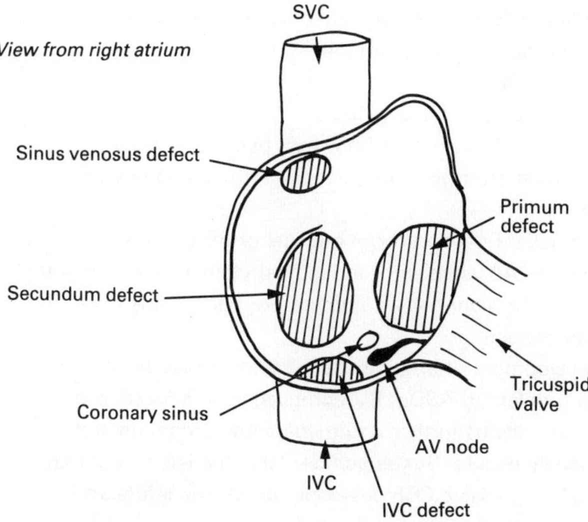

Fig. 2.2 The sites of the common ASDs are shown. The lower panel shows the LV cineangiogram in the RAO projection diagrammatically. In the secundum ASD this may be normal or show a prolapsing mitral valve. The typical 'goose neck' of primum ASDs or AV canal is shown with a horizontal outflow tact, grossly abnormal LV shape and cleft mitral valve.

Pathophysiology and symptoms

Left-to-right shunting at atrial level occurs during the first months of life as the RV becomes more compliant than the LV (which becomes thicker and stiffer in response to systemic pressures). High pulmonary flow results with flow murmurs audible over pulmonary and tricuspid valves. Pulmonary flow may be five times the systemic.

In young adults the development of pulmonary hypertension is not common but it results in RV pressure approaching systemic levels and the start of shunt reversal (Eisenmenger ASD). It does not occur in infancy.

Secundum ASD patients are often asymptomatic in childhood and may not be diagnosed until 40–50 years old. Primum ASDs are picked up earlier.

Symptoms or reason for diagnosis:

- The chesty child: resulting from high pulmonary flow.
- Dyspnoea on effort and occasionally orthopnoea (stiff lungs, not LVF).
- Symptomatic. Routine school medical or mass x-ray.
- Palpitations. All varieties of atrial dysrhythmias are common especially in the older patient and are not necessarily cured by closing the defect.
- The development of atrial fibrillation and cardiac failure. This is a serious problem in ASDs. RV compliance is reduced, the tricuspid ring dilates further and tricuspid regurgitation and hepatomegaly occurs. Systemic flow falls, the left atrium may enlarge as progressive CCF develops. (In SR the left heart is small in secundum ASD).
- Paradoxical embolism or cerebral abscess may occur in patients with high RV pressures and shunt reversal.

Infective endocarditis is not a problem with an ASD *per se*, unless there is an associated mitral valve lesion.

Physical signs of secundum ASD

More common in females. May occur as part of the Holt–Oram syndrome (triphalangeal thumbs, ASID or VSD).

Right heart signs are dominant:

- Raised JVP with equal 'a' and 'v' waves.
- RV prominence with precordial bulge in children and large pulmonary conus and flow.
- Pulmonary systolic ejection murmur (flow).
- Fixed split A2 and P2 on any phase of respiration is typical although occasionally very slight movement of P_2 can be detected.
- Tricuspid diastolic flow murmur with large left-to-right shunts.
- Systolic thrill in the pulmonary area may occur from high flow and does not necessarily mean additional pulmonary stenosis
- With AF signs of tricuspid regurgitation.
- Pulmonary hypertension results in a softer ejection systolic murmur, often an ejection click, the tricuspid flow murmur disappears and P_2 is loud. Pulmonary regurgitation may occur (Graham–Steell early diastolic murmur).

Differential diagnosis

In the simple secundum ASD is with mild pulmonary stenosis (P_2 delayed, softer and moves with respiration).

With larger hearts pulmonary hypertension and the development of cardiac failure, the conditions confused with an ASD include: mixed mitral valve disease (see Fig. 3.2); pulmonary hypertension and/or cor pulmonale; congestive cardiomyopathy.

Patients with ASDs are usually in SR with right heart signs most obvious. In AF with low output it is more difficult, but on CxR the pulmonary artery is very large in ASDs and there is pulmonary plethora.

Associated lesions

- *Floppy mitral valve* (often overdiagnosed on angiography).
- *Pulmonary stenosis*. This will cause right-to-left shunting if severe.
- *Anomalous venous drainage*. The sinus venosus defect is almost always associated with anomalous drainage of the right upper pulmonary vein to the right atrium. However more than one pulmonary vein may be involved. This is checked at cardiac catheter.
- *Mitral stenosis* (Lutembacher's syndrome). Probably rheumatic mitral stenosis associated with an ASD. Congenital mitral stenosis is a rare possibility.
- As part of more complex congenital heart disease, e.g. TAPVD, TGA, tricuspid atresia, pulmonary atresia with intact ventricular septum.

The sinus venosus defect behaves as a small secundum ASD with its associated right upper lobe anomalous venous drainage.

Chest x-ray

- *Small aortic knuckle*. Large pulmonary artery conus.
- *Pulmonary plethora*. Cardiac enlargement is due to RV dilatation. Right atrial enlargement common.
- Progressive enlargement of both atria once in AF.

ECG

Incomplete or complele RBBB.
Right axis deviation.

Echocardiography

This is all that may be needed in children when PVR is usually normal.

Cardiac catheterisation

Cardiac catheterisation is performed to document the diagnosis, assess the shunt with a saturation run, check pulmonary and coronary sinus drainage, check RV function, and the mitral valve with an LV injection. Thus LV, RV and PA angiograms with follow through are usually required.

Oximetry is performed early in the catheter prior to angiography. If the oxygen step up is high in the RA there may be a sinus venosus defect. In secundum ASD the step up is in mid RA. If the oxygen step up is very low in the RA near the tricuspid valve and the ASD cannot be crossed with the catheter, consider the possibility of anomalous pulmonary veins draining into the coronary sinus.

In secundum ASD the LV is small and normal. The mitral valve may appear to prolapse. In primum ASD there is the so-called 'goose-neck' appearance with a cleft in the mitral valve (see Fig. 2.2) plus some mitral regurgitation which may fill the RA if severe. In complete AV canal the cleft becomes a large gap and the LV has a characteristic appearance in the RAO view. The LAO views visualise the septum.

The aorta is small, shifted to the left (large RA).

Treatment

Surgical closure is usually recommended between the ages of 5 and 10 years to avoid late onset pulmonary hypertension, RV failure and hopefully to reduce and delay the onset of atrial arrhythmias. The calculated left-to-right shunt on saturations should be 2:1 at atrial level or greater to recommend closure. In the older patient closure is still often worthwhile, symptomatic improvement being associated with a reduction in RV size (especially if there is a low voltage on RV leads on the ECG preoperatively).

Primum ASD

A more complex and serious lesion than the secundum ASD, it forms part of the spectrum of AV canal defects. It is due to maldevelopment of the septum primum and endocardial cushions. Its most simplified subdivisions are:

• *Primum ASD*. No VSD component. Mitral valve (anterior leaflet) is cleft with associated mitral regurgitation of varying degrees, from none to severe. Sometimes called 'partial AV canal'

• *Complete AV canal*. Primum type ASD plus VSD component. Mitral and tricuspid valves are abnormal with abnormally short chordae and bridging leaflets stretching across the VSD and joining mitral and tricuspid valves

It accounts for only 3–5% of congenital heart disease in the first year of life, and less than a tenth of all ASDs.

Associated lesions

• Down's syndrome (very common), Klinefelter's syndrome, Noonan's syndrome. Renal and splenic abnormalities

• Cardiac abnormalities: common atrium; unroofed coronary sinus (left SVC to LA); pulmonary stenosis; coarctation

Presentation

Primum ASD usually presents in childhood, and the complete AV canal in infancy (heart failure and failure-to-thrive in infancy with signs of VSD, early childhood with dyspnoea with chest infections and central cyanosis if pulmonary vascular disease develops).

Chest x-ray

CxR of a simple primum defect resembles a secundum ASD. The AV canal CxR has a large globular heart with pulmonary plethora.

ECG

• RBBB

• left axis deviation (cf. right axis in secundum defect)

• long PR interval

Conduction defects are common (the AV node is in the inferior portion of the defect), especially junctional rhythms or

	Secundum ASD	**Primum ASD**	**AV canal**
Presentation	Child or adult	Usually childhood	Infancy
Appearance	Normal	Normal	Mongoloid
Colour	Normal	Normal	Cyanosis
Signs	2°ASD	As 2° ASD ± MR	As VSD, but S_2 split
Ventricular septum	Intact	Intact	VSD component
Pulmonary hypertension	–	–	+
ECG	RBBB + RAD	RBBB + LAD	RBBB. LAD Long PR or worse
Mitral valve	Occasionally prolapsing, usually normal	Cleft anterior leaflet, varying degrees of MR	Severe MR, grossly abnormal MV and TV

complete AV block. If right axis deviation develops it suggests the development of pulmonary hypertension or additional pulmonary stenosis.

Treatment

Primum ASD. 50% reach surgery before age 10 years. Early surgery may help prevent RV dysfunction. The cleft mitral valve is repaired if there is significant mitral regurgitation and the defect closed with a patch.

Complete AV canal. 50% die within 1 year if untreated. Options in infancy are banding the pulmonary artery or closure of ASD and VSD components dividing the bridging leaflets. Subsequent mitral valve replacement may be necessary, as well as permanent pacing for AV block. The presence of pulmonary hypertension makes operative mortality high.

Rarer defects

The IVC defect may be large and allow shunting of IVC blood into LA with children becoming slightly cyanosed on effort. It may also occur following surgical closure of a primum ASD.

Unroofed coronary sinus with a left SVC draining to LA usually occurs as part of a more complex lesion (e.g. common atrium).

2.3 The patent ductus arteriosus (PDA)

In fetal life the duct allows flow from the pulmonary circuit to the aorta. It normally closes spontaneously within the first month after birth. In premature babies it is more likely to remain patent for longer or permanently. Up to 50% of premature babies have a PDA, especially those with respiratory distress syndrome. The duct responds less well to a rise in Po_2 in prematurity and the duct may be silent.

The PDA is more common in

- children born in high altitudes
- females
- history of maternal rubella in the first trimester of pregnancy

(PDA is the commonest congenital heart lesion following maternal rubella)

Pathophysiology and symptoms

Most children with a PDA are asymptomatic, the condition being diagnosed at school medical, etc. With larger ducts a significant left-to-right shunt occurs causing an increased LV volume load similar to a VSD. Symptoms of LVF are similar. Irreversible pulmonary hypertension may develop in a few cases causing an Eisenmenger syndrome (approx. 5%).

Differential cyanosis and clubbing may be noticed by the patient with shunt reversal (blue feet, pink hands) with preferential flow of pulmonary arterial blood down the descending aorta.

In rare instances death is due either to CCF or infective endocarditis.

Physical signs to note

Very small ducts have few signs except the continuous machinery murmur in the second left interspace.

Signs to note in a moderate PDA are;

- collapsing pulse with wide pulse pressure (feel the feet in babies)
- thrill, second left interspace, systolic and/or diastolic
- LV +. Hyperdynamic ventricle
- machinery murmur. Loud continuous murmur obscuring second sound in second left interspace and just below the left clavicle, louder in systole. It is not present in the neonate (with the high PVR), but appears as the PVR falls in the first few days
- mitral diastolic flow murmur at apex
- the second sound is usually inaudible

Pulmonary hypertensive ducts

The diastolic component of the murmur may disappear, and the systolic become shorter and ejection in quality. The second sound is single (loud P_2). Occasionally it is reversed audibly (prolonged LV ejection).

Dilatation of the pulmonary trunk causes an ejection sound, and sometimes pulmonary regurgitation.

Associated lesions

- VSD
- pulmonary stenosis
- coarctation
- as part of more complex lesions: e.g. pulmonary atresia with intact septum. If collaterals are poor pulmonary flow is duct-dependent. Drug control in this instance is important. In interrupted aortic arch or hypoplastic left heart syndrome the PDA maintains flow round the body.

Pharmacological control of the PDA

Helping to close the duct in neonatal LVF

Important points are: avoiding fluid overload; normal blood

glucose and calcium; diuretics rather than digoxin (AV block in babies). Then use indomethacin 0.2 mg/kg via nasogastric tube given at 6 hourly intervals for a maximum of 3 doses. An i.v. preparation is not generally available.

There is a risk of renal damage (unlikely with this regime) but the drug should be avoided if there is an elevated serum creatinine (> 150 mmol/l or 1.7 mg/100 ml). Also avoid indomethacin if there is a bleeding disorder.

Helping to keep the duct patent in pulmonary atresia
This is more difficult as sudden deaths have been reported following the use of prostaglandin E_1 (PGE_1), and the cause is unknown.

PGE_1 is infused at 0.1 μg/kg/min via an umbilical artery catheter. The Po_2 rises. Vasodilatation may drop the mean aortic pressure and increase the right-to-left shunt if there is one already. After a few minutes the dose is reduced to 0.05 μg/kg or even to 0.025 μg/kg/min.

Other side-effects include fever, irritability. Orally the drug produces troublesome diarrhoea. *It should not be tried except in experienced neonatal centres.*

Differential diagnosis
Includes
- A–P window
- VSD with aortic regurgitation
- coronary AV fistula
- pulmonary AV fistula
- ruptured sinus of Valsalva
- innocent venous hum
- mammary souffle (pregnancy)
- surgical shunts (Waterston, Blalock, etc.)

Cardiac catheterisation
This is performed if additional lesions are suspected. The right

heart catheter follows a characteristic course from PA down the descending aorta. Associated lesions are excluded by a saturation run (VSD). Aortography indicates duct size and site. LV cine is necessary if a VSD is suspected in addition.

Treatment

The PDA should be closed surgically in the pre-school year to avoid infective endocarditis and the Eisenmenger reaction. Occasionally if the duct is ligated a continuous machinery murmur recurs. This is not due to so-called recanalisation, but to inadequate ligation.

Recently the Rashkind PDA occluder has been developed and is a startling advance in the management of the PDA. This is a device inserted percutaneously in the catheter laboratory and avoids the need for a thoracotomy. It is like a pair of miniature back to back umbrellas which are positioned across the duct under screening and when in the correct position the insertion catheter is withdrawn leaving the device *in situ*. Angiography confirms the correct positioning of the device and the occlusion of the duct.

2.4 Coarctation of the aorta

A congenital narrowing or shelf-like obstruction of the aortic arch. The constriction is usually eccentric, distal to the left subclavian artery, opposite the duct and termed 'juxtaductal'. In extreme form the arch may be interrupted. Recognised types are:

Infantile type

Associated with hypoplasia of the aortic isthmus (a diffuse narrowing of the aorta between left subclavian artery and duct) this was called 'pre-ductal' coarctation. Presentation is in the first month of life with heart failure and associated lesions which are extremely common.

Adult type
This coarctation is juxtaductal or slightly post-ductal. The obstruction develops gradually and presentation is commonly between the ages of 15 and 30 years with complications. Associated cardiac lesions are much less common than with the infantile type, apart from a bicuspid aortic valve.

Pseudocoarctation
This is just a tortuosity of the aorta in the region of the duct. There is no stenosis, just a 'kinked' appearance. It is not of haemodynamic significance.

Other severe stenotic lesions may occur in the aorta (e.g. supravalvar aortic stenosis, descending thoracic or abdominal stenoses). The abdominal and descending thoracic aorta stenoses may be due to an aortitis. Classic coarctation may be due to abnormal duct flow *in utero* associated with other anomalies, and the two types are not strictly comparable.

Children with coarctation are usually male. Female coarctation is suggestive of Turner's syndrome.

Associated lesions
These are very common.

- *bicuspid aortic valve* (which may become stenotic and/or regurgitant). Approximately 50% of cases, but series vary enormously
- PDA. The commonest associated shunt

Post-ductal coarctation + PDA. Usually left-to-right shunt into the pulmonary artery. If the duct is large, pulmonary hypertension may occur

Infantile coarctation + PDA. High pulmonary vascular resistance results in right-to-left shunt, with distal aorta, trunk and legs supplied by right ventricular flow through the PDA.

Differential cyanosis results (blue legs, pink hands), and heart failure

- VSD. In isolation or with:

Transposition of the great arteries, + VSD + PDA. Complex lesion with differential cyanosis (blue hands, pink feet)
Mitral valve disease. Congenital mitral valve anomalies, stenosis or regurgitation
Other complex lesions. Primitive ventricle, primum ASD or AV canal.
Aortic arch anomalies. Hypoplastic left heart with hypoplastic aortic root. Aortic atresia. Aortic root aneurysms
Non-cardiac associations. Berry aneurysms, renal anomalies (especially Turner's syndrome)

Symptoms

• infantile heart failure is expected in > 50% pre-ductal coarctation. It may also occur with post ductal coarctation plus a large PDA (see above).

Post ductal coarctation may be missed in childhood presenting in adolescence or early adult life with one or more of the following:

• noticing a vigorous pulsation in the neck or throat
• hypertension. May be symptomless. Routine medical
• tired legs or intermittent claudication on running
• subarachnoid haemorrhage from a Berry aneurysm
• infective endocarditis on coarctation or bicuspid aortic valve
• left ventricular failure
• rupture or dissection of the proximal aorta. Distal aortic rupture has occurred (e.g. into the oesophagus). Aortic rupture is more common in pregnancy
• angina pectoris. Premature coronary disease occurs

Physical signs to note

• blood pressure in both arms (? left subclavian involved or not). Hypertension with wide pulse pressure in right ± left arm
• weak, delayed, anacrotic, or even absent femoral pulses compared to right radial. Low blood pressure in legs
• prominent carotid and subclavian pulsations

• collaterals in older children (not before age 6 years) and adults. Bend the patient forward with arms hanging down at the sides. Feel round the back with the palm over and around the scapulae, and around the shoulders. Collaterals do not develop in pre-ductal coarctation with PDA as distal aorta supply is from the pulmonary artery
• tortuous retinal arteries. Frank retinopathy is not common
• JVP is usually normal
• LV hypertrophy
• *Murmurs*
due to bicuspid aortic valve (p. 90)
from the coarctation itself: a continuous murmur with small, tight coarctation (<2 mm) heard over the thoracic spine or below the left clavicle. With a larger coarctation the murmur is ejection systolic only

From collaterals. Ejection systolic, bilateral, front or back of chest. In interrupted aorta (complete coarctation) the murmurs are due to collaterals

From an associated PDA or VSD

From lower thoracic or abdominal coarctation

It may be difficult to decide the source of an ejection systolic murmur in coarctation!
• second sound. A_2 is usually loud, but not usually delayed beyond P_2

Chest x-ray

Rib notching occurs from the age of 6–8 years (dilated posterior intercostal arteries). They do not occur in the first and second ribs. (The first two intercostals do not arise from the aorta.)

The heart is usually normal in size unless there are associated lesions.

The typical aortic knuckle is absent, and is replaced by a double knuckle (in post ductal coarctations). The upper part is the dilated left subclavian, the lower the post stenotic dilatation of the descending aorta.

ECG

Shows left ventricular hypertrophy; RBBB is common.

Echocardiography

May obviate the need for cardiac catheter in the infant with no associated lesion.

Cardiac catheterisation

Is required in children with atypical signs or associated lesions. Babies can be catheterised from the right heart via a PFO, or from a right axillary cut-down in older children. Additional lesions are checked (bicuspid aortic valve, PDA, VSD, etc.) and aortography performed in the LAO projection to show the coarctation. A coarctation gradient of 40 mmHg is highly significant. The size of the descending aorta is noted and the site and size of collaterals.

Surgery

The prognosis without surgery is poor: most patients die before the age of 40 years with complications. Severe preductal coarctation in infancy or interrupted aortic arch (usually with PDA + VSD) may require urgent reconstructive surgery.

In post-ductal coarctation surgery is performed between 5 and 10 years or at the time of diagnosis which may be later. Patients with both coarctation and aortic stenosis have the coarctation resected first, and a subsequent aortic valve replacement if necessary.

Balloon angioplasty

In some paediatric units is now an alternative to surgery as first line treatment. Redilatation may be necessary, but so far long term results seem good.

Follow-up

Post-operative hypertension is expected usually requiring nitroprusside, trimetaphan and/or chlorpromazine in the immediate post-operative phase.

Long term hypertension is also common. All patients should be followed up for life following coarctation resection to check:

- continued hypertension
- the possibility of premature coronary artery disease
- repeat cardiac catheter in infants or early adult life is often performed to check the coarctation site and possible residual gradient, especially if hypertension persists

2.5 Transposition of the great arteries (TGA) (complete transposition, D-transposition)

In its commonest form the aorta arises from the right ventricle and the pulmonary artery from the left ventricle. The aorta is anterior and to the right of the pulmonary artery (D-loop). There is thus atrioventricular concordance, and ventriculoarterial discordance. Unless there is an associated shunt (ASD, VSD, PDA) the two circuits are completely separate and life is impossible once the duct closes.

TGA occurs in approximately 1 per 4500 live births (100–200 cases per year in the UK). It s commoner in males. Untreated mortality is high (10% one year survival).

Presentation

At birth with cyanosis which increases in the first week as the PDA closes. Birth weight is normal or high. Progress is poor and progressive cardiac enlargement occurs. As PVR declines in the first weeks of life high pulmonary flow develops and LVF occurs. Congestive cardiac failure is the commonest cause of death.

Physical signs to note

- the commonest cyanotic congenital heart disease causing cyanosis at birth
- initially hyperdynamic circulation: bounding pulses in a blue baby

• loud (palpable) A_2 retrosternally from anterior aorta. P_2 not heard
• murmurs often absent: high pulmonary flow may cause a soft mid-systolic ejection murmur, ejection sound may arise from either aorta or pulmonary artery, right-to-left shunt through VSD may cause a soft early systolic murmur; left-to-right shunt through VSD (high PVR or LVOTO) does not usually cause a murmur

The signs depend on the level of the PVR, the presence or absence of LVOTO and/or a VSD.

ECG

Is very variable. Usually shows RA + RV + and RAD. Additional LV + and LA + occurs with high pulmonary flow and LV volume overload. It is not so prevalent in patients with additional pulmonary stenosis.

Chest x-ray

Shows pulmonary plethora. Heart has 'egg on its side' appearance and the pedicle is small (aorta In front of PA). The left heart border is convex.

Differential diagnosis

All causes of cyanosis and pulmonary plethora (see Table p. 20) but TGA is the commonest.

Also consider Eisenmenger VSD.

If there is LVOT obstruction, lung fields are not plethoric, and the condition may then resemble Fallot's tetralogy or DORV with pulmonary stenosis.

Associated lesions

• PDA may be life saving if there is no VSD. Differential cyanosis occurs
• VSD
• VSD + LVOT obstruction (fibrous shelf or fibromuscular

tunnel beneath pulmonary valve) = TGA + VSD + LVOTO. These patients have poor pulmonary flow and may have frank cyanotic spells

- ASD. Usually without PS, and high pulmonary flow occurs
- coarctation
- juxtaposed atrial appendages

Prognostically the best situations are TGA + ASD, or TGA + VSD + moderate pulmonary stenosis. The child can survive the early months and does not get the irreversible pulmonary vascular changes (usually present by one year of age) in children with TGA + large VSD but no protective pulmonary stenosis.

Cardiac catheterisation

Confirms normal AV connections, but RV injection fills anterior aorta. The associated shunt is identified. It is important to reach PA (often via aorta through RV→VSD→LV→PA) to check PVR and the possible presence of LVOT obstruction.

Options for treatment

1 *Rashkind balloon septostomy*. May be lifesaving in the neonate. Performed at diagnostic catheterisation. A PFO is enlarged by inflating the balloon catheter carefully in the left atrium, and sudden traction of the balloon into RA increases atrial mixing. Approx 70% babies can be helped through the first year with this technique, and atrial septectomy is not generally needed.

2 *Intra-atrial reconstruction*. Senning or Mustard operation. Usually performed between 6 months and 1-year-old these operations separate systemic venous and pulmonary venous return at atrial level.

In the Mustard operation systemic venous return is diverted through the mitral valve via an intra-atrial baffle into LV thence to PA. Pulmonary venous return is diverted through the tricuspid valve to the right ventricle, thence to the aorta.

Advantages:
• circuits are separated
• cyanosis disappears
• child grows with reasonable exercise tolerance.
Disadvantages:
• RV bears load of systemic circulation. Both RV muscle and tricuspid valve may not be up to it with RV failure or TR
• It is not strictly anatomical total correction
• Post-operative supraventricular dysrhythmias are common (especially with the Mustard procedure)
• Baffle obstruction may occur.

3 *Rastelli procedure for TGA, VAS and LVOTO.* These patients may be shunted early (Blalock). Then at age 3–4 years the Rastelli procedure is performed. The VSD is enlarged, the pulmonary valve closed, and the pulmonary artery ligated just above the pulmonary valve. The LV is connected to the aorta by means of an intra-cardiac patch. Then an extra-cardiac valve conduit connects the anterior RV to the pulmonary artery.

This is total correction with the LV bearing the systemic load.

Problems are a residual VSD, tricuspid regurgitation, conduit compression by the sternum, and conduit valve degeneration.

4 *Anatomical correction.* Switching the great arteries to their correct ventricles. This is also physiological correction. Cases reported recommend early surgery in the first few weeks of life while the LV is still capable of generating systemic pressures (otherwise a two-stage procedure is suggested with preliminary pulmonary artery banding to 'tone up' the left ventricle).

Problems are primarily surgical with the delicate surgery of coronary artery relocation.

Most children with TGA are managed by initial Rashkind balloon septostomy, later having a Senning or Mustard intra-atrial reconstruction.

2.6 Corrected transposition (l-transposition)

In its commonest form the aorta lies anterior and to the left of the pulmonary artery (l-loop). It is physiologically corrected in that the circulation proceeds on a normal route although the ventricles are 'switched', i.e.

RA→Morphological LV but in RV position→PA
→LA→Morphological RV but in LV position→Ao

There is thus atrioventricular discordance and ventriculoarterial discordance. There is usually situs solitus with the atria normally placed. Rarely the condition presents with situs inversus and dextrocardia.

A few cases of corrected transposition have no associated lesions and live a normal adult life with no symptoms, the RV coping well with systemic load. The presence of associated lesions usually results in presentation in childhood, and the condition is not particularly benign.

Associated lesions: the four most common (Fig. 2.3)

- VSD. Shunt from systemic (RV) to venous (LV) ventricle. Occurs in 70–90% cases depending on series. A 'malalignment' defect: as there is malalignment between the atrial and ventricular septum
- pulmonary stenosis in 40%. Often sub-valvar due to an aneurysm of the membranous septum bulging out beneath the pulmonary valve
- AV valve regurgitation. Usually a problem with the tricuspid valve (left-sided) not coping with systemic pressures produced by the RV. Also it is often dysplastic with a typical Ebstein malformation. Mitral (right-sided) prolapse also may occur
- complete AV block. The AV node is anterior and the bundle runs beneath the pulmonary valve and anterior to the VSD.

Pulmonary valve or VSD surgery run the risk of inducing AV block (which may occur spontaneously anyway)

2.6 Corrected transposition

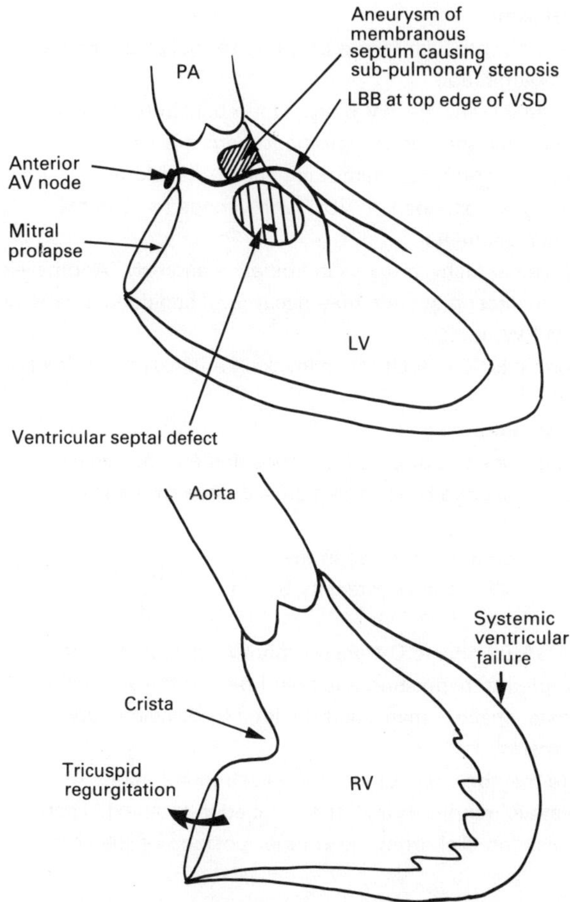

Fig. 2.3 Problems in corrected transposition. The upper diagram shows the left (venous) ventricle and the position of the VSD in relation to the bundle. An aneurysm of the membranous septum is shown causing sub-pulmonary obstruction. The lower diagram shows the right (systemic) ventricle which is trabeculated. Dysplastic tricuspid valve associated with tricuspid regurgitation. Systemic (RV) ventricular failure is a common cause of death.

2.6 Corrected transposition

Presentation

• systemic ventricular failure (RV) due to tricuspid (left AV valve) regurgitation

• congenital complete AV block. Not a benign type of AV block, children may be symptomatic from this alone

• cynotic heart disease mimicking Fallot's tetralogy (subpulmonary stenosis + VSD with venous to systemic ventricular shunting)

• paroxysmal tachycardia as in Ebstein's anomaly. Anomalies of the conducting system may occur (e.g. additional posterior AV node, WPW, etc.)

• abnormal ECG in adult life: mimicking anteroseptal infarction

Physical signs

The best clues to corrected transposition are the clinical findings of second or third degree AV block in a child.

e.g. cannon 'a' waves in the JVP, variable intensity S_1 } in third degree block

As in TGA (complete D-transposition) A_2 is loud and palpable. In corrected transposition it is heard best in the second left intercostal space – mimicking the loud P_2 of pulmonary hypertension.

There may be signs of left AV valve regurgitation (pansystolic murmur from left sternal edge to apex). There may be an ejection click from the anterior position of the aortic valve.

Chest x-ray

The left-sided aorta produces a 'duck's back' appearance with a straight left heart border, AV valve regurgitation causes the respective ventricles and atria to enlarge. The left pulmonary artery may be hidden behind the heart and aorta.

ECG

Long PR interval. Higher degress of AV block. Prominent Q waves in right chest leads (V_{1-3}) but absent Q waves in left precordial leads. Left axis deviation. Q wave in standard lead 3, but no Q wave in lead 1.

Treatment

Patients may require medical treatment for heart failure if the systemic (RV) ventricle fails to cope with systemic work loads. Congestive cardiac failure is the commonest cause of death in cases with no additional anomalies.

Patients may require left AV valve (tricuspid) replacement or repair plus VSD closure. The latter risks the development of complete AV block with the conducting system in the roof of the VSD (see Fig. 2.3).

Intra-cardiac mapping helps identify and avoid bundle damage. Unusual coronary artery anatomy may make ventriculotomy of the venous (LV) ventricle difficult.

Even with the greatest care permanent pacing may be needed. The establishment of a permanent system is not without problems either. The transvenous wire must grip the endocardial surface of the non-trabeculated (venous) left ventricle.

2.7 Fallot's tetralogy

This is the most common cyanotic congenital heart disease presenting after one year of age. It forms part of a spectrum of complex cyanotic congenital heart disease, and is very similar in many respects to double outlet right ventricle with pulmonary stenosis (DORV + PS). VSD with severe infundibular stenosis, and pulmonary atresia with VSD.

Development of Fallot's tetralogy

In Fallot's tetralogy there is a failure of the bulbus cordis to rotate properly so that the aorta is more anterior and to the right (dextroposed) than normal. The aorta moves nearer the tricuspid valve and over-rides the septum with a 'malalignment' VSD beneath the aortic valve.

Infundibular stenosis develops with hypertrophy of the septal and parietal bands of infundibular muscle which form part of the crista (Fig. 2.4). Obstruction to RV outflow is usually a combination of infundibular and valve stenosis, but may be either alone. In addition RV outflow obstruction may be due to the small size of the pulmonary valve ring or main pulmonary trunk. Peripheral pulmonary stenoses are common.

The original tetralogy described by Fallot in 1888 (Fig.2.4) is:

- pulmonary stenosis
- VSD
- over-riding of the aorta
- right ventricular hypertrophy

Additional anomalies or problems commonly associated are:

- right-sided aortic arch (in 25%)
- absent or hypoplastic left pulmonary artery (more common if arch is right-sided)
- aortic regurgitation due to large aortic ring plus subaortic VSD
- ASD

Pathophysiology and symptoms

With the large VSD both ventricles are at the same (systemic) pressure. Pulmonary flow and the degree of right-to-left shunt across the VSD depend on the severity of pulmonary stenosis and the level of systemic vascular resistance (SVR). Increasing SVR will reduce the right-to-left shunt and increase pulmonary flow. Mild pulmonary stenosis may be associated with the 'acyanotic Fallot'. Pulmonary blood flow may be increased by a patent ductus arteriosus although the association is not that common. Bronchial collaterals develop with increasingly severe pulmonary stenosis.

Infundibular stenosis is a variable obstruction. It increases

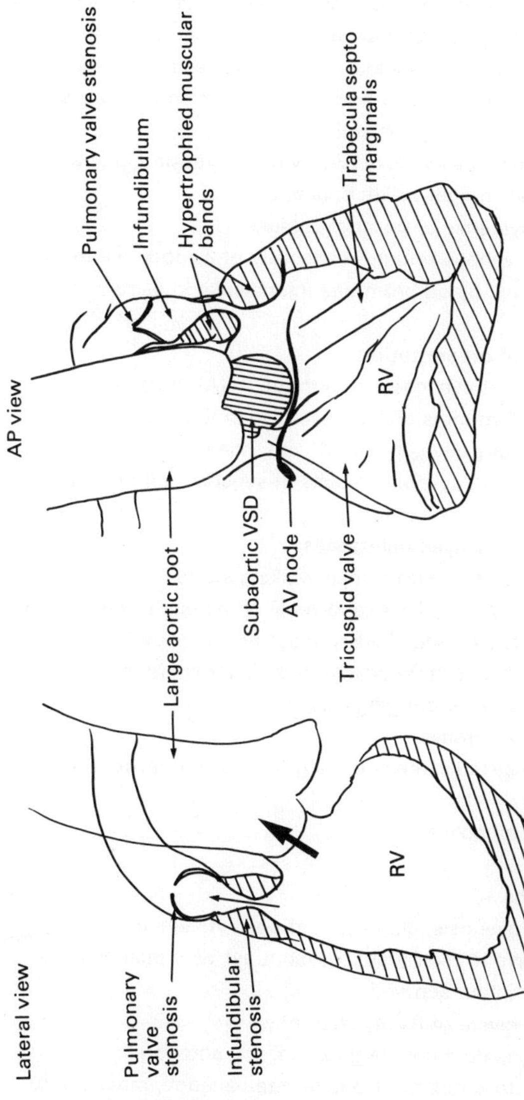

Fig. 2.4 Fallot's tetralogy. The left diagram shows a lateral view of the right ventricle with the large aorta overriding the VSD. The severe infundibular stenosis results in diversion of RV blood straight up into the aorta (heavy arrow). The right panel shows the right ventricle in the AP projection. The VSD is subaortic. Note the hypertrophied bands of the infundibulum. The bundle lies immediately beneath the VSD and is at risk during VSD closure.

with time (muscle and fibrous tissue accumulation) and also with hypoxia or acidosis which may result in cyanotic attacks (infundibular spasm). Infundibular shutdown results in a severe reduction in pulmonary flow and an increased right-to-left shunt of blood from RV straight into the aorta.

Squatting helps cyanosis in two ways, increasing pulmonary flow and reducing right-to-left shunting:

- increasing systemic vascular resistance
- reduction in venous return—especially of acidotic blood from the legs (acidotic blood promotes infundibular spasm)

Typical clinical presentation

- patients are not cyanosed at birth (cf. TGA). It usually appears at 3–6 months and increases with time
- cyanotic attacks develop. Often with 'stress', crying or feeding. Increasing cyanosis results in syncope, and convulsions (see p. 436)
- poor growth. Delayed milestones
- squatting after mild effort once walking starts
- symptoms of polycythaemia: arterial or venous thromboses, particularly cerebral, and children must not be allowed to get dehydrated, which can precipitate this. Later in life: gout, acne, kyphoscoliosis, recurrent gingivitis
- infective endocarditis
- cerebral abscess (absence of lung filter with right-to-left shunt)
- paradoxical embolism

Physical signs

- developing cyanosis, clubbing and polycythaemia
- JVP: 'a' wave is usually absent (contrast with pulmonary stenosis with intact septum)
- parasternal heave of RV hypertrophy
- palpable A_2 is common (large aorta, too anterior)
- ejection systolic murmur from left sternal edge, radiating up

to pulmonary area. Systolic thrill
- Single second sound (A_2 only)

The systolic murmur is due to pulmonary stenosis, not the VSD. With cyanotic attacks the murmur becomes quieter or may disappear.

Chest x-ray

The classical heart shape is *coeur en sabot* (heart in a boot) appearance with the apex lifted off the left hemidiaphragm by RV hypertrophy. Lung fields are oligaemic and pulmonary arteries small. A right aortic arch may be visible.

EGG

Shows sinus rhythm, right axis deviation and RV hypertrophy with incomplete or complete RBBB. Ventricular ectopics are common, and paroxysmal ventricular tachycardia may be found on 24-hour ECG taping.

Cardiac catheterisation (Fig. 2.5)

Is needed to assess the anatomy of the RVOT and the main pulmonary artery branches, RV and LV function, site and size of VSD, competence of the aortic valve, coronary anatomy to exclude a PDA or coarctation and to visualise any previous shunt.

This is best managed with biplane RV cine (and craniocaudal tilt on the AP projection helps visualise the main pulmonary trunk and its bifurcation). An LV cine in the LAO projection will show the VSD and LV function. An aortogram is essential in Fallot's tetralogy.

The most difficult differential diagnosis is from double outlet right ventricle with subaortic VSD and pulmonary stenosis. In Fallot's tetralogy less than half the aortic valve should straddle the VSD, and in DORV more than half. The final arbiter may be the surgeon.

Medical treatment of cyanotic attacks and management of polycythaemia: see **10.4** and **2.9**.

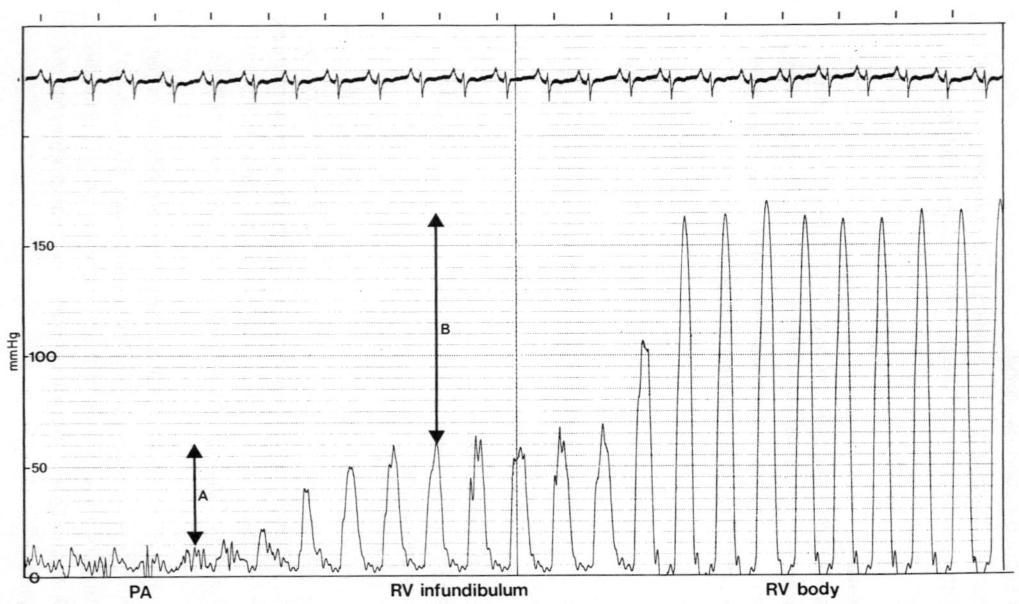

Fig. 2.5 Fallot's tetralogy. Right heart withdrawal. PA pressure is normal. The RVOT gradient is both at valve level and sub-valve level (infundibular). Valvar gradient (A) = 45 mmHg, and the infundibular gradient (B) = 105 mmHg. Total gradient 150 mmHg.

Surgery

Initial enthusiasm for complete one stage repair in the first year of life was tempered by high mortality in many cases: especially those needing a trans-annular patch on the RV outflow tract.

Total correction under the age of one year is usually reserved for those infants who do not need an outflow trans-annular patch. A Blalock shunt is performed (Fig. 2.6) if the anatomy is unfavourable. Under the age of about three months a Waterston shunt is preferred as the subclavian artery is too small for a good Blalock. A second stage total correction can be performed

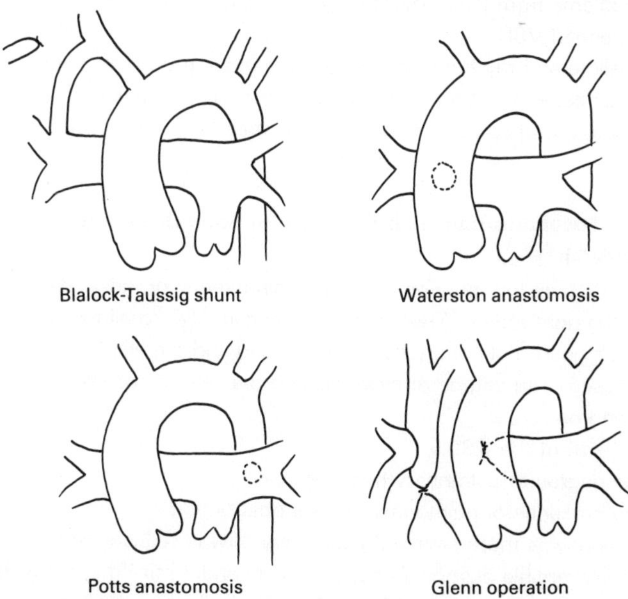

Fig. 2.6 Shunt operations for cyanotic congenital heart disease. Blalock Taussig shunt: either subclavian artery to respective pulmonary artery. Waterston shunt: back of ascending aorta to pulmonary artery. Potts anastomosis: back of pulmonary artery to descending aorta. Glenn operation: SVC to right pulmonary artery. The Potts and Glenn operations are rarely used now.

when the child is larger (age 5–10 years). Conditions favouring an initial shunt include:
hypoplastic pulmonary arteries, single pulmonary artery, virtual pulmonary atresia and anomalous coronary anatomy.

Following total correction there may be further problems:

- RV failure
- tachyarrhythmias
- heart block (see position of bundle just beneath VSD)
- pulmonary regurgitation
- RVOT aneurysm
- problems from initial shunt
- reopened VSD

RV failure and rhythm problems are the most important. Repeat cardiac catheterisation is sometimes necessary in patients following total correction to assess all these factors.

2.8 Total anomalous pulmonary venous drainage (TAPVD)

In TAPVD all four pulmonary veins drain directly or indirectly into the right atrium. There is an associated ASD to allow flow to the left heart. Pulmonary flow is increased and the child is cyanosed. The degree of cyanosis and the severity of symptoms depend on:

- the size of the ASD
- the degree of pulmonary hypertension
- the presence of pulmonary venous obstruction

Cyanosis is more severe if pulmonary flow is reduced (e.g. with irreversible pulmonary hypertension) and if mixing in the atria is poor (e.g. with small ASD or PFO). The child with the least cyanosis is the one with high pulmonary flow, low PVR and good atrial mixing (large ASD). Pulmonary venous obstruction reduces pulmonary flow and increases cyanosis, and is most common with infra-cardiac TAPVD (see below).

2.8 Total anomalous pulmonary venous drainage

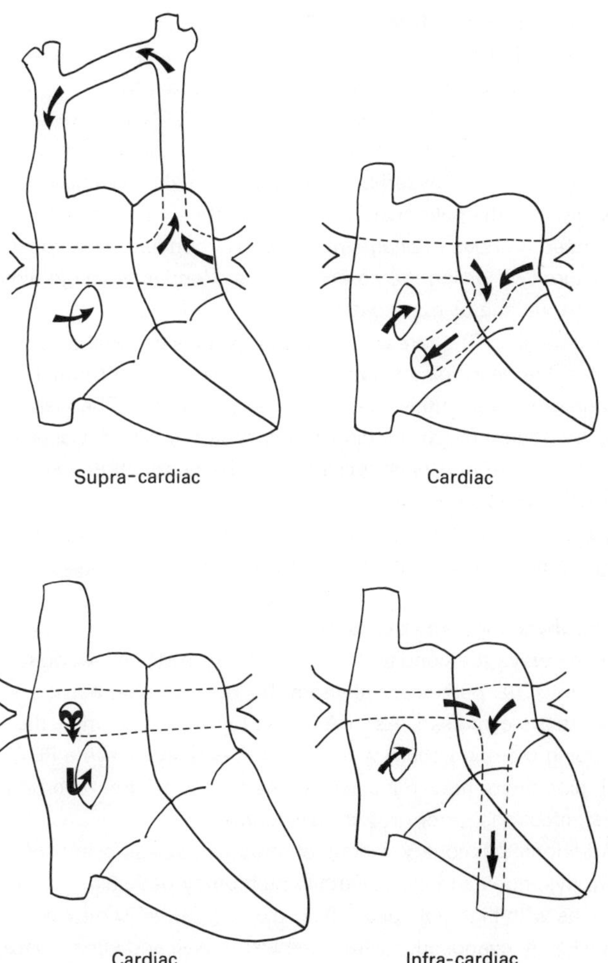

Fig. 2.7 Total anomalous pulmonary venous drainage. An ASD is part of the lesion.

2.8 Total anomalous pulmonary venous drainage

Anatomical possibilities (Fig. 2.7)
A variety of venous pathways can conduct pulmonary venous blood to the right atrium. They can be divided into:

- *Supra-cardiac*. Venous drainage to a left SVC which joins the left innominate vein thence to the right SVC. This vein may be occasionally compressed between the left main bronchus (behind) and the pulmonary trunk (in front).
- *Cardiac*. Venous drainage into a venous confluence (a sort of miniature LA) joining the coronary sinus. Venous drainage directly into RA via one or more ostia.
- *Infra-cardiac*. The rarest variety. The venous confluence at the back of the heart joins a vertical vein passing down through the diaphragm to join either the IVC or the portal vein. The vein may be obstructed at the diaphragm, or at the liver if it drains into the portal system. Crying will increase the obstruction and increase cyanosis.

Various combinations of these three are possible (e.g. left lung to vertical vein, right lung direct to RA).

Pathophysiology and symptoms
In many ways the condition is similar to an ASD (left-to-right shunt into RA, pulmonary plethora, RV hypertrophy) but the patients are cyanosed. As in ASD the LV is usually small, the RV doing the extra shunt work. Most infants also have a PDA. High pulmonary flow in a child causes cardiac failure, recurrent chest infections, poor growth development.

Additional pulmonary venous obstruction causes cyanosis at birth, dyspnoea and early death in pulmonary oedema.

Cases with high pulmonary flow plus a large ASD may be only slightly cyanosed, tolerate the lesion well and survive into adult life.

Physical signs
In patients with no venous obstruction (usually supra-cardiac TAPVD) similar to those in ASD (p. 31) with additional:

- cyanosis (mild-to-moderate depending on pulmonary flow)
- a continuous murmur (hum) either high up the LSE or in the aortic area. This is the venous hum of high flow in the SVC with TAPVD to the left innominate vein (supra-cardiac)

In patients with venous obstruction (usually infra-cardiac TAPVD) look for:

- prominent 'a' wave in JVP with pulmonary hypertension, but difficult to see in babies
- sick infant, vomiting, deeply cyanosed, tachypnoea, CCF
- no murmus. Loud P_2. Gallop rhythm

Chest x-ray

The supra-cardiac type shows the 'cottage loaf' heart. Dilated SVC and anomalous vein (left SVC) to the left innominate forming the wide upper mediastinal shadow. There is pulmonary plethora although this may not be obvious in the neonate. With additional pulmonary venous obstruction there are additional signs of pulmonary oedema. The left ventricle and left atrium are small, however, so that marked cardiomegaly is not common.

ECG

Similar to a secundum ASD in mild cases. With pulmonary hypertension marked RAD, and RV hypertrophy occur with P pulmonale, and RV strain pattern (T wave inversion V_{1-4}).

Echocardiography

May be useful in defining cases with pulmonary venous obstruction. Septal motion is paradoxical in patients with high pulmonary flow and unobstructed pulmonary veins (RV volume overload). In children with pulmonary hypertension and pulmonary venous obstruction septal motion is usually normal. Two-dimensional echocardiography is useful in defining pulmonary venous anatomy, the venous confluence and the site of drainage.

Differential diagnosis

In cyanosed children with pulmonary plethora on the CxR consider: TGA, primitive ventricle, truncus arteriosus, single atrium.

In patients with gross pulmonary venous obstruction other causes have to be considered, e.g. cor triatriatum, congenital mitral stenosis.

Cardiac catheterisation

Pulmonary angiography with follow through is necessary to detect the pulmonary venous anatomy. A saturation run is needed with sampling also in low IVC and left innominate vein. All pulmonary veins must be identified.

If infants are less than 2 months old, Rashkind balloon septostomy may help by increasing ASD size and allowing better mixing, with reduction in cyanosis and an increased PaO_2.

Surgery

Supra-cardiac type. The common pulmonary vein is anastomosed to the back of the LA. The ASD is closed and the left SVC ligated.

Cardiac type. The inter-atrial septum is refashioned depending on the exact anatomy to include the drainage site of the pulmonary veins into the LA. The coronary sinus may be included in the LA.

Infra-cardiac type. The common pulmonary vein is anastomosed to the back of the LA. The ASD is closed and the descending anomalous vein ligated.

Recurrence of pulmonary venous obstruction post-operatively may be a problem.

Cases with high pulmonary flow and good mixing tolerate the lesion well without surgical intervention.

2.9 Cyanotic congenital heart disease in the adult

In adults, inoperable cyanotic congenital heart disease is usually due to the Eisenmenger situation with PA pressure at systemic level and bidirectional shunting through an ASD, or VSD, or patent ductus arteriosus. It may also be caused by incompletely corrected Fallot's tetralogy or more rarely Ebstein's anomaly, pulmonary atresia, or truncus.

In a few young patients, heart lung transplantation has offered the only hope of a cure for the Eisenmenger syndrome. Early results are good and at least one woman has had a child following heart lung transplantation.

Careful follow up of these patients is essential as there are many non-cardiac problems to be considered.

Polycythaemia

A persistent haemoglobin level over 20 mg/100 ml carries a risk of thrombosis. Patients may also complain of headaches, transient visual disturbances, dizzy turns or even pruritus. Regular venesection may be necessary with simultaneous exchanges of whole blood with a plasma expander. Patients must not become hypotensive during venesection. Iron deficiency may keep the haemoglobin low with patients rapidly becoming polycythaemic if put on oral iron.

Dental hygiene

Frequent dental visits are often necessary as adults may get periodontal disease and gingivitis. A dental brace is a particular hazard for this group with the risks of infected gums seeding the circulation and causing a cerebral abscess.

Skin

Acne is a common problem and septic foci must be treated early. Long-term tetracycline therapy may be indicated.

2.9 Cyanotic congenital heart disease in the adult

Cerebral abscess
This is a recognised hazard of dental or skin sepsis with the passage of bacteria across a septal defect due to the bidirectional shunt. The development of neurological symptoms or signs, drowsiness or a PUO require urgent investigation and a neurological expert.

Gout
A common problem which can usually be managed with long term allopurinol 100–300 mg od. Renal function must be checked in these patients.

Contraception
Pregnancy is poorly tolerated in this condition and spontaneous abortion is very common. Contraception must be discussed with all women with cyanotic heart disease. The pill is contra-indicated (thrombosis risk) and the IUCD best avoided (infection risk). Sterilisation must be seriously considered and is probably safer using a mini laparotomy and tubal ligation rather than laparoscopic sterilisation.

High altitudes
Should be avoided.

Antibiotic prophylaxis
Routinely given prior to any dental or surgical procedure.

General anaesthesia
Is not contra-indicated but may be hazardous. Hypotension must be avoided with the risk of increasing the right-to-left shunt.

3 Valve disease

3 Valve disease

3.1 Mitral stenosis

This is almost always secondary to rheumatic fever, although only half the patients have a positive history. The incidence is declining although many cases from the third world are severe. Two-thirds of patients are female.

Aetiology

Valvar

1 Rheumatic. Almost all cases. All the rest are rare.
2 Congenital: isolated lesion or associated with ASD (Lutembacher's syndrome). Some of these cases may be rheumatic mitral stenosis plus a patent foramen ovale.
3 Mucopolysaccharidoses. Hurler's syndrome. Glycoprotein deposition on the mitral leaflets.
4 Endocardial fibroelastosis spreading on to the valve.
5 Prosthetic valve. Usually only in mechanical valves (e.g. Starr – Edwards, Bjork – Shiley).
6 Malignant carcinoid.

Inflow obstruction

Conditions which mimic mitral stenosis, e.g.

- left atrial myxoma
- left atrial ball valve thrombus
- hypertrophic obstructive cardiomyopathy (p. 117)
- cor triatriatum (stenosis of a common pulmonary vein).

Pathogenesis

Group A (usually Type 12) streptococci have cell wall antigens which cross react with structural glycoproteins of the heart valves. Very small nodules (macrophages and fibroblasts) develop on the valve edge and the cusp gradually thickens. Stenosis occurs at three levels:

- commissures: these fuse with the valve cusps still mobile
- cusps: the valve leaflets become thick and eventually they become calcified

• chordae: these fuse, shorten, and thicken
A combination of all three results in a 'fish mouth' button hole orifice.

Pathophysiology and symptoms

1 Dyspnoea on effort: orthopnoea and PND
A rising left atrial pressure is transmitted to pulmonary veins. Secondary pulmonary arterial hypertension results.
Pulmonary oedema may be precipitated by:
• development of uncontrolled AF
• pregnancy
• exercise
• chest infection
• emotional stress
• anaesthesia.

2 Fatigue: due to low cardiac output in moderate to severe stenosis. A doubling of cardiac output quadruples the mitral valve gradient. The loss of atrial transport when AF develops results in a fall in cardiac output. Exercise tolerance on the basis of four classes is based on the New York Heart Association criteria (see p. 5).

3 Haemoptysis: may be due to:
• bronchial vein rupture: 'pulmonary apoplexy'. Large haemorrhage but not usually life threatening
• alveolar capillary rupture: pink frothy sputum in pulmonary oedema
• pulmonary infarction: in low output states and immobile patients
• blood stained sputum: in chronic bronchitis associated with attacks of dyspnoea.

4 Systemic emboli: in 20–30%.
Thrombus develops in large 'stagnant' left atrium and atrial appendage, mainly in patients with AF, low output and large atria. It may be the presenting symptom. Mesenteric, saddle and ilio-

femoral emboli are common. Ball valve thrombus may occur in LA.

5 Chronic bronchitis: common in MS. Due to oedematous bronchial mucosa.

6 Chest pain: like angina. In patients with RV hypertrophy secondary to pulmonary hypertension—even with normal coronaries. Coronary embolism may occur.

7 Palpitations: paroxysmal AF with fast ventricular response.

8 Symptoms of right heart failure: pulmonary hypertension and possible functional tricuspid regurgitation: hepatic pain on effort (hepatic angina), ascites, ankle and leg oedema.

9 Symptoms of left atrial enlargement compressing other structures:

- left recurrent laryngeal nerve. Hoarseness (Ortner's syndrome)
- oesophagus. Dysphagia (beware potassium replacement tablets causing oesophageal ulceration)
- left main bronchus. Very rarely causing left lung collapse.

10 Infective endocarditis: (p. 336). Rare in pure mitral stenosis.

Physical signs (Fig. 3.1)

1 S_1 loud as mitral valve is open throughout diastole and is suddenly slammed shut by ventricular systole. It indicates mobile leaflets.

2 A_2–OS interval shortens with increasing severity of stenosis. LA pressure 'climbs' up LV pressure curve approaching in time aortic valve closure. (See cardiac catheterisation.)

3 The length of the diastolic murmur is an indication of the severity of stenosis.

Differential diagnosis

1 Causes of inflow obstruction (HOCM, LA myxoma, ball valve thrombus).

2 Causes of rumbling mitral or tricuspid diastolic murmur

- aortic regurgitation (p. 99) (Austin–Flint)

3.1 Mitral stenosis

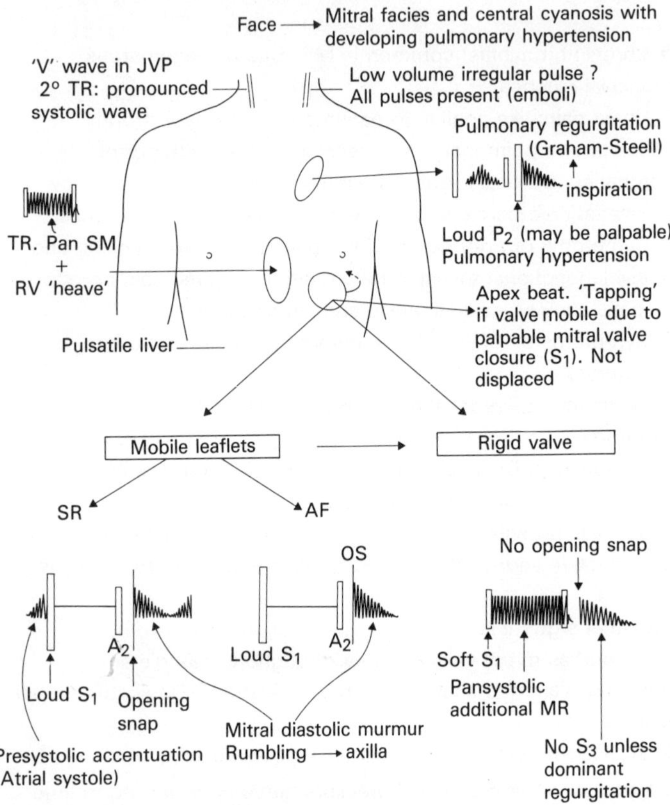

Fig. 3.1 Physical signs of mitral stenosis.

- flow murmur in ASD. This may be confusing (see Fig. 3.2)
- tricuspid stenosis. Diastolic murmur accentuated by inspiration. Best sign is slow 'y' descent on JVP.

3 Causes of early diastolic sound resembling opening snap:

- constrictive pericarditis } sudden cessation of early
- restrictive myopathy } rapid ventricular filling.

3.1 Mitral stenosis

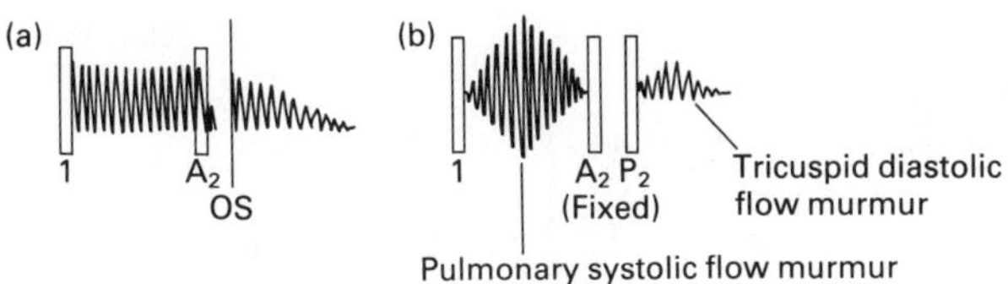

Fig. 3.2 Similarity on ausculation between mixed mitral valve disease (a) and ASD (b).

4 Causes of loud S_1: Tachycardia and hyperdynamic states (valve still open at end-diastole, and forceful closure by hypercontractile LV).

ECG

Atrial fibrillation (in sinus rhythm P mitrale). RV hypertrophy. Small voltage in lead V_1. Progressive right axis deviation.

Echocardiography (see 10.3)

In pure mitral stenosis with mobile leaflets this obviates the need for cardiac catheterisation. It may show:

- thickened mitral leaflets with the posterior leaflet moving anteriorly in diastole. Mitral opening coincides with snap on phonocardiogram
- reduced diastolic closure rate (E–F) slope of mitral anterior leaflet
- small LV (unless additional MR present)
- pulmonary valve may be flat with absent 'a' wave opening (in pulmonary hypertension)
- calcification of mitral leaflets or mitral annulus

Echocardiography is also very useful in distinguishing the 'mimics' of mitral stenosis. It will diagnose a left atrial myxoma, HOCM, and aortic regurgitation. It is very useful as a guide to the severity of mitral stenosis, and to document the results of mitral valvotomy. The mobility of the mitral leaflets is easily seen.

3.1 Mitral stenosis

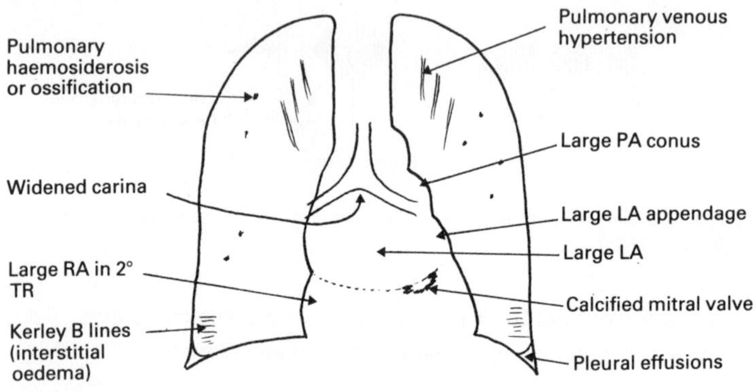

Fig. 3.3 Chest x-ray in mitral stenosis.

Cardiac catheterisation

Should be unnecessary in young patients with a mobile valve and no signs of mitral regurgitation. It is contraindicated in pregnancy when echocardiography is essential. A patient with atrial myxoma diagnosed by echo should not be catheterised. (The LV catheter may knock fragments off a prolapsing myxoma.) A myxoma requires urgent surgery.

Cardiac catheterisation is necessary in patients who have had a previous valvotomy to assess the mitral valve and the degree of regurgitation. It is necessary in patients with signs of mitral regurgitation. This cannot be measured by conventional M-mode echo. Doppler echocardiography can be diagnostic. See **10.3**.

Catheterisation is also required in patients with signs of other valve disease, symptoms of angina (coronary angiography), signs of severe pulmonary hypertension and when the mitral valve is calcified on CxR. If mitral valve replacement is envisaged, coronary angiography is usually performed (especially in the elderly).

The mean mitral gradient is calculated at rest and if this is low also on exercise (straight leg raising). The mitral valve area can be calculated if the cardiac output is measured (p. 441).

Medical treatment

1 Digoxin: In atrial fibrillation only. If fast AF is not slowed by standard doses either a small dose of Verapamil or β-blocking agent should be added. There is no evidence that digoxin prevents the development of AF in patients still in sinus rhythm.
2 Diuretics: are necessary to reduce preload and pulmonary venous congestion. They may help delay the need for surgery.
3 Anticoagulants: are still controversial. They should be used in patients who:
• have had a previous systemic/pulmonary embolism
• have a mitral prosthesis (tissue or mechanical)
• have low output states with right heart failure
• are in AF with moderate mitral stenosis and who have not had an atrial appendicectomy.

Anticoagulants are not of proven benefit in sinus rhythm. They should be avoided in pregnancy. Patients who have had a mitral valvotomy and atrial appendicectomy can probably be managed without anticoagulants provided they do not fall into the above categories.

Cardioversion

May be attempted if the development of AF is recent and the patient is anticoagulated. If not there is a risk of systemic emboli.

Heparinisation for 24 hours prior to cardioversion is not adequate. There is nothing to be gained by repeated cardioversions. AF should be accepted and the ventricular rate slowed. Quinidine or amiodarone may help prevent the development of AF in patients who have been successfully cardioverted.

Infective endocarditis (p. 331) is rare in pure mitral stenosis.

Acute rheumatic fever should be thought of in any young patient presenting for the first time with mitral stenosis. Histology of the atrial appendage will help in diagnosis. Prevent further attacks with penicillin 250 mg b.d. or sulphadimidine 500 mg b.d. It should be continued in young women to age 40 years.

Surgical considerations

There is still no perfect mitral valve prosthesis and surgery aims to preserve the native valve if possible, especially in the younger patient. It is necessary to consider surgery in the following:

- patients with moderate symptoms (functional NYHA Class III or IV)
- patients unable to work because of symptoms
- systemic emboli
- calculated valve area of $< 1\ cm^2$
- serious symptoms developing in pregnancy

1 Closed mitral valvotomy: (closed commissurotomy). Performed through left thoracotomy without bypass. Used in younger patients with mobile non-calcified valves with no regurgitation. The operation splits the commissures and with a successful operation benefit should last 10–15 years. It can sometimes be repeated, but usually with a shorter period of symptomatic relief. May be performed in mid trimester of pregnancy.

2 Open mitral valvotomy: (open commissurotomy). Performed through median sternotomy with bypass. Used in patients who may have already had a closed valvotomy and in whom there are other features, e.g. mild regurgitation or mild valve calcification, or in whom there is some evidence of 'sub-valvar' stenosis or a history of systemic emboli.

3 Mitral valve replacement. In heavily calcified valves, rigid fibrosed valves, severe chordal thickening and fusion, or unacceptable mitral regurgitation.

Mitral restenosis occurs over a period of years due to turbulent flow through thickened valve leaflets resulting in platelet and fibrin deposition. It is least likely to occur where a good commissurotomy with pliable leaflets results in good mitral flow.

Early restenosis (symptoms after 5 years) usually means inadequate valvotomy and patients may do well with a second (open) valvotomy. Late restenosis may need valve replacement due to degenerative change plus calcification.

Mitral valvuloplasty
Balloon mitral valvuloplasty is now a possibility as an alternative to surgery in patients suitable for a closed valvotomy. One or two balloons are inserted via the trans-septal route across the mitral valve and stabilised by guide wires advanced into the aorta. It is a complex technique not yet available in every cardiac centre.

3.2 Mitral regurgitation

This may be due to abnormalities of the mitral annulus, the mitral leaflets, the chordae or the papillary muscles. Chordal or papillary muscle dysfunction is subvalvar mitral regurgitation. Many disease processes affect the valve at more than one level.

Aetiology (see table on p. 76)

Functional mitral regurgitation
Is probably a combination of mitral annulus dilatation and papillary muscle malalignment. It occurs in LV dilatation from any cause, commonly in congestive cardiomyopathy (COCM) and ischaemic heart disease.

Annulus calcification
Occurs in the elderly and is more common in females, diabetics, and patients with Paget's disease. It commonly affects the posterior part of the mitral annulus and is often visible as a calcified band at the back of the heart on the lateral chest x-ray with calcium in the posterior AV groove. The calcium may involve the mitral leaflets causing mitral regurgitation and eventually the conducting system. Very severe ring calcification

may make mitral valve replacement impossible. In its milder form it causes no mitral valve problem and may be a chance finding on CxR or echocardiography.

Valvar regurgitation
Is commonly due either to rheumatic fever, infective endocarditis or the floppy valve. In rheumatic causes the cusps are thickened, with fused commissures and often a 'fish mouth' orifice. Patients commonly have combined MS and MR.

Aetiology of mitral regurgitation

Mitral annulus	**Mitral leaflets**			**Chordae**	**Papillary muscles**
Senile calcification Degeneration Functional dilatation Ring abscesses Marfan	*Infective*	*Congenital*	*Connective tissues disorders*	*Elongation rupture*	*Dysfunction rupture*
	SBE Rheumatic	1° ASD A–V canal Clefts Perforations Absence (2° ASD)	Marfan PXE Osteo-genesis imperfecta Ehlers-Danlos	Marfan Ischaemia SBE Trauma Rheumatic Idiopathic Ehlers-Danlos Parachute MV	Ischaemia Infarction Abscess Infiltrations Sarcoid Amyloid Myocarditis Hurlers
	Floppy valve				*Malalignment* *LV* dilatation LV aneurysm HOCM EFE Corrected TGA

Chordal rupture
Is often idiopathic. Myxomatous degeneration in the floppy valve syndrome may also involve the chordae which stretch and eventually rupture. Ischaemia may cause chordal rupture.

Papillary muscle dysfunction
Inferior infarction commonly causes posterior papillary muscle dysfunction with characteristic signs (see below). Anterior papillary muscle dysfunction is much rarer and signifies a large anterior infarct with probable additional right coronary artery disease.

The floppy valve
This forms a spectrum of conditions from an asymptomatic patient with a mid-systolic click, to one with severe mitral regurgitation from chordal rupture. (It has also been called: mitral leaflet prolapse, mitral click systolic murmur syndrome, Barlow's syndrome, myxomatous degeneration of the mitral valve, billowing mitral valve syndrome). It occurs as the following:
• an isolated lesion often in symptomatic patients
• associated with other conditions, e.g. secundum ASD; Turner's syndrome; PDA; Marfan's syndrome; osteogenesis imperfecta; pseudoxanthoma elasticum; cardiomyopathy; WPW syndrome

It occurs in approximately 4% of the normal asymptomatic population. It has been grossly overdiagnosed echocardiographically and is a cause of cardiac neurosis. It is due to progressive stretching of the mitral leaflets with weakening due to acid mucopolysaccharide deposition in the zona spongiosa. The chordae are also involved. Tricuspid prolapse may coexist.
• most patients are asymptomatic. Some have non-specific atypical chest pain (non-anginal) and palpitations
• infective endocarditis prophylaxis is necessary for those patients with a murmur. An isolated mid-systolic click does not merit them

3.2 Mitral regurgitation

Rarely complications develop, e.g. progressive mitral regurgitation requiring MVR; cerebral emboli; dysrhythmias may be ventricular with re-entry and pre-excitation associated pathways; sudden death.

Pathophysiology and symptoms

Mild cases of MR may be asymptomatic for many years. Most patients fall into one of two groups depending on the time course of events, and the size/compliance of the left atrium.

In acute MR the small LA cannot absorb the regurgitant fraction and the systolic wave is transmitted to the pulmonary veins, with resulting acute pulmonary oedema. In long-standing MR the LA is large, it can absorb the regurgitant fraction and the 'v' wave transmitted to the pulmonary veins is small.

Symptoms are similar to mitral stenosis in the chronic state. Haemoptysis and systemic emboli are less frequent.

Acute	Chronic
Sudden onset dyspnoea and pulmonary oedema	Chronic dyspnoea and fatigue
Small LA. 'Non compliant'	Large LA. 'Compliant'
Usually still in SR	Usually in AF
?Apical thrill if chordal rupture	?Associated mitral stenosis
Often ejection quality systolic murmur	Pansystolic murmur
Pulmonary hypertension	Pulmonary hypertension less severe
Large 'v' wave on wedge trace	Lower 'v' wave in wedge trace except on effort
Common causes	
Chordal rupture	Rheumatic valve
Acute inferior infarction with posterior papillary muscle dysfunction (rupture is rarer)	Floppy valve
Infective endocarditis	Functional MR

Generally pulmonary hypertension and right heart symptoms are not as frequent in MR as in pure MS. Infective endocarditis is more common in MR however.

Physical signs in the floppy valve syndrome
These vary with the degree of mitral regurgitation. With mild or moderate degrees of mitral regurgitation signs peculiar to the floppy valve syndrome are shown below. With severe regurgitation physical signs are less specific.

Apex beat
A double apex may be noted in some patients with a floppy valve. Tensing of the chordae in mid-systole may cause this mid-systolic dip. It is best felt with the patient lying on his or her left side.

Murmurs
As LV volume diminishes in mid-systole the floppy valve starts to prolapse and a mid-systolic click (tensing of chordae) often precedes the murmur of mitral regurgitation (there may be more than one click). In very mild cases a mid-systolic click with no murmur is common.

The smaller the ventricle the earlier the systolic click and the longer the murmur, which gets louder up to S_2. The signs may be altered by various manoeuvres in a similar way to HOCM (p. 121) (Fig. 3.4).

Differential diagnosis
1 *Aortic valve stenosis*: The floppy valve has a normal or slightly collapsing pulse. The mid-systolic click occurs after the carotid upstroke.
2 HOCM: This is more difficult as both may have similar pulses, double apex beats, and murmurs getting louder on amyl nitrate inhalation. HOCM does not have a mid-systolic click, and more LV+.

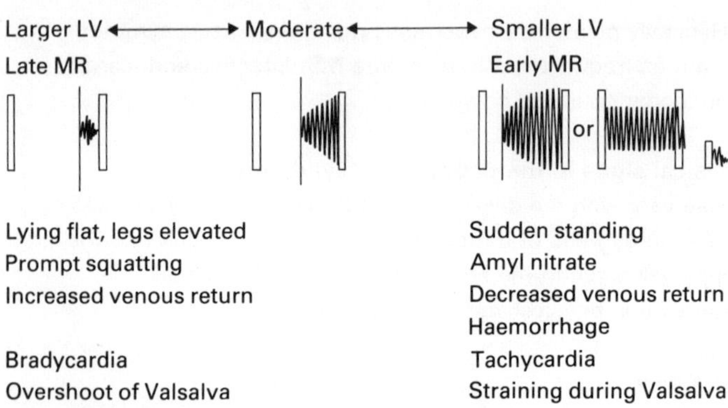

Fig. 3.4 Mitral regurgitation in the floppy valve syndrome.

3 VSD: Here the murmur is usually pansystolic with a thrill both maximum at the left sternal edge. Differentiation from subvalvar regurgitation with posterior chordal rupture may be impossible clinically, especially if associated with myocardial infarction.

4 *Papillary muscle dysfunction*: Classically post-inferior infarct. The murmur may be late systolic but without a click. In more severe cases the murmur is pansystolic.

5 *Tricuspid regurgitation*: An 'inspiratory' murmur loudest at the left sternal edge. Best sign is prominent systolic waves in the JVP.

Physical signs in chronic valvar mitral regurgitation (Fig. 3.5)

1 Sudden premature ventricular emptying due to MR results in early aortic valve closure. The murmur may continue through A_2. S_2 is thus more than normally split and P_2 may be loud if additional pulmonary hypertension is present.

2 Features to suggest chordal rupture as opposed to valvar regurgitation

- sinus rhythm
- apical thrill in systole

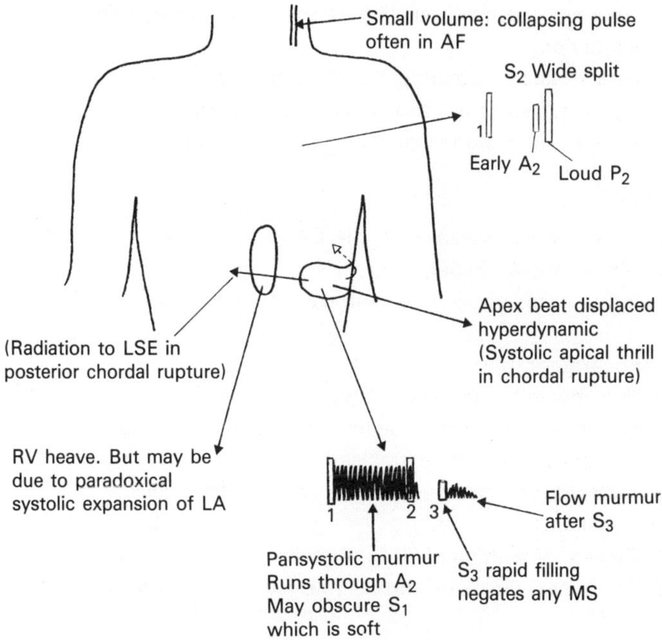

Fig. 3.5 Physical signs in chronic valvar mitral regurgitation.

• murmur is more ejection in quality and sometimes mid- to late-systolic.

3 In posterior chordal rupture the jet is directed to the anterior wall of the left atrium. The murmur is often loudest at the left sternal edge. In anterior chordal rupture the jet is directed posteriorly and the murmur may be loudest in the back.

Important points in mitral regurgitation clinically

• the intensity of the systolic murmur is absolutely no guide to the severity of the regurgitation. Prosthetic valve regurgitation may be inaudible

• a murmur maximal at the left sternal edge may be mitral regurgitation
• mitral regurgitant murmurs may be pansystolic, late-crescendo-systolic or ejection systolic in quality
• check P_2 moves on inspiration to exclude ASD

ECG
1 AF in chronic disease. If in SR: LA +.
2 Left ventricular hypertrophy.
3 A few cases show right ventricular hypertrophy in addition.

Echocardiography
1 To show left atrial size with systolic expansion.
2 May show a flail mitral leaflet with chaotic movement.
3 May show posterior mitral leaflet prolapse—late or pansystolic: vegetations on mitral valve, mitral annulus calcification.
4 Dilated LV with rapid filling. Dimensions relate to prognosis.
5 Rapid diastolic mitral closure rate (steep E–F slope) due to rapid filling.
6 Mean VCF (circumferential fibre shortening) often increased with good LV function.
7 Possibly additional floppy tricuspid or aortic valves.
8 Doppler will establish size and site of regurgitation jet.

Chest x-ray
• left ventricular dilatation enlarging the ventricular mass and left heart border
• LA dilatation in chronic cases. Rarely giant left atrium may occur with calcified wall
• mitral valve calcification, signs of pulmonary venous congestion, Kerley B lines as in mitral stenosis

Cardiac catheterisation
Is necessary to confirm the diagnosis and exclude other valve

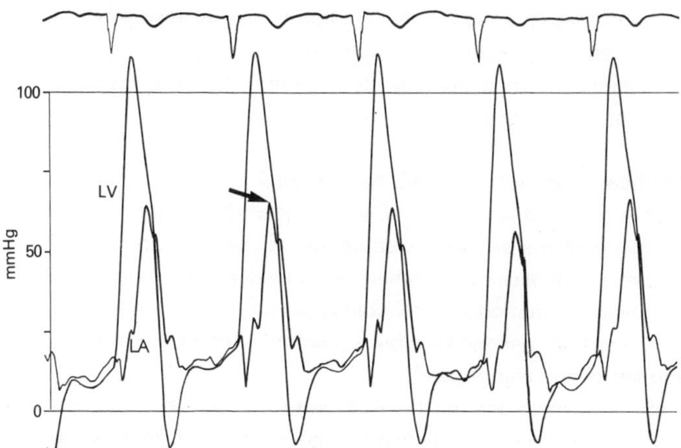

Fig. 3.6 Mitral regurgitation. Simultaneous recordings of left ventricualr and left atrial (recorded from PA wedge position) in a patient with actue mitral regurgitation from ruptured chordae. The 'v' wave reaches 60 mmHg due to the severe regurgitation and the small left atrium. The patient is still in sinus rhythm. The peak of the 'v' wave is arrowed.

disease. Left ventricular function is assessed. Coronary angiography is also performed.

The size of the 'v' wave in the pulmonary wedge or left atrial pressure trace depends on the severity of mitral regurgitation and the size of the left atrium. In severe cases of acute mitral regurgitation the 'v' wave may reach 50 mmHg or more. The height of the 'v' wave increases sharply with effort (Fig. 3.6).

Left ventricular angiography in the 30° right anterior oblique projection will show the severity of the regurgitation. In severe cases the regurgitant jet fills the pulmonary veins in one systole. The angiogram will also help identify the cause. In rheumatic mitral regurgitation there is usually one or more discrete jets through an immobile valve with associated stenosis.

In the floppy valve or chordal rupture the regurgitant jet is over a broad front, and the prolapsing leaflet can usually be seen.

Posterior papillary muscle dysfunction is usually associated with inferior hypokinesia. Spurious mitral regurgitation may be produced by ectopic beats or by a catheter too near the mitral valve or sub-valve apparatus.

Medical treatment (p. 192, heart failure)

- as in mitral stenosis fast AF is treated with digoxin
- anticoagulants are not indicated unless there is: a history of systemic embolism; a prosthetic mitral valve, either xenograft or mechanical; additional mitral stenosis with a low output
- diuretics are needed to reduce pulmonary venous congestion and left ventricular preload
- afterload reduction has been shown to reduce the regurgitant fraction and may even abolish it. Acute cases can be treated with i.v. nitroprusside, chronic ones with oral hydralazine
- in acute mitral regurgitation with chordal rupture and pulmonary oedema artificial ventilation and full monitoring as in cardiogenic shock may be necessary (p. 218)
- infective endocarditis should be considered (p. 333)

Prognosis

As in chronic aortic regurgitation chronic mitral regurgitation is a relatively well tolerated lesion if left ventricular function is preserved. Approximately 60% of patients with chronic MR are alive 10 years later. Prognosis depends on LV function.

Poorer prognostic features are:

- symptomatic history longer than one year
- atrial fibrillation
- patients aged over 60 years
- angiographic ejection fraction $< 50\%$
- angiographic LVEDV $> 100\ \mathrm{ml/m^2}$
- echocardiographic dimensions of left ventricle: end systolic dimension > 5 cm; end diastolic dimension > 7 cm

Surgery

Mitral valve replacement (MVR) for pure MR has been less successful than for pure mitral stenosis, possibly because MVR has been delayed until LV function is irreversibly impaired. Overall operative mortality is 5–10%.

1 *Acute mitral regurgitation with chordal rupture*: Surgery is necessary as medical treatment alone carries a poor prognosis. Mitral valve repair may be possible in some cases (e.g. plication of mitral cleft or commissure, advancement of posterior cusp in floppy valve). Annuloplasty is not usually satisfactory. Recurrent mitral regurgitation may occur following mitral repair. Most patients need MVR.

2 *Chronic mitral regurgitation*: MVR should be performed before LV function deteriorates irreversibly. Surgery is indicated for symptoms of increasing fatigue and dyspnoea (NYHA grades III and IV). Also in patients with Grade II symptoms who have enlarging heart on CxR and increasing dyspnoea.

3 *Post infarct mitral regurgitation*: papillary muscle infarction or rupture usually require urgent MVR without delay. Intensive vasodilator therapy or IABP may hold the situation for a few hours but are no substitute for surgery.

3.3 Aortic stenosis

Levels of aortic stenosis

Aortic stenosis may occur at three levels and the three are not mutually exclusive.

1 Valvar aortic stenosis.

2 Supravalvar aortic stenosis.

3 Subvalvar aortic stenosis. This may be due to:

- discrete fibromuscular ring
- hypertrophic obstructive cardiomyopathy (HOCM)
- tunnel subaortic stenosis
- anomalous attachment of anterior mitral leaflet: e.g. in AV

canal, or parachute deformity of mitral valve with fused papillary muscles

Various anatomical combinations may occur: a discrete fibromuscular ring with supravalve stenosis and/or a grossly hypertrophic upper septum. In severe cases in childhood the term 'higgledy-piggledy' left heart has been used to describe pathology in the subvalve region, the valve and aorta occurring together.

The term 'fixed subaortic' stenosis has been used to describe a group of conditions: discrete fibromuscular ring and tunnel subaortic stenosis as opposed to variable obstruction due to muscular hypertrophy in HOCM. The division is artificial as the conditions may coexist, and 'fixed' obstruction may be gradually acquired.

Valvar aortic stenosis

The commonest cause of aortic stenosis. It does not have a single aetiology (Fig. 3.7).

1 *Congenital valvar abnormality*

The commonest cause of isolated aortic stenosis, 72% in one series. Commoner in males (4:1).

- bicuspid valve (approx 1% of the population). The commonest form of congenital heart disease
- other degrees of commissural fusion: Unicommissural with eccentric hole, or even diaphragm (3 fused cusps) with central orifice. Unicuspid aortic valve is the commonest cause of aortic stenosis presenting under the age of one year. It often presents as part of the hypoplastic left heart syndrome. Both types become increasingly fibrotic and calcified with age, the bicuspid valve being the commonest cause of aortic valve stenosis in the age group 40–60 +

2 *Senile calcification of a normal valve*

Occurs in the age group 60 +. The valve is tricuspid. The commissures are not fused, but the cusps are immobilised by heavy calification. This often causes an ejection systolic

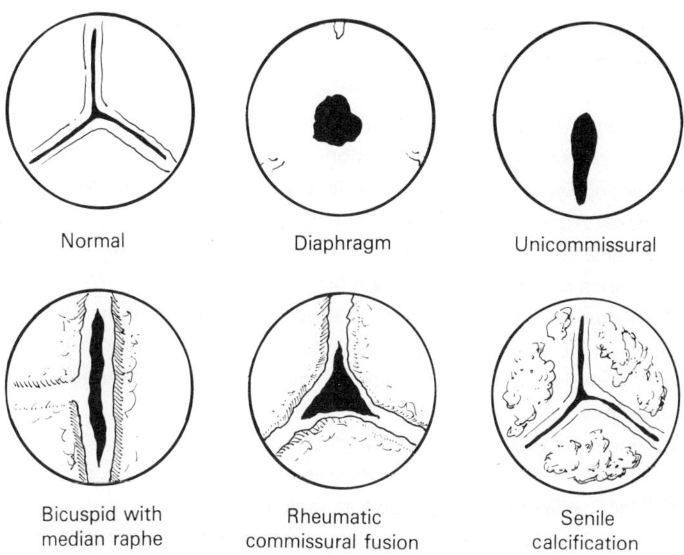

Fig. 3.7 Diagrammatic summary with valve viewed from above.

murmur, but frank aortic valve stenosis is not so common.

3 *Inflammatory valvulitis*

Rheumatic fever results in commissural fusion of a tricuspid valve. The valve is usually regurgitant also (Fig. 3.8). Rheumatoid arthritis may cause nodular thickening of aortic valve leaflets and rarely a degree of aortic stenosis usually with regurgitation.

4 *Atherosclerosis*

Severe hypercholesterolaemia in homozygous type II hyperlipoproteinaemia. Gross atheroma involves aortic wall, major arteries, aortic valve and coronary arteries.

Disease progression

Valvar obstruction gradually increases even in children who may be asymptomatic. Progressive valve calcification occurs, and may be visible on the chest x-ray from about the age of 40 years onwards. The severity of the calcification correlates roughly with the degree of stenosis.

Pathophysiology and symptoms

1 Compensated: good LV function with valve area >1 cm^2 May be asymptomatic. Children may be asymptomatic with severe disease. Adults may not present until age 60 +.

2 Angina: occurs with normal coronary arteries. Due to imbalance of myocardial oxygen supply/demand.

3 Dyspnoea: occurs due to high diastolic pressures in the left ventricle increasing with exercise. As LV function deteriorates (or AF occurs) orthopnoea and paroxysmal nocturnal dyspnoea supervene.

4 Giddiness or syncope on effort: possible reasons are:

• high intramural pressure on exercise firing baroreceptors to produce reflex bradycardia and vasodilatation

• skeletal muscle vasodilatation on exercise with no increase in cardiac output or additionai rhythm disturbance

Increased demand	Decreased supply
↑Cardiac work	Prolonged systole with shorter diastole.
↑Muscle mass from hypertrophy	
↑Wall stress from high intra-cavity pressure: both in systole and diastole	Reversed coronary flow in systole from venturi effect of narrow valve orifice. High intramural pressure in systole preventing systolic coronary flow. Low aortic perfusion pressure in diastole with high LVEDP. Rarely calcification extending to coronary ostia.

• development of complete AV block with aortic ring calcium extending into the upper ventricular septum.

5 Systemic emboli: often retinal or cerebral. Amaurosis fugax may be the presenting symptom especially when the valve is calcified. Small flecks of calcium and/or platelet emboli may be seen wedged in retinal arterioles on opthalmoscopy.

6 Sudden death: may occur in 7.5% of cases, even before severe ECG changes develop, e.g. in children.

7 Infective endocarditis: p. 331.

8 Congestive cardiac failure: severe aortic stenosis may present for the first time as CCF with a large heart, very low pulse volume and soft murmurs.

Physical signs. See Fig. 3.8.

Coexisting lesions

In addition to the fact that an aortic valve abnormality may coexist with subvalve stenosis, both lesions may occur with certain other congenital cardiovascular defects, e.g.

• aortic valve stenosis (bicuspid valve) + coarctation of the aorta (e.g. Turner's syndrome)

• aortic valve stenosis + coarctation + PDA

• VSD ± pulmonary stenosis

• as part of the hypoplastic left heart syndrome

• corrected TGA

• supra-valve stenosis with pulmonary artery branch stenosis

ECG in aortic valve stenosis

1 Should be in sinus rhythm. If in AF suspect additional mitral valve disease or ischaemic heart disease.

2 P mitrale with prominent negative P wave component in V_1 (due to high LVEDP).

3 LV hypertrophy.

4 'Strain pattern' in lateral chest leads. In children T wave inversion in inferior leads often occurs first. Severe aortic stenosis

3.3 Aortic stenosis

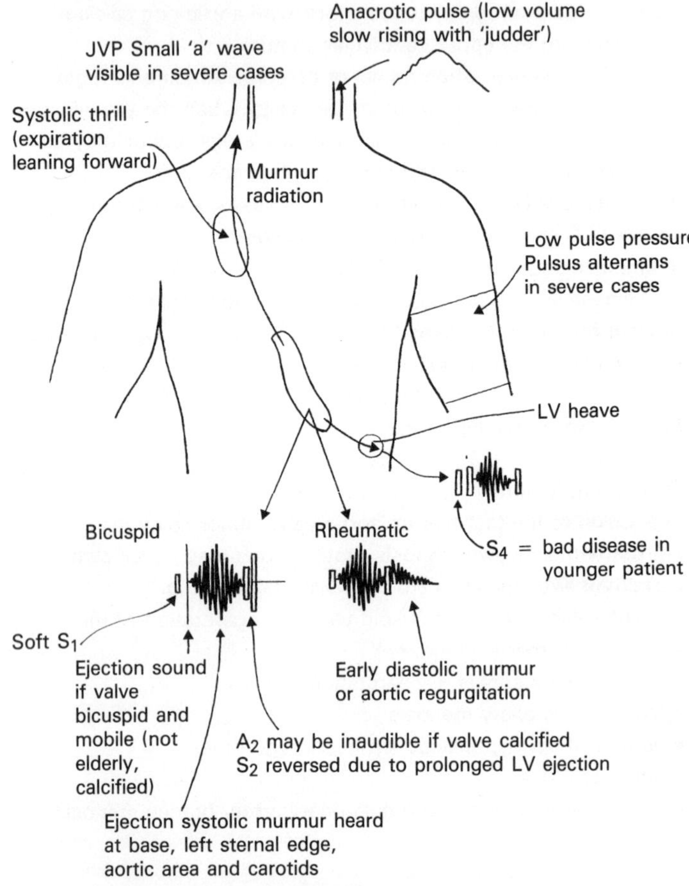

Fig. 3.8 Typical signs in valvar aortic stenosis.

may occur with a normal ECG in children.

5 Left axis deviation (due to left anterior hemiblock).

6 Poor R wave progression in anterior chest leads.

7 LBBB or complete heart block with calcified ring (in approx 5% cases).

Following aortic valve replacement there is often a reversion of the P and T wave changes gradually over the years, and a reduction in LV voltage as the LV mass is reduced.

Chest x-ray

May show:

- left ventricular hypertrophy
- calcified aortic valve (in age 40+). Calcium on lateral view will be above and anterior to oblique fissure
- post-stenotic dilatation of ascending aorta (not specific for valvar stenosis, e.g. may occur with fibromuscular ring in subvalvar stenosis)
- pulmonary venous congestion and signs of LVF
- *NB*. Check for rib notching and small or 'double' aortic knuckle in coarctation

Echocardiography

May show:

- bicuspid valve (eccentric 'closure' line) with reduced valve opening
- calcified valve (multiple echo-bands)
- LV hypertrophy. Assess LV function
- diastolic fluttering of anterior mitral leaflet if additional aortic regurgitation is present

Attempts to assess aortic valve gradient from Doppler echocardiography may be a substitute for cardiac catheterisation in the younger patient. 2-D echocardiography gives more information about the valve and LV function, but cannot provide coronary artery anatomy.

Cardiac catheterisation

May be performed to:

1 Document the aortic valve gradient (Fig. 3.9) or calculate the valve area (see Fig. 10.30). Peak systolic gradient of > 100 mmHg and valve area <0.5 cm^2 = severe aortic stenosis.

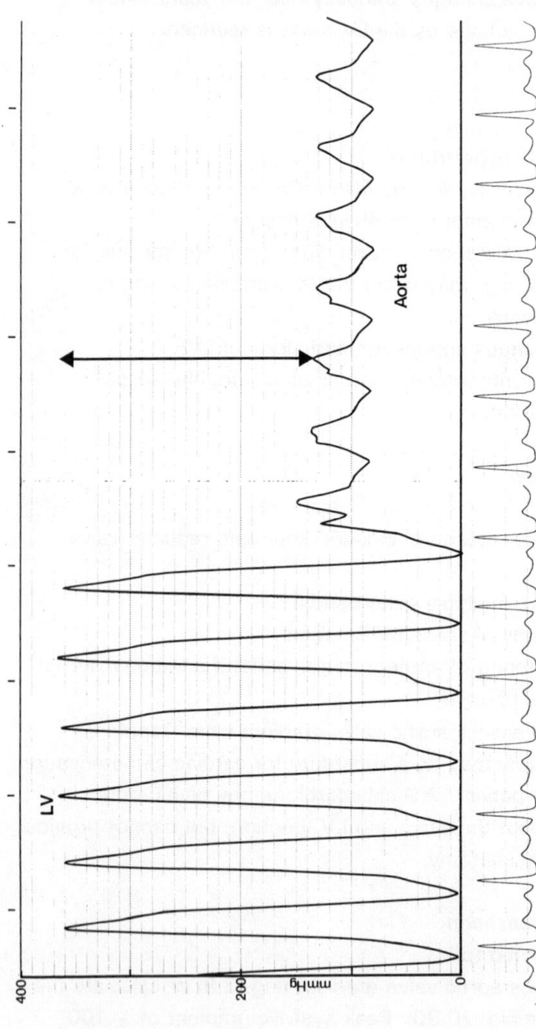

Fig. 3.9 Severe aortic valve stenosis. Withdrawal of catheter from left ventricle to aorta in a man with severe aortic valve stenosis due to a calcified bicuspid aortic valve. LV pressure is 360/0–40 and aortic pressure is 130/80. Peak-to-peak valve gradient is 230mmHg (arrowed).

2 Assess LV function.

3 Perform coronary angiography to document possible CAD and check the coronary ostial anatomy. Bicuspid aortic valve is associated with a dominant left coronary artery and short main stem.

4 Check the aortic root.

Indications for surgery

1 In children aortic valvotomy is performed in symptomatic patients or in asymptomatic ones with severe stenosis.

2 In adults aortic valve replacement is recommended once symptoms develop. The natural history of medically treated patients who are symptomatic is poor. (Average survival is 2–3 years with angina or syncope, 1½ years with cardiac failure.)

In patients who are asymptomatic but have documented severe stenosis and a deteriorating ECG, valve replacement is also recommended.

3 The decision to operate on the elderly patient must depend on:

- adequate hepatic and renal function
- adequate lung function (FEV_1 preferably >0.8–1 litre)
- reasonable adult weight (>40 kg)
- the severity of additional coronary disease or LV dysfunction.

Average operative mortality for isolated aortic valve replacement is now < 5%. The need for additional coronary revascularisation or the presence of poor LV function increases the risk (10–20%). Long-term survival post AVR depends on presence of:

- additional CAD and history of infarction
- heart size increasing pre-operatively
- low cardiac output
- pulmonary hypertension

Aortic valvuloplasty

This technique is proving useful in a very small group of elderly patients with severe aortic stenosis, who are considered inoperable (very poor LV function, poor lung function, renal failure, etc.). It is performed percutaneously in the catheter laboratory. The technique involves insertion of one or two balloons across the aortic valve via a guide wire(s). The balloon can usually be advanced across the valve retrogradely but the distal end of the balloon may damage the left ventricular septum and cause arrhythmias. The balloon is usually inflated for 4–9 atmospheres for up to 1 minute. The procedure usually causes an abrupt reduction in cardiac output during inflation and the patient should be well atropinised and not hypovolaemic.

Following valvuloplasty there is a gradient reduction, and usually an increase in aortic valve area. Long term results vary, and some workers have found only a temporary improvement in aortic valve area. Complications include profound bradycardia, hypotension, tamponade, systemic emboli, and death in a few cases. In addition there is a significant problem with entry site complications, some patients needing femoral artery repair. This problem is receding with use of a long arterial sheath.

Aortic valvuloplasty cannot be considered an alternative to aortic valve replacement. It is of value in a very small group of infirm patients, but its benefits may only be temporary.

Supra-valvar aortic stenosis

This is caused by a constricting ridge of fibrous tissue at the upper margin of the sinuses of Valsalva. The coronary ostia are below the stenosis. Rarely the obstruction is a more generalised hypoplasia of the ascending aorta.

Associated conditions

Williams' syndrome (autosomal dominant with variable penetration)

Children with:

- elfin facies (large mouth with protruding upper lip, high forehead, epicanthic folds, recessed nasal bridge, mental retardation, strabismus, low set ears)
- hypervitaminosis D and hypercalcaemia
- other cardiac lesions: peripheral pulmonary artery stenoses;

3.3 Aortic stenosis

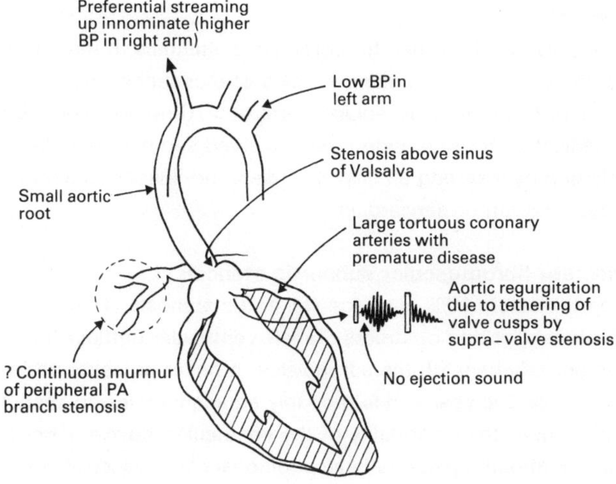

Fig. 3.10 Diagrammatic summary of supra-valvar aortic stenosis.

valvar pulmonary stenosis; aortic valve regurgitation.

- mesenteric artery stenoses, thoracic aortic aneurysms.
- rubella syndrome.

Cardiac lesion and signs

Supra-valve aortic stenosis should also be considered in a child who has additional aortic regurgitation, no ejection sound, and blood pressure in the left arm lower than the right. The CxR does not show post-stenotic dilatation of the ascending aorta.

Symptoms are those of valve stenosis. Coronary arteries are characteristically large but tend to have premature arterial disease due to the high pressure below the supra-valve stenosis.

The supravalve shelf and the adherent aortic cusps may rarely isolate the coronary artery orifice ('house martins nest' appearance on angiogram) and acute myocardial infarction or sudden death occur.

Surgery
Is less satisfactory than for aortic valve stenosis. It may only be possible if the ascending aorta is of reasonable size. A gradient from LV to ascending aorta of >70 mmHg would be an indication for operation. The narrowed segment may be enlarged by inserting an ellipse or diamond-shaped patch of woven dacron or pericardium.

Discrete fibromuscular subaortic stenosis
Approximately 10% of congenital aortic stenosis. The fibromuscular ring obstructs the left ventricular outflow tract immediately beneath the aortic valve. It never presents under the age of one year and is probably an acquired lesion associated with congenital abnormality of the ventricular muscle. About half the affected patients have additional cardiovascular lesions.

Distinction from valvar aortic stenosis
This may be very difficult. Discrete fibromuscular subaortic stenosis is a possibility if:
• there is aortic regurgitation (thickening of valve due to high velocity jet through obstruction or even attachment to the right coronary cusp)
• absent ejection sound (Fig. 3.11)
• no valve calcification
Post-stenotic dilatation of ascending aorta may or may not occur and is not reliable diagnostically.

Echocardiography
Is invaluable in establishing the diagnosis. On M-mode it may show the following:
• very early systolic closure of aortic valve (right coronary cusp especially), and systolic fluttering of aortic leaflets
• cluster of subaortic echoes above anterior mitral leaflet
Two dimensional echocardiography may show the subaortic shelf clearly in the long axis view in older children. The

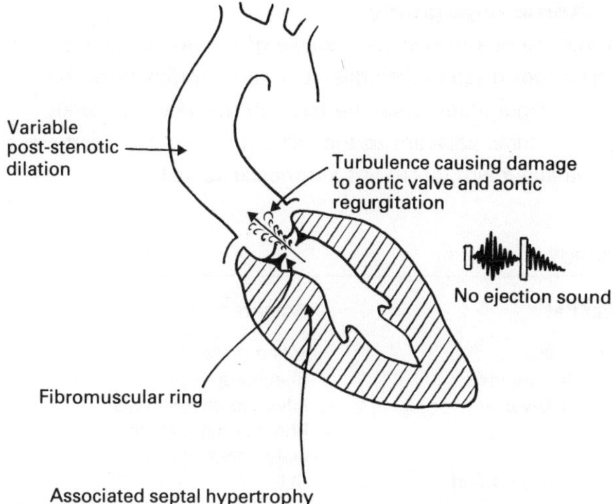

Fig. 3.11 Diagrammatic summary of discrete fibromuscular subaortic stenosis.

differentiation of the echoes from the aortic valve itself in younger children may be difficult.

Cardiac catheterisation

Confirms subaortic obstruction. The ring is visualised on LV angiography. The degree of the obstruction can be measured and additional aortic regurgitation assessed.

Surgery

Excision of the fibromuscular ring is possible, but often residual abnormal LV muscle remains (very similar to HOCM). The ring is excised through the aortic valve. There is usually a small residual gradient and sometimes mild aortic regurgitation. Follow up with repeat cardiac catheterisation is necessary to exclude recurrent obstruction. Occasionally eventual aortic valve replacement is required later for aortic regurgitation.

3.4 Aortic regurgitation

This may be due to primary disease of the aortic valve or due to aortic root disease with dilatation and stretching of the valve ring. The regurgitation may be through the valve, or rarely down a channel adjacent to the valve ring (e.g. ruptured sinus of Valsalva aneurysm, aorto-left ventricular tunnel).

Aetiology

Congenital	Acquired
Bicuspid valve Supra-valve stenosis Discrete sub-valvar fibromuscular ring Supra-cristal VSD with prolapse of right coronary cusp Ruptured sinus of Valsalva aneurysm	*Valve disease* Rheumatic fever Infective endocarditis Rheumatoid arthritis (valve nodules) SLE Pseudoxanthoma elasticum Hurler's syndrome and other mucopolysaccharidoses *Aortic root disease* Dissection (types I and II) Syphilis Cystic medial necrosis, e.g. Marfan's syndrome, Osteogenesis imperfecta Giant cell aortitis Arthritides with aortitis, e.g. ankylosing spondylitis, Reiters syndrome, Psoriasis Hypertension Trauma

Pathophysiology

Often moderate aortic regurgitation is tolerated with no symptoms.

- aortic regurgitation results in an increase in left ventricular end-diastolic volume (LVEDV) and end systolic volume (LVESV)

- the stroke volume (SV) is high in compensated cases
- left ventricular mass is raised with LV hypertrophy
- compensatory tachycardia reduces the regurgitant flow per beat by shortening diastole, and allows an increase in cardiac output

As the regurgitation increases and LV function deteriorates:

- LVEDP rises and may eventually equal aortic diastolic pressure
- premature mitral valve closure occurs preventing diastolic forward flow through the mitral valve
- LVEDV rises further but stroke volume falls

Symptoms

As in aortic stenosis, but angina and syncope are much less common. Unlike aortic stenosis, aortic regurgitation is a well tolerated lesion if gradual compensatory mechanisms can occur. Even moderate aortic regurgitation may be tolerated for years. However, acute valvar aortic regurgitation or ruptured sinus of Valsalva is poorly tolerated and quickly produces LVF or congestive cardiac failure. Intensive medical therapy followed by investigation and surgery is often necessary.

Eponyms associated with aortic regurgitation

1 Austin–Flint murmur. Due to vibrations in diastole of anterior mitral leaflet: oscillating between regurgitant jet and antegrade blood flow from left atrium. Very similar to mitral stenosis, but S_1 is quiet and there is no opening snap.

2 Duroziez's sign: to and from murmur audible over femoral arteries.

3 Quincke's pulse: capillary pulsation in finger tips or mucous membranes.

4 Traube's sign: 'pistol shot' sound audible over femoral arteries.

5 De Musset's head bobbing due to collapsing pulses.

Presence of additional aortic stenosis is detected by the bisferiens carotid pulse.

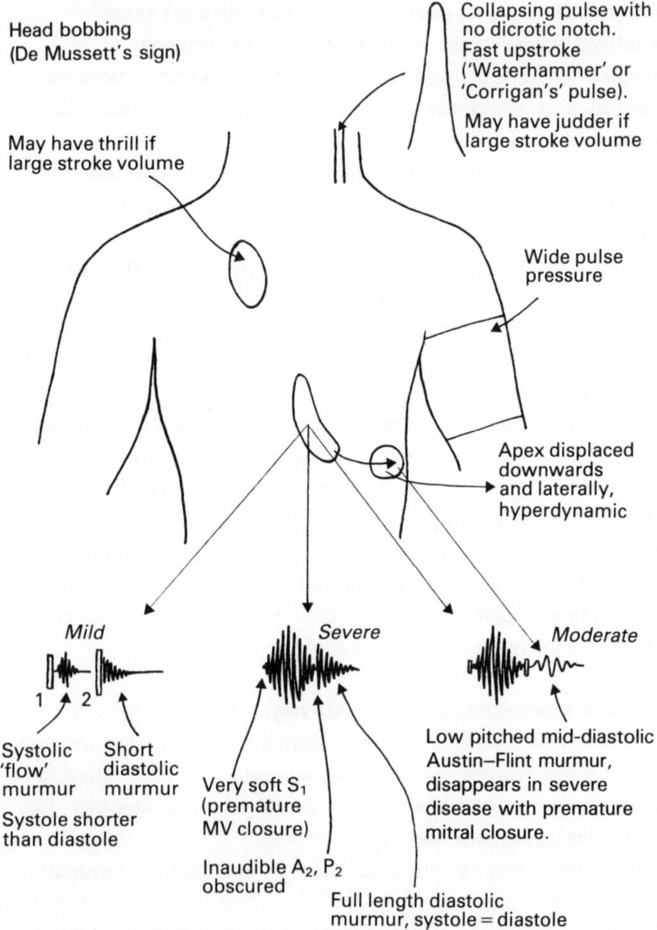

Fig. 3.12 Typical signs of aortic regurgitation. Left sternal edge: use diaphragm with patient sitting forward and breath held in expiration. Apex (to hear S_3 and Austin–Flint murmurs): use Bell with patient lying on left side.

Differential diagnosis of valvar aortic regurgitation

• pulmonary valve regurgitation, e.g. in patients who have had total correction of Fallot's tetralogy or post-pulmonary valvotomy. Patients with pulmonary hypertension secondary to mitral valve disease (Graham–Steel murmur)

• patent ductus arteriosus. Machinery murmur usually loudest in second left interspace

• VSD with aortic regurgitation. Usually right coronary cusp prolapses into or through a supracristal VSD. The prolapsing cusp may cause right ventricular outflow tract obstruction. (Retrosternal thrill, harsh pansystolic murmur, early diastolic murmur)

• ruptured sinus of Valsalva aneurysm. Usually right coronary sinus ruptures into RV outflow tract or RA. Sudden onset chest pain and CCF with high JVP

More rarely:

• coronary AV fistula. This presents during adult life with LVF due to left-to-right shunt (into RA, RV or coronary sinus)

• Pulmonary AV fistula. e.g. in patients with Osler–Rendu–Weber syndrome. + bronchiectasis, cyanosis and 2° polycythaemia

• aorto-pulmonary window. Usually large communication with resultant pulmonary hypertension. Rarely survive to adult life

• aorto-left ventricular tunnel

• persistent truncus arteriosus. Again rarely survive to adult life (early pulmonary hypertension, cyanosis, VSD + truncal valve regurgitation)

ECG

Left ventricular hypertrophy with diastolic overload pattern (prominent Q waves in anterolateral leads). ST depression and T wave inversion occur as the condition deteriorates.

Echocardiography

May show:

- LV function and dimensions. Exercise may detect early LV dysfunction
- aortic valve thickening. Possible 'vegetations' on aortic valve
- diastolic fluttering of anterior mitral leaflet (may be audible as the Austin–Flint murmur)
- premature mitral valve closure. Occasionally only the 'a' wave opens the mitral valve at all in severe cases

More rarely:

- aortic root dimensions and possible 'double' wall in aortic dissection
- flail aortic leaflet prolapsing into LV outflow tract

Chest x-ray

May show:

- aortic valve calcification uncommon in pure AR
- large LV
- ascending aorta may be very prominent (e.g. dissection) or aneurysmal (e.g. Marfan's syndrome, syphilis)
- calcification of ascending aorta (syphilitic AR)
- signs of pulmonary venous congestion or pulmonary oedema

Cardiac catheterisation

Is necessary to document:

1 The severity of the aortic regurgitation

- Grade I — dye just regurgitant. Not filling the ventricle
- Grade II — dye gradually accumulating to fill the whole ventricle
- Grade III — dye filling the whole ventricle, but cleared each systole
- Grade IV — dye filling the ventricle in one diastole. Never cleared.

2 The anatomy of the aortic root, and to check the

regurgitation is valvar and not ruptured sinus of Valsalva. To exclude dissection. To check for rarer congenital defects mimicking aortic regurgitation.
3 To assess LV function. With severe aortic regurgitation the LVEDP equals the aortic end-diastolic pressure.
4 To check coronary arteries and coronary ostia.
5 Additional valve disease.

Indications for surgery
1 Symptoms of increasing dyspnoea and LVF.
2 Consider AVR if:
- enlarging heart on CxR
- pulse pressure >100 mmHg (especially if diastolic <40 mmHg)
- ECG deterioration with T wave inversion in lateral chest leads

65% of patients with all three of these criteria will either die or develop CCF within three years.
3 Ruptured sinus of Valsalva aneurysm.
4 Post infective endocarditis if not responding to medical treatment.

3.5 Pulmonary stenosis

Obstruction to RV outflow may be at several levels as in aortic stenosis.

Peripheral pulmonary artery stenosis. Stenoses of main trunk of pulmonary artery or more distal stenoses. These stenoses may be localised or diffuse. Commonly associated with supravalvar aortic stenosis and infantile hypercalcaemia. Also part of the rubella syndrome associated with PDA.

Pulmonary valve stenosis. A common isolated lesion (7% of congenital heart lesions). Also occurs as part of Noonan's syndrome, Fallot's tetralogy, rubella syndrome. It is rarely acquired, e.g. carcinoid syndrome.

Pulmonary infundibular stenosis. Rare as an isolated lesion. Usually associated with a VSD, or as part of Fallot's tetralogy or just in association with pulmonary valve stenosis.

Sub-infundibular stenosis. This rarest form has been described. It may occur as part of right-sided HOCM.

Pathophysiology and symptoms

The effects of pulmonary stenosis depend on its severity and the structure and function of the rest of the right heart, i.e. RV function (systolic and diastolic), competence of the tricuspid valve, presence or absence of a VSD, presence or absence of an ASD/PFO, maintenance of sinus rhythm.

With good RV function and a competent tricuspid valve plus sinus rhythm, moderate pulmonary stenosis can be tolerated with no symptoms.

Very severe 'pin-hole' pulmonary stenosis is virtual pulmonary atresia and may lead to early infant death, especially if the duct closes.

The additional presence of an ASD or PFO may lead to right-to-left shunting (e.g. on effort) with cyanosis.

RV failure is the commonest cause of death with gross cardiac enlargement.

Common symptoms are thus:

- dyspnoea and fatigue (low cardiac output). Not orthopnoea or PND
- cyanosis (if ASD or PFO)
- RV failure with ascites, leg oedema, jaundice, etc.
- retarded growth in children

Symptoms which are uncommon (unlike aortic stenosis) are angina, syncope on effort, and symptoms from infective endocarditis. Patients may be aware of pulsation in the neck from the giant 'a' wave in the JVP.

3.5 Pulmonary stenosis

Physical signs to note

Characteristic facies may be

- rounded plump face with isolated pulmonary valve stenosis
- Noonan's syndrome ('male Turner')
- Williams' syndrome (hypercalcaemia + supravalvar aortic stenosis + pulmonary artery stenoses). Elf-like facies.

JVP: Prominent or giant 'a' wave.
RV hypertrophy. Palpable RVOT thrill.

Valve stenosis (Fig. 3.13)
With mild valve stenosis there is an ejection sound, ejection systolic murmur, and A_2 and P_2 clearly heard and widely split. As the stenosis becomes more severe the murmur is longer and obscures A_2. P_2 is delayed still further and is softer. With severe stenosis P_2 become inaudible, and the ejection sound disappears as the valve calcifies. The murmur radiates towards the left shoulder, and over the left lung posteriorly.

With infundibular stenosis there is no ejection sound and the murmur may be more prominent at the left sternal edge.

Differential diagnosis

Differential diagnosis is from aortic valve or subvalve stenosis, VSD, Ebstein's anomaly, ASD, and innocent RVOT murmurs in children.

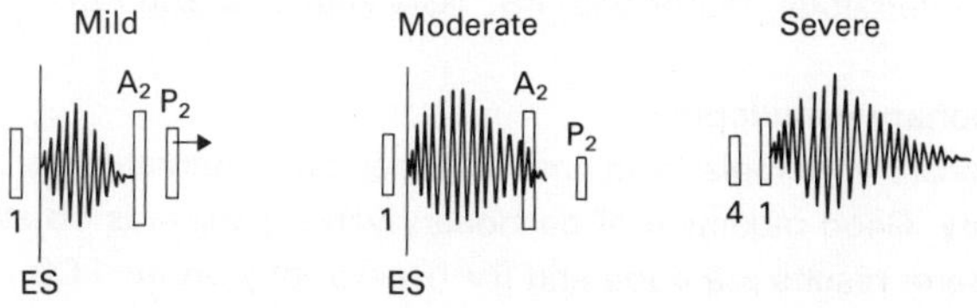

Fig 3.13 Grades of pulmonary stenosis. ES = ejection sound.

ECG

Shows right axis deviation, right atrial hypertrophy, 'P pulmonale', right ventricular hypertrophy, incomplete or complete RBBB.

Chest x-ray

There is post-stenotic dilatation of the pulmonary artery, but lung fields are oligaemic in contrast to the ASD. RV hypertrophy causes some cardiac enlargement with the apex lifted off the left hemidiaphragm.

With severe long standing pulmonary stenosis the heart may be very large with an enormous right atrium. (The wall-to-wall heart.) This appearance is seen in:

- severe pulmonary stenosis in the adult
- Ebstein's anomaly
- large pericardial effusion (chronic)
- mitral stenosis with giant atria
- congestive cardiomyopathy
- Uhl's anomaly (RV hypoplasia)

Cardiac catheterisation

Is necessary to document the gradient and site of the stenosis.

The size of the pulmonary arteries and possible additional stenoses in them. Additional lesions must be excluded — especially PDA, VSD, ASD, and left-sided obstructive lesions. RV function is important. The position and comparative size of the great vessels is important in more complex lesions (e.g. Fallot's tetralogy, DORV with PS, TGA with VSD and PS).

Pulmonary valvuloplasty

Pulmonary valvuloplasty is now an acceptable alternative to surgery. Good reduction of pulmonary valve gradient is obtained, long term results are good and RV hypertrophy on the ECG regresses.

Surgery

Pulmonary valvotomy and/or infundibular resection should be considered if there is RV failure, or if peak systolic gradient at valve/subvalve level is >70 mmHg. Emergency surgery may be needed in infants. An additional PFO/ASD or VSD is closed usually. With severe valve stenosis a trans-annular patch may be needed.

3.6 Tricuspid valve disease

The commonest tricuspid valve disease is functional regurgitation secondary to pulmonary hypertension. Tricuspid valve destruction from infective endocarditis is increasingly seen in drug addicts. Other forms of tricuspid valve disease are uncommon:

Congenital lesions	**Acquired lesions**
Tricuspid atresia Tricuspid hypoplasia Ebstein's anomaly (p.109) Cleft tricuspid valve (AV canal)	Functional regurgitation Destruction from infective endocarditis (p.331) Rheumatic involvement Floppy valve Endocarditis due to hepatic carcinoid

Tricuspid regurgitation (TR)

Dilatation of the tricuspid valve ring with deteriorating right ventricular function is common in patients with pulmonary hypertension from any cause. It often occurs in patients with rheumatic mitral valve disease and pulmonary hypertension. The development of atrial fibrillation in ASDs is associated with tricuspid regurgitation. AF is expected with any significant degree of TR, both RA and RV dilate with the change to AF and the regurgitation worsens.

Symptoms
There may be none. However, there may be fatigue, hepatic pain on effort, pulsation in the throat and fullness in the face on effort, ascites, and ankle oedema.

Signs
Systolic 's' wave in the JVP with rapid 'y' descent; if still in sinus rhythm (rare) prominent 'a' wave also; RV heave; soft inspiratory pansystolic murmur at LSE; pulsatile liver; ankle oedema and possible ascites and jaundice; peripheral cyanosis.

Treatment
Some degree of TR can be tolerated in the ambulant patient by conventional diuretic therapy and digoxin. Spironolactone, amiloride or an ACE inhibitor should be part of the regime. Support stockings may help prevent troublesome ankle oedema and venous ulceration.

In more severe and symptomatic patients a period of bed rest and i.v. diuretic therapy is needed. The symptoms quickly recur usually once the patient is mobilised. In these cases tricuspid valve replacement must be considered. Tricuspid annuloplasty does not often result in any lasting benefit.

Tricuspid stenosis (TS)
This is rare, almost always rheumatic, and associated with additional mitral or aortic valve disease. Symptoms are as in TR.

Signs
Slow 'y' descent in JVP; prominent 'a' wave if in SR; RV heave absent; tricuspid diastolic murmur at LSE best heard on inspiration and after effort.

At cardiac catheterisation even a gradient of 3–4 mmHg across the tricuspid valve is highly significant. RV angio usually shows additional TR. The only treatment is valve replacement.

Ebstein's anomaly

A tricuspid valve dysplasia with downward displacement of the valve into the body of the ventricle. The tricuspid leaflets are abnormal: they may be fused, perforated or even absent and their chordae are abnormal. The clinical picture depends on:

- severity of tricuspid regurgitation
- RV function. The atrialised portion of the RV is thin walled and functions poorly
- rhythm disturbances. These are frequent. Both SVT and VT. There is often an abnormal conducting system with Type B (right-sided) WPW syndrome
- associated lesions, commonly ASD or PFO; pulmonary stenosis; corrected transposition. Less commonly mitral stenosis, Fallot's tetralogy

Presentation

Infancy. Heart failure from severe tricuspid regurgitation with chronic low output. Cyanosis from right-to-left shunting at atrial level (PFO or ASD). This may increase when a PDA closes as pulmonary flow is reduced still further. Prognosis at this age is poor.

Older child or young adult. This may be with a murmur at school medical, or paroxysmal SVT. Mild forms may be asymptomatic.

Physical signs

Depend on above lesions. Usually the child is cyanosed, with elevated JVP, and hepatomegaly.

At LSE listen for pansystolic murmur (TR), S_3 (RV), tricuspid diastolic murmur.

Chest x-ray

Shows very large right atrium in symptomatic cases often with oligaemic lung fields. With large globular hearts consider:

pericardal effusion, pulmonary stenosis, congestive cardiomyopathy as alternatives.

ECG
Shows RBBB. RAD. RA + (P pulmonale). Sometimes Type B WPW.
Echocardiography is diagnostic, see p.420

Treatment
Is medical initially to control symptoms of right heart failure and arrhythmias if present.

RV angiography is diagnostic, but frequently produces rhythm disturbances which may be difficult to control. Simultaneous measurement of intracardiac electrogram and pressure shows at one point an RA pressure, but an RV cavity electrogram.

Tricuspid valve replacement plus closure of an ASD is possible but results are generally not good.

4 The cardiomyopathies

4 The cardiomyopathies

These heart muscle diseases of unknown cause are divided into three functional categories:

- congestive (dilated) cardiomyopathy (COCM)
- hypertrophic obstructive cardiomyopathy (HOCM)
- restrictive cardiomyopathy

The restrictive group now includes patients with endomyocardial fibrosis and/or eosinophilic heart disease. These were once known as a fourth group of obliterative cardiomyopathies in which the apex of either or both ventricles is obliterated by fibrous tissue. However the functional result is a small stiff ventricle and they are now classified with the restrictive group.

These three groups do not include rare specific heart muscle diseases (e.g. connective tissue diseases, haemochromatosis, metabolic and endocrine disease) in which cardiac involvement occurs as part of a systemic disease.

4.1 Congestive (dilated) cardiomyopathy

A dilated flabby heart with normal coronary arteries. The definite diagnosis can only be made following cardiac catheterisation, as ischaemic heart disease may sometimes present as heart failure in patients who have never had angina.

Factors incriminated as a possible cause include: alcohol, undiagnosed hypertension, viral infection, autoimmune disease and puerperal heart failure. Thyrotoxicosis may rarely present as a congestive cardiomyopathy. There is a rare form of X-linked dilated cardiomyopathy.

Pathophysiology and symptoms

Progressive dilatation of both ventricles (usually LV > RV) with a low cardiac output and tachycardia produces fatigue, dyspnoea, and later oedema and ascites typical of congestive cardiac failure.

Additional problems result from:

- functional valvar regurgitation. Dilated mitral and tricuspid

valve rings plus poor papillary muscle function
- Systemic or pulmonary emboli. Mural thrombus is common in either ventricle
- Atrial fibrillation: especially in COCM secondary to alcohol. A further reduction in cardiac output occurs with the development of AF
- Paroxysmal ventricular tachycardia
- Secondary renal failure or hepatic failure. Further salt and water retention, secondary hyperaldosteronism and hypoalbuminaemia all contributing to the oedema

Typical signs

A cool, peripherally cyanosed patient with very poor exercise tolerance or a bed-ridden patient.

- BP: Low. Small pulse pressure (e.g. 90/75)
- pulse: small volume. Thready. May be in AF. If in sinus rhythm may have pulsus alternans. Usually rapid (> 100/min)
- JVP: Raised to the angle of the jaw. May have prominent 'v' wave of tricuspid regurgitation
- apex: displaced to anterior or mid-axillary line. Diffuse
- ausculation. Gallop rhythm (summation if in SR) with functional mitral regurgitation and/or tricuspid regurgitation
- pleural effusions and possible crepitations
- hepatomegaly. Mild jaundice. Ascites. Oedema of legs and sacrum

Check also for signs of hypercholesterolaemia, excessive alcohol intake, previous hypertension (fundi), or collagen disease. Check thyroid for bruit.

Investigations

Chest x-ray shows moderate-to-gross cardiac enlargement with signs of left ventricular failure, pleural effusions or pulmonary oedema.

ECG shows sinus tachycardia usually, with non-specific T wave changes. Poor R wave progression in anterior chest leads may be mistaken for old anterior infarction.

Echocardiography: shows large left and right ventricles with very poor septal and posterior wall movement. 2D echo may show mural thrombus. There is often a small pericardial effusion. Ejection fraction is very low. Doppler studies may quantitate the degree of mitral regurgitation.

Cardiac catheterisation may be dangerous in patients with very poor LV function and precipitate acute pulmonary oedema, systemic emboli or arterial occlusion. It may be necessary once a patient has been 'dried out' to:

- confirm the diagnosis and document normal coronaries
- exclude LV aneurysm
- check on the severity of associated mitral regurgitation

Ventricular biopsy is rarely useful. There may be some hypertrophy and fibrosis. Numerous electron microscopic and histochemical abnormalities occur, but there are usually no clues to aetiology. It is only indicated if the history suggests an acute myocarditis.

Recently DNA probes have been developed to several viruses implicated in congestive cardiomyopathy (e.g. to Coxsackie B and enterovirus) and can be used to detect virus RNA within myocardial biopsy specimens. The virus may persist within the myocardium after the acute phase of the disease.

Blood tests: Viral titres (especially Coxackie B group), and an autoimmune screen are routine. HLA typing and blood grouping are necessary if transplantation is considered. T_4 if in AF.

Management

Complete prolonged bed rest with careful fluid balance monitoring, daily weight, and some fluid restriction are required. Intravenous diuretics are usually needed. Digoxin is indicated in AF or if a loud S_3 persists in spite of diuretics and bed rest. There is rarely enough afterload to reduce. Beta-blockers are not used even with an inappropriate tachycardia. An ACE inhibitor is usually necessary. Anticoagulation is very important in all patients with COCM even if in sinus rhythm. Only small doses of warfarin may be needed (hepatic congestion) 24 hour ECG monitoring is performed to check for AF or VT.

Cardiac transplantation
Conventional cardiac surgery has little to contribute. Mitral valve replacement is considered if mitral regurgitation is severe but carries an increased risk if the ejection fraction is very low. Cardiac transplantation in the younger patient carries the only hope of long term survival and good life style. Transplantation centres vary in their top age limit for accepting cases. This is usually between 50 and 60. It is important that the patient is referred early before the development of renal failure, recurrent chest infections, and cardiac cachexia which greatly influence operative risks and post-operative survival.

Patients with systemic disease may not necessarily be refused. Insulin dependant diabetics have been transplanted successfully. Specific conditions must be discussed in advance with the transplant centre.

Exclusions
In patients with suspected COCM it is important to exclude conditions which resemble it and may respond to surgery:
- pericardial constriction
- severe aortic stenosis with LVF
- severe mitral regurgitation
- LV aneurysm
- severe pulmonary stenosis
- severe Ebstein's anomaly

In low output states these conditions may produce few or no murmurs. Echocardiography is important in these exclusions.

4.2 Hypertrophic obstructive cardiomyopathy (HOCM)

First described in 1958 by Teare who noted asymmetric septal hypertrophy in nine adults, eight of whom died suddenly. It is known by other terms, such as IHSS (idiopathic hypertrophic subaortic stenosis), familial hypertrophic subaortic stenosis, ASH (asymmetric septal hypertrophy) and DUST (disproportionate upper septal thickening), although the last two are really just echocardiographic terms.

Although the pathology, haemodynamics and natural history of the condition are well described we are ignorant of the causes of sudden death and have made little difference to the progression of the disease with medical treatment.

Inheritance

Autosomal dominant with high degree of penetrance. Equal sex distribution. The evidence of a second (non-familial) form of disease is poor.

Pathogenesis

Unknown. It has been suggested the abnormal arrangement of myocardial cells in the septum may be the result of excessive catecholamine stimulation due to a genetic abnormality of neural crest tissue (cf. association of HOCM with hypertension, with lentiginosis, and phaeochromocytoma). A very similar lesion occurs in Friedreich's ataxia.

Pathology

Hypertrophy of the ventricular septum compared with the LV free wall. The abnormal muscle fibres are short, thick and fragmented. There is fibrosis. The nuclei are large and the fibres are arranged in whorls. These findings may be patchy but are concentrated in the septum. The pathological changes have been found in the RV outflow tract in patients with a VSD, and in the RV of infants with pulmonary atresia. The subvalve obstruction occurs between the thickened interventricular septum

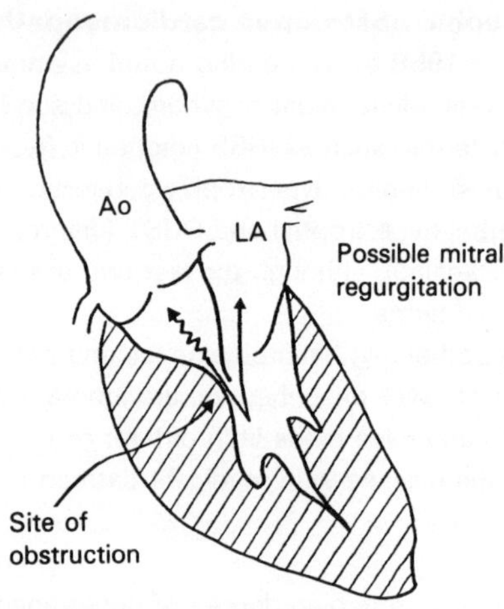

Fig. 4.1 Site of obstruction in HOCM.

and the anterior leaflet of the mitral valve and its apparatus:

The mitral apparatus is either sucked forward in systole (Venturi effect of high velocity jet), or pulled by malaligned papillary muscles. The mitral valve becomes thickened, and may be regurgitant.

It is possible to have ASH without obstruction. Hypercontractile ventricles may look like HOCM on LV angiography but have no gradient at rest or on provocation (sometimes seen in first degree relatives of patients with HOCM). Occasionally the obstruction seems more apical in site. The condition is similar to true HOCM.

Pathophysiology and symptoms

The symptoms may be identical to aortic valve stenosis. It may present at any age.

1 Angina, even with normal coronaries

• possibly due to excessive muscle mass exceeding coronary supply. High diastolic pressures producing high wall tension

preventing diastolic coronary flow. High systolic stress increasing myocardial oxygen demand. Excessive internal work for any level of external work due to increased frictional and viscous drag. The disarrayed hypertrophy results in inefficient transfer of rising muscle tension to muscle shortening
• abnormal narrowing of small coronary vessels.

2 Dyspnoea
• due to poor LV compliance, resulting in a stiff ventricle in diastole. LVEDP is high. Atrial transport is vital. Symptoms become rapidly worse if AF supervenes. Thick papillary muscles may result in 'inflow obstruction'
• due to associated mitral regurgitation.

3 Syncope and sudden death: as in aortic valve stenosis. But also
• extreme outflow obstruction due to catecholamine stimulation (effort or excitement)
• known association with Wolff–Parkinson–White syndrome, Rapid AV conduction down accessory pathway leading to VF in patients who develop AF or sinus tachycardia
• massive myocardial infarction.

Poor prognostic features

Young age at diagnosis (under 14 years)
• syncope as a symptom at diagnosis
• family history of HOCM with sudden death
• surgery (operative mortality 10–25%)

These features are more useful than prognosis from haemodynamic measurements.

Natural history

Annual mortality in children (under 14 years) is 5.9%. Generally children are less symptomatic (apart from syncope). Annual mortality rate in those aged 15–45 years is 2.5%.

Symptom severity is not closely related to haemodynamic estimates of LVOT obstruction. Some patients may develop

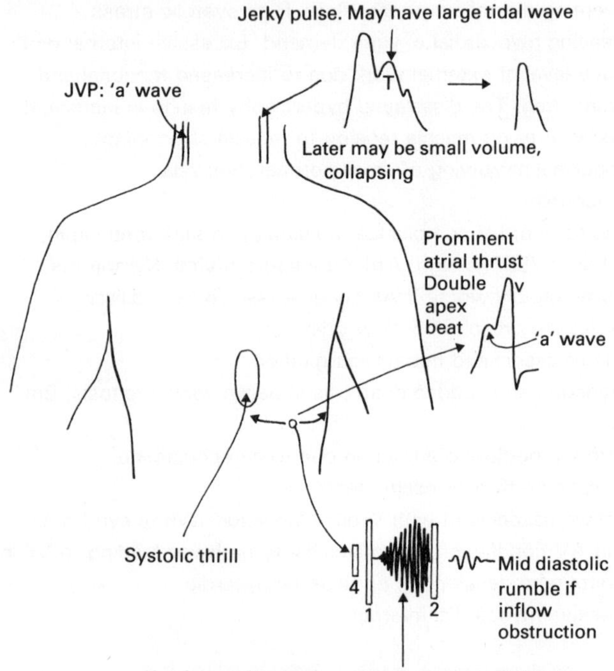

Fig. 4.2 Clinical signs of HOCM.

endstage congestive cardiac failure with rapidly enlarging heart and reduction in LVOT gradient (post-myotomy patients are said to do this more frequently).

Differentiation from aortic valve stenosis

The three conditions most likely to be confused with HOCM are:

1 Aortic valve stenosis.

2 'Sub-valve' mitral regurgitation (e.g. chordal rupture).

3 VSD.

	Valve stenosis	HOCM
Carotid pulse	Anacrotic	Jerky
Thrill	Second right interspace	Lower sternum to left
Ejection sound	May be present	Absent
Aortic EDM	Often present	Rare (post-surgery)
Manoeuvres to vary obstruction	Fixed	Variable

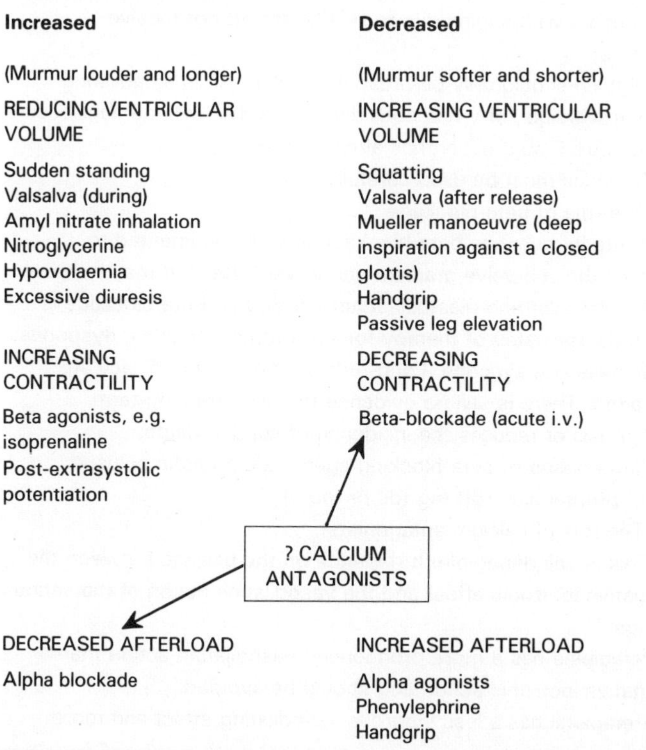

Variation in LV outflow obstruction
Increased
Decreased
(Murmur louder and longer)
(Murmur softer and shorter)
REDUCING VENTRICULAR VOLUME
Sudden standing
Valsalva (during)
Amyl nitrate inhalation
Nitroglycerine
Hypovolaemia
Excessive diuresis
INCREASING VENTRICULAR VOLUME
Squatting
Valsalva (after release)
Mueller manoeuvre (deep inspiration against a closed glottis)
Handgrip
Passive leg elevation
INCREASING CONTRACTILITY
Beta agonists, e.g. isoprenaline
Post-extrasystolic potentiation
DECREASING CONTRACTILITY
Beta-blockade (acute i.v.)
? CALCIUM ANTAGONISTS
DECREASED AFTERLOAD
Alpha blockade
INCREASED AFTERLOAD
Alpha agonists
Phenylephrine
Handgrip

'Sub-valve' mitral regurgitation, VSD and HOCM may have small volume 'jerky' pulses, a harsh ejection systolic murmur and a systolic thrill. The thrill in mitral regurgitation is usually apical in chordal rupture (but may be more anterior in posterior chordal rupture).

Therefore the demonstration of variable obstruction is very important.

Some of these manoeuvres can be performed at the bed side and are therefore useful in the differentiation from aortic valve stenosis.

Relevance to medical therapy

1 Patients with angina due to HOCM should not receive nitrates.

2 Digoxin should only be prescribed when AF is established and irreversible, or when considerable cardiac enlargement occurs when LVOT obstruction has already fallen.

3 Diuretics must be used carefully.

4 The role of beta-blockade:

• Acute intravenous beta-blockade is well documented to reduce the sub-valve gradient and lower LVEDP. It may increase left ventricular end-diastolic volume (LVEDV). Beta-blockade is thus the mainstay of therapy for symptoms of angina, dyspnoea, giddiness and syncope. Long-term studies of its efficacy are awaited. There is still no evidence that it alters long-term prognosis or reduces the incidence of sudden death.

• Large doses of beta-blocking agents are sometimes used (e.g. propranolol 160 mg tds or more)

5 The role of calcium antagonists:

• This is still debatable. It depends on the balance between the negative inotropic effect and the vasodilating action of the various drugs.

• Nifedipine has a more pronounced vasodilating action than a negative inotropic action and should be avoided.

• Verapamil has a less vigorous vasodilating effect and more pronounced negative inotropic effect. The claims that it reduces septal thickness have not been substantiated. It should be avoided in patients on beta-blockade. It is not as effective an antiarrhythmic drug as amiodarone In HOCM. It can be used as alternative to beta-blockade.

6 Dysrhythmias

AF: should be cardioverted as soon as possible even in large hearts. Patients who will not revert should be digitalised. Amiodarone taken orally may induce version to sinus rhythm.

Ventricular dysrhythmias are very common in HOCM and the likeliest cause of sudden death. VT occurs in over 20% on ambulatory monitoring. Propranolol and verapamil are not effective in abolishing these. Amiodarone should be tried. Alternatives are flecainide or mexiletine. Recently a small trial of intravenous disopyramide has been shown to reduce the LVOT gradient in acute studies and this drug may prove useful in long-term management, but further trials are needed.

7 Pregnancy with HOCM is generally well tolerated. Beta-blocking agents should be withdrawn if possible (small-for-dates babies and fetal bradycardia may occur as side-effects of beta-blockade). Vaginal delivery is possible but excessive maternal effort should be avoided. Haemorrhage may increase the resting gradient and volume replacement should be available. Ergometrine may be used. Epidural anaesthesia is probably best avoided as it may cause vasodilatation and hence an increased gradient. Antibiotic prophylaxis for delivery is advised. There is a strong chance the child will be affected.

8 Infective endocarditis may occur in HOCM. Routine antibiotic prophylaxis should be given for dental and surgical procedures (p. 348):

9 Systemic emboli may occur and require anticoagulation.

Echocardiography (p. 416)

Several features in association are diagnostic:

1 Mid-systolic aortic valve closure (occurring later than discrete

fibromuscular ring obstruction). Mid-systolic fluttering of aortic valve.
2 ASH. Grossly thickened septum compared with posterior LV wall, with reduced motion of the septum. Angulation of the echc beam may produce false positives on M-mode.
3 Small LV cavity with hypercontractile posterior wall.
4 SAM. Systolic anterior movement of the mitral apparatus. This may demonstrate contact between the anterior mitral leaflet and septal wall in systole. This contact has been used to quantitate the severity of the obstruction.
5 Reduced diastolic closure rate of anterior mitral leaflet. This is due to slow LV filling in diastole with low LV compliance
Echocardiography is useful in assessment of the results of drug treatment.

Electrocardiography (Fig. 10.7)
Usually abnormal even in asymptomatic patients (only about 25% have no symptoms plus a normal ECG).
Commonest abnormalities:
• LV hypertrophy plus ST and T wave changes. Progressive and steeper T wave inversion with time
• deep Q waves in inferior and lateral leads (septal hypertrophy and fibrosis)
• pre-excitation and Wolff–Parkinson–White syndrome
• ventricular ectopics
• ventricular tachycardia on ambulatory monitoring

Cardiac catheterisation
M-mode and 2D echocardiography have reduced the need for diagnostic catheterisation. The LV is very irritable and entering the LV with a catheter often provokes ventricular tachycardia. The procedure should document:
• the severity of the resting gradient, or provocation of a gradient if none at rest. A typical withdrawal gradient is seen in Fig. 4.3.

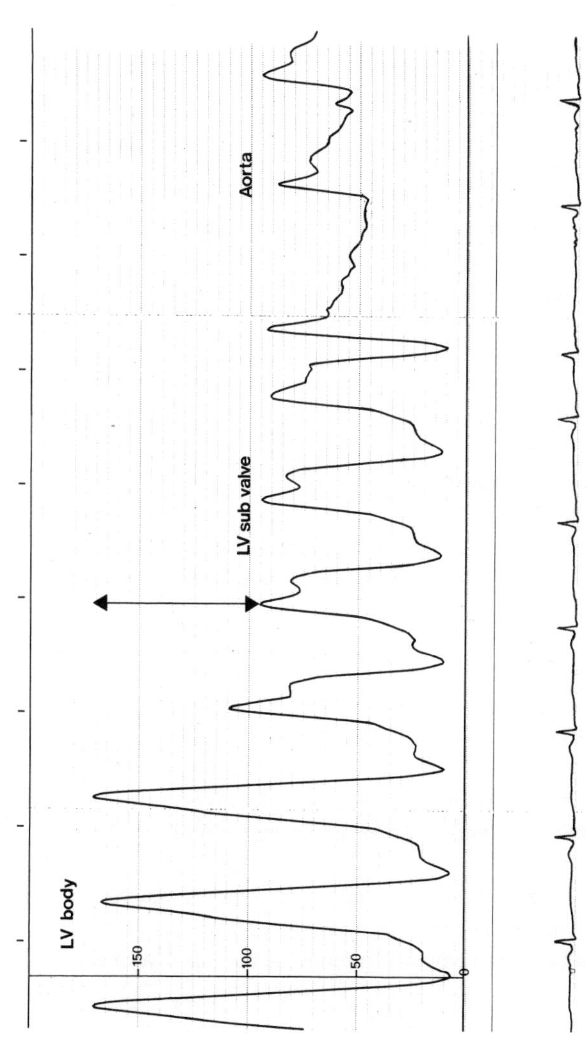

Fig. 4.3 Subaortic stenosis. Withdrawal of catheter from LV body to aorta in a patient with hypertrophic obstructive cardiomyopathy. The gradient (arrowed) is between the body of the LV and the subaortic chamber: 70 mmHg. The LVEDP is high at 25 mmHg.

- the presence of mitral regurgitation
- the possibility of an additional fibromuscular ring
- the state of the coronary arteries
- electrophysiological investigation may be needed in patients with WPW syndrome
- post-operative assessment

Indications for surgery

Reserved for severely symptomatic patients (angina, dyspnoea and syncope) in spite of vigorous medical treatment.

A myotomy/myomectomy is performed (through the aortic valve). This reduces the LVOT gradient. The development of LBBB post-operatively may help reduce the obstruction. Surgery carries some risk (10–27% mortality in various series) usually due to malignant post-operative ventricular dysrhythmias. Less commonly complete heart block may result.

4.3 Restrictive cardiomyopathy

Clinically this may be identical to constrictive pericarditis. Whereas surgery is necessary for pericardial constriction it is of no benefit to and possibly harmful to patients with restriction (see pp. 326–329).

Causes

- iron storage diseases
- scleroderma
- amyloidosis
- Loffler's eosinophilic endocarditis and endomyocardial fibrosis (EMF), both known as 'eosinophilic heart disease'
- Sarcoidosis

Patients with amyloid heart disease or sarcoidosis may have additional mitral or tricuspid regurgitation. Q waves on chest leads of the ECG are common and may be confused with old infarction.

Differentiation of constrictive pericarditis from amyloid heart disease

This is difficult. Both restrictive myopathy and constrictive pericarditis may have:

- raised JVP with prominent 'x' and 'y' descents
- normal systolic function
- LVEDV > 110ml/m^2
- absence of LV hypertrophy
- rapid early diastolic filling with diastolic dip and plateau wave form (Fig. 7.1)

The best technique to differentiate the two conditions is at cardiac catheter:

- LVEDP and RVEDP are different especially at end expiration in restriction usually by > 7 mmHg (identical in constriction)
- cardiac biopsy is usually diagnostic
- the search for amyloid elsewhere, e.g. urinary light chains; gum or rectal biopsy may help but cannot prove cardiac amyloid
- technetium pertechnetate scanning is positive in amyloid heart disease, with extensive uptake in the infiltrated muscle

5 Coronary artery disease

5.1 Pathophysiology of angina

Relevance to medical therapy

Ischaemia develops if myocardial oxygen demand exceeds supply. Cellular acidosis and lactate release occur before ST segment depression on the ECG, which in turn precedes angina. ST depression occuring in the absence of pain is called silent ischaemia (see below). Oxygen supply is increased by increasing coronary flow (autoregulation) rather than by increasing oxygen extraction from coronary artery blood. Coronary A–V O_2 difference remains constant at approx 11 ml/100 ml blood. Coronary dilatation in response to ischaemia is probably mediated via adenosine, which is the ideal messenger having a very short half life. Adenosine may be the cause of anginal pain when released from the ischaemic cell, acting as a self protecting mechanism. Determinants of the O_2 supply/demand ratio are shown in the table below. Angina therapy works by improving this ratio.

Mechanisms of angina therapy

↑O_2 supply	↓O_2 demand
Length of diastole ↑: beta-blockade	Heart rate ↓: beta-blockade
Coronary tone ↓:nitrates, calcium antagonists	Contractility ↓: beta- blockade
LV diastolic pressure ↓: nitrates	Wall tension ↓: LV pressure, LV cavity radius^2 } nitrates
O_2 capacity of blood ↑: transfusion if anaemic	
Aortic perfusion pressure: improve if hypotensive or hypovolaemic	
Coronary atheromatous stenoses: angioplasty or surgery	

Coronary tone

Coronary tone is under neurogenic and humoral control

5.1 Pathophysiology of angina

(Fig. 5.1). Coronary arterial smooth muscle contains α, β_1, dopamine and parasympathetic receptors. Beta-blockade is avoided in patients with proven coronary spasm (unopposed α-receptor activity). Cardioselective agents are used with care in patients with angina plus possible vasospasm (Raynaud's phenomenon or migraine).

The coronary endothelium is now realised to be very important in the release of vasoactive substances, some causing constriction, and others dilatation (see table). Many vasodilators act by releasing endothelial derived relaxant factor

Regulation of coronary artery tone

Constriction	**Dilatation**
Systolic compression LV>RV Muscle bridge over epicardial artery	Metabolites from ischaemic myocardium *adenosine*. Lactate, H^+, CO_2, bradykinin
α-receptor stimulation ? β-receptor blockade	α-receptor blockade β-receptor stimulation ($\beta_1 > \beta_2$)
Dopamine (> 15 μgm/kg/min) via nor-adrenaline	Dopamine (< 5 μg/kg/min)
Cold pressor test	Parasympathetic (vagal) receptors Vagal stimulation via acetyl choline
Ergot alkaloids	Calcium antagonists Nitrates and nitrites
Thromboxane A_2 (platelet derived)	Prostacyclin (PGI_2)
Prostaglandin F series	Prostaglandin E series
Neuropeptide Y	Endothelial derived relaxant factor (EDRF probably nitric oxide (NO)) α-calcitonin gene related peptide (CGRP) Vasoactive intestinal peptide (VIP) Substance P

5.1 Pathophysiology of angina

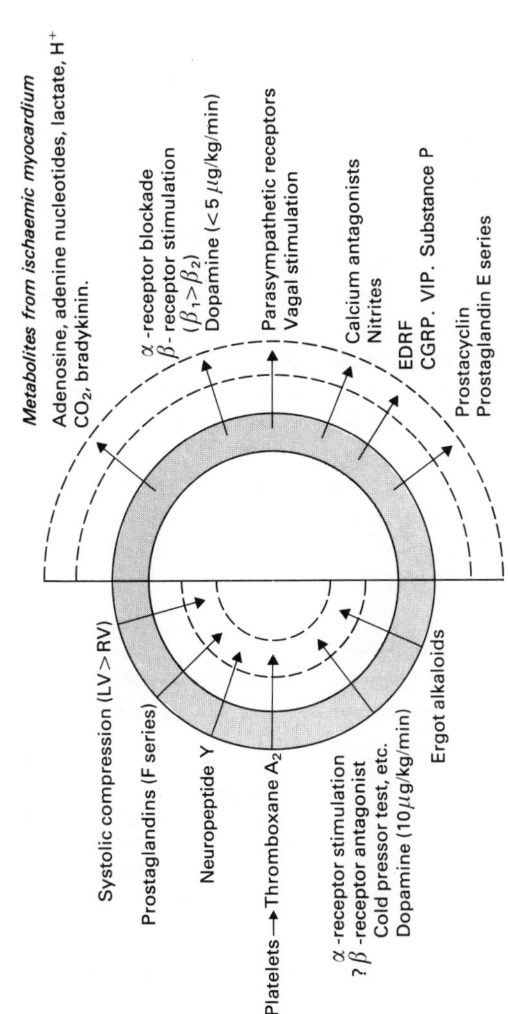

Fig. 5.1 Regulation of coronary artery tone.

(EDRF) from the endothelial cell which in turn increases intra-cellular cyclic guanylate cyclase (cGMP) which results in muscle relaxation. EDRF is probably nitric oxide. Some vasodilators only work in the presence of an intact endothelium (e.g. acetyl choline) but others are independant of an intact endothelium (e.g. nitrates and isoprenaline). If the endothelium is denuded, acetyl choline may even cause coronary constriction.

The role of prostaglandins in coronary tone is still poorly understood. Prostacyclin (PGI_2) is derived from intact endothelium and acts locally to cause dilatation, by increasing intra-cellular cyclic AMP. It acts in opposition to platelet derived thromboxane A_2 (TXA_2), a potent vasoconstrictor.

Nitrates probably work by forming nitric oxide which stimulates guanylate cyclase, increasing intra-cellular cylic GMP.

The action of nitrates and beta-blockers is shown in Figs 5.2 and 5.3.

In spite of our increasing knowledge of vasoactive substances released by the coronary endothelium, a few patients still present with absolutely typical angina but angiographically normal coronary arteries.

Angina with normal coronary arteries

There are many causes of chest pain which may mimic angina in patients with angiographically normal coronary arteries.

Non cardiac	**Cardiac**
Bad history	Angiogram misinterpretation,
Musculo-skeletal pain	e.g. ostial stenosis
Thoracic root pain	coronary arteritis
Cervical root pain	Coronary spasm
Anaemia	Small vessel disease
Thyrotoxicosis	Coronary emboli { atrial myxoma, mural thrombus, valve vegetation
Hyperventilation	
Gastritis/peptic ulcer	
Oesophageal spasm	Aortic valve stenosis
	HOCM
	Syndrome X

Syndrome X

This label has been applied since 1981 to a group of patients (often middle aged women) who have:

- typical angina pectoris
- a positive treadmill stress test
- angiographically normal coronary arteries

They probably represent a heterogeneous group and the cause of their angina is completely unknown. There is evidence to suggest their angina is ischaemic and related to abnormal perfusion reserve: i.e. failure of the smaller coronary arteries (approx 100 μm diameter) to dilate properly on effort—a form of microvascular spasm. Slow flow of dye down the larger epicardial coronary arteries is often seen on the angiograms. Other cardiac abnormalities found in some Syndrome X patients include:

- abnormal intramural arteries (100 μm) on cardiac biopsy
- abnormal systolic function
- abnormal diastolic function (abnormal LV filling rates, high LVEDP)
- ischaemia proven on coronary sinus lactate studies with atrial pacing
- myocardial damage: conduction abnormalities, mitochondrial swelling, etc.

Whatever the cause of angina in Syndrome X, it responds well to nitrates and calcium antagonists. Beta-blockade should be avoided. Patients should be reassured that with normal arteries their prognosis is good. Their symptoms should not be dismissed as of no consequence. Regular follow-up may in time provide more clues to the cause of their angina.

Silent myocardial ischaemia

Episodes of ST depression occurring without chest pain are termed silent ischaemia. This may be documented on an exercise test or during 24 hour Holter monitoring using FM recording equipment (Fig 5.2). Silent asymptomatic ST depression has been

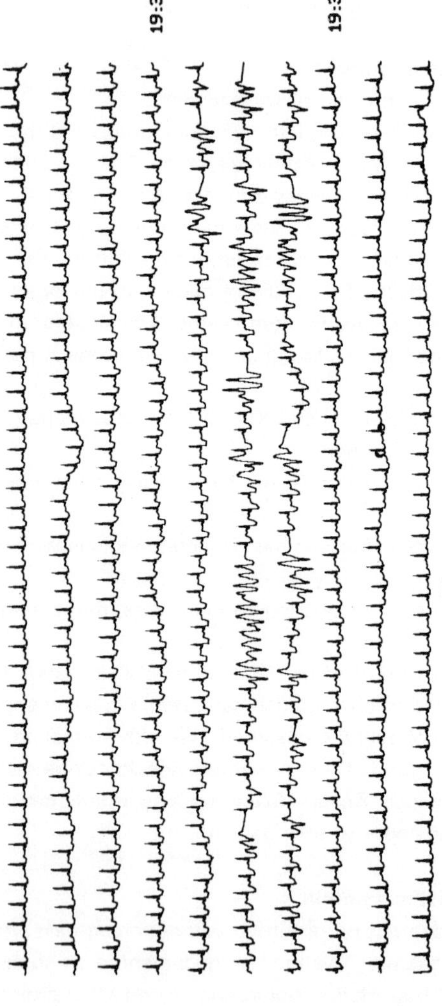

Fig. 5.2 Sample from a continuous 24 hr ECG recording, showing the development of silent ST segment depression followed by a burst of non-sustained ventricular tachycardia. The silent ischaemia gradually resolves.

found to occur in 2.5% of the male population.

It is now appreciated that silent ischaemia represents impaired myocardial perfusion. It occurs in patients with chronic stable angina and up to 75% of episodes of ST depression on 24 Holter monitoring may be silent. Generally the more severe the ST depression the more likely it is to be felt by the patient as angina. The frequency of silent ischaemia on the 24 hour tape parallels the exercise test result: the more positive the exercise test and the worse the exercise tolerance, the greater the incidence of silent ischaemia.

Silent ischaemia on Holter monitoring occurs more commonly in the morning. This circadian rhythm is mirrored by the increased incidence of myocardial infarction in the morning. It occurs in about 10% patients following myocardial infarction and has prognostic significance in this group.

Patients with frequent episodes of silent ischaemia should be investigated along conventional lines with exercise testing and subsequent coronary angiography if indicated. Conventional medical treatment for stable angina reduces episodes of silent ischaemia. Beta-blockade will reduce the episodes of silent ischaemia and will abolish the early morning peak of silent ST depression.

5.2 Management of angina

This involves alteration of life style, exclusion or treatment of precipitating factors, drug treatment, and possibly surgery or angioplasty if medical treatment fails.

Alteration of life style

This involves a reduction of physical activity at work and in the home. It may require a change in job (heavy goods vehicle drivers, airline pilots, divers) or a change within employment (miners, furniture removers, etc). Smoking must be stopped. Weight reduction may be needed. Many activities (e.g. gardening, sex) can be continued with medical treatment and nitrates taken prophylactically.

Driving may be continued provided traffic does not induce angina, that angina is stable, and that it is a private car only. PSV or HGV licence holders should not drive their respective vehicles.

Rarely attention to climate or altitude may help. Patients may be helped by moving to warmer climates during winter months.

Flight as an airline passenger is not contraindicated provided angina is stable. The airline medical personnel should be informed before the flight, the patient should not carry heavy luggage and should be well insured for hospital care abroad.

Vigorous competitive sports should be stopped (e.g. squash, rugby). Regular daily exercise within the anginal threshold is important. Swimming is allowed if angina is stable. Patients should not swim alone, should not dive into cold water, and should get into the water within their depth. Heated pools are obviously preferable.

Skiing is not recommended (high altitude, physical effort, cold air and emotional factors).

Exclusion and treatment of precipitating factors

These include anaemia; high output states, thyrotoxicosis, etc.; diabetes mellitus; hypercholesterolaemia.

The most important cardiac precipitating factors are hypertension; obstruction to LV outflow, aortic valve stenosis, HOCM; paroxysmal arrhythmias.

Angina in aortic valve stenosis may be cured by aortic valve replacement. Patients with angina and aortic regurgitation should have a VDRL/TPHA checked (ostial stenosis). 24-hour ECG monitoring should be performed if the history suggests arrhythmias precipitating angina.

Investigation and medical treatment

Exercise testing is performed on patients with stable angina provided there are no contraindications (see **10.2**). This helps confirm the diagnosis, assess the severity of symptoms, and is a guide to the need for coronary angiography. Patients who cannot complete stage 2 of the standard Bruce protocol because of symptoms or who develop positive ST changes, hypotension or arrythmias need angiography.

Drug therapy involves three groups of drugs: nitrates, beta-blocking agents, and calcium antagonists. Additional diuretic or anti-hypertensive therapy may be needed. Stable angina is treated initially with a beta-blocking agent and glyceryl trinitrate. Calcium antagonists are the drugs of first choice when beta-blockers are contraindicated, i.e.

- low output state. Borderline LVF
- prinzmetals variant angina
- high degree AV block
- severe peripheral vascular disease, claudication, gangrene
- asthma, moderate or severe bronchospasm
- depressive psychosis in the history

Unstable angina is controlled initially medically and then investigated with a view to surgery. Nocturnal or decubitus angina may respond to a diuretic taken in the evening, or a calcium antagonist taken at night.

5.3 Beta-blocking agents

The choice of beta-blocker

The table (pp. 142–3) shows the currently available agents in the UK. Personal preference and experience mostly dictate the choice. Most of the ancillary properties of beta-blockers (e.g. membrane stabilising effect, intrinsic sympathomimetic activity (ISA)) matter little clinically. Drugs with ISA prevent a resting bradycardia. The membrane-stabilising effect (quinidine-like) may play a role in the anti-arrhythmic action, as may the reduction in platelet stickiness which occurs with beta-blockade. Additional non-cardiac conditions are considered in the choice.

- Patients with cool peripheries, peripheral vascular disease, diabetes mellitus, or mild bronchospasm should start with a cardioselective drug (acebutolol, atenolol, metoprolol).

• Patients complaining of bad dreams (e.g. on propranolol) should receive a non-fat-soluble drug (atenolol, nadolol or sotalol).

• Hypertensive patients may be best managed with a single dose schedule taken in the morning (atenolol, sustained action metoprolol, propanolol). Alternatively they should start labetalol, a combined α- and β-receptor antagonist. Many beta-blockers can be used as single dose schedules for hypertension. More frequent dose schedules are usually required for angina.

• Renal failure. Dose of beta-blocker should be reduced. Reduction of cardiac output lowers renal plasma flow (there are claims that nadolol does not do this).

• Elderly patients. Start with a very small dose (e.g. propranolol 10 mg bd or metoprolol 50 mg bd).

• Liver disease. First pass metabolism occurs with fat-soluble drugs (e.g. propranolol, labetolol, acebutolol). Patients with liver disease should have the dose of fat-soluble drugs reduced or switched to a non-fat-soluble drug (e.g. pindolol, nadolol) which are excreted only by the kidneys.

• Diabetes mellitus is not a contraindication to beta-blockade, even if the patient is on insulin. Beta-blockade prevents the sympathetic reaction to hypoglycaemia. Muscle glycogenolysis is mediated via beta-2-receptors. Hence the cardioselective drugs are preferable in diabetic patients.

• Pregnancy. The evidence that beta-blockade during pregnancy results in small-for-dates babies is largely retrospective. Prospective trials have shown that beta-blockade as treatment for hypertension in pregnancy confers a benefit to the fetus compared with methyldopa or hydralazine.

• Overdose of beta-blocking agents is treated by intravenous beta-agonists in competitive doses, e.g. dobutamine (10–15 μg/kg/min or more as required), or atropine 1.2 mg i.v. (Complete AV block may occur and not be reversed by atropine.) Temporary pacing is often necessary.

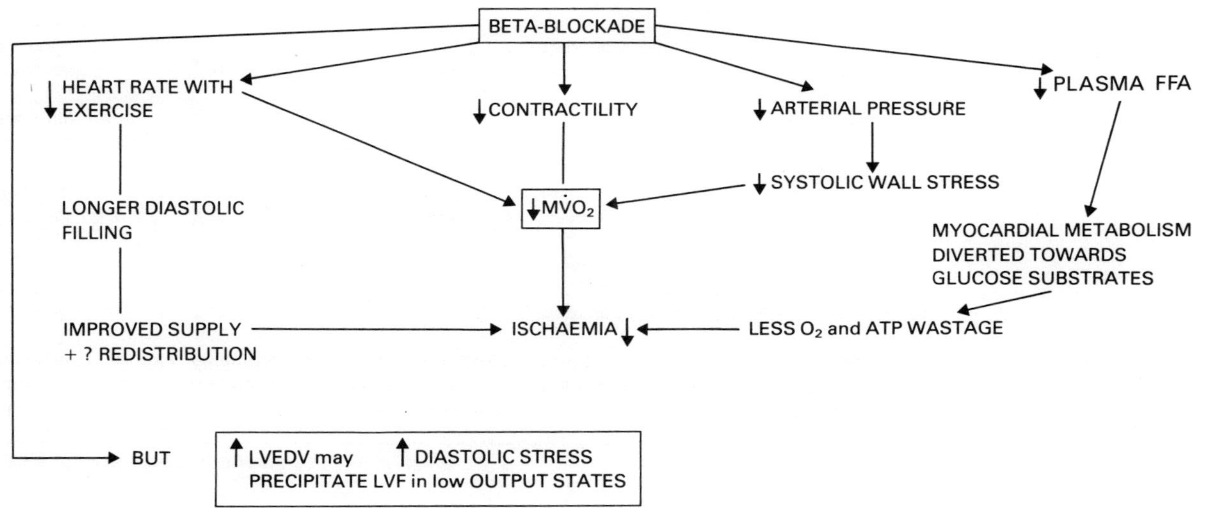

Fig. 5.3 Mode of action of beta-blockade in reducing myocardial oxygen consumption.

Table of beta-blocking agents

Drug (trade name/s)	Fat soluble	Cardio-selective	ISA	Plasma half life (hours)	Plasma protein binding%	Elimination route	Starting oral dose for angina	?Single schedule for hypertension	IV Dose (slowly over 5 minutes)
Acebutolol (Sectral)	+	Yes	Yes	3	15	Hepatic 60% 1st pass renal	200 mg tds	200–400 mg od	10–50 mg
Atenolol (Tenormin)	–	Yes	No	6–9	10	Renal only	100 mg od	100 mg od	–
Betaxolol (Kerlone)	–	Yes	No	15–22	50	Renal	10 mg od	Yes	–
Bisoprolol (Emcor, Mononcor)		Yes	No	10–12	30	Renal 50% Hepatic 50%	10 mg od	Yes	–
Labetalol (Trandate)	+ +	No	No	3–4	85	Hepatic 90% metabolised	100 mg tds	No	50 mg repeated if necessary

Metoprolol (Lopresor) (Betaloc)	+	Yes	No	3	15	Hepatic and renal	50–100 mg tds	Durules 200 mg od	–
Nadolol (Corgard)	–	No	No	16–24	20	Renal only	40 mg od	40–80 mg od	–
Oxprenolol (Trasicor)	+	No	Yes	2	75	Hepatic	40 mg tds	Slow oxprenolol 160 mg od	1–10 mg
Pindolol (Visken)	–	No	Yes	3–4	60	Hepatic and renal	5 mg tds	No	
Propranolol (Inderal)	+ + +	No	No	3–6	90	Hepatic 95% 1st pass metabolism	40 mg tds	Propranolol L.A. 160 mg od	1–10 mg
Sotalol (Betacardone) (Sotacor)	–	No	No	12–15	5	Renal only	80 mg bd	No	10–20 mg
Timolol (Betim) (Blocadren)	+ –	No	No	4–6	65	Hepatic and renal	10 mg bd	No	0.5–1 mg

5.4 Nitrates

Sub-lingual preparations

Preparations	Effective time
Glyceryl trinitrate 0.5 mg	10 sec – 30 min
Isosorbide dinitrate 5 mg	10 sec – 1 hour
Pentaerythritol tetranitrate 10 mg	10 sec – 45 min

Isosorbide dinitrate preparations dissolve particularly quickly in the mouth and are often preferred by patients to standard GTN. Nitrates may relieve the pain of oesophageal spasm, and renal or biliary colic.

They are contra-indicated in angina due to HOCM as they increase the outflow tract gradient.

Patients should be told:

- to renew the tablets every 6 months. Shelf life is limited.
- a GTN spray may be preferred
- to take them prophylactically and concurrently
- tablets taken in hot atmospheres may induce postural hypotension or even syncope
- to expect a headache and/or facial flushing. If these symptoms are intolerable, GTN may be swallowed and absorption is reduced. The tablet may of course be spat out. Isosorbide is absorbed from mouth and gut
- the tablets are not addictive. Tolerance is not a problem. Patients should not limit their intake to a fixed number daily. (Methaemoglobinaemia is possible with very high tablet consumption but is rare in clinical practice)
- chewing the tablets will speed absorption in severe angina

Patients with additional beta-blocking therapy will not develop a reflex tachycardia.

Care must be taken on prescribing nitrates to patients with cerebral arteriosclerosis. Hypotension may provoke cerebral ischaemia.

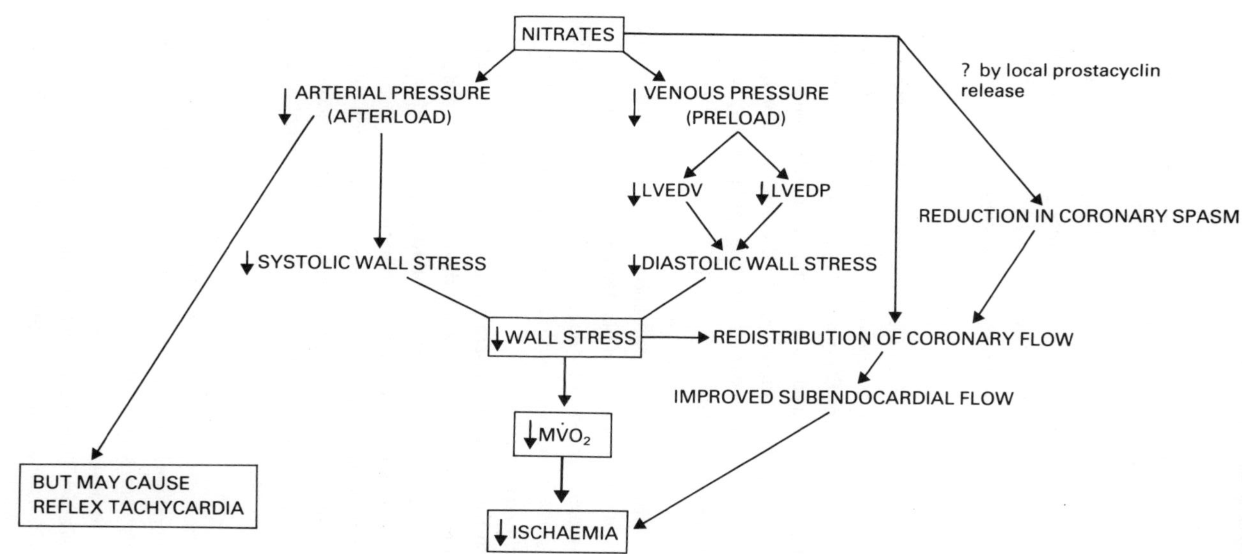

Fig. 5.4 Mode of action of nitrates in reducing myocardial oxygen consumption.

Amyl nitrite

Ampoules of amyl nitrite are used in echocardiography or in the catheter laboratory to provoke outflow tract gradients in patients with labile LVOT obstruction. They cause headaches with both patients and operators and are only used diagnostically.

Transdermal nitrates

Nitropaste 2% (Percutol, Nitro Bid). This ointment is absorbed through the skin and has a prolonged action (3–4 hr). Ointment is usually contained in 30 or 60 g tubes and one inch is squeezed onto the chest and covered by an occlusive plaster. Absorption occurs and if the patient becomes hypotensive or develops severe headache it can be wiped off. It is rather messy and dosage control is uncertain.

Transiderm-Nitro. This is a preparation of glyceryl trinitrate (25 mg) contained beneath a small plaster with a rate-limiting membrane which controls its release. In 24 hours approximately 5 mg is absorbed and only one plaster is needed daily. The plaster is waterproof.

With both transdermal preparations it is important to make sure that the area of skin used each day is different. Inflamed cracked or icthyotic skin should not be used (too rapid absorption). Skin sensitivity is not common.

Steady state plasma levels can be achieved with the once-daily preparation (0.1–0.2 ng/ml) which, although much lower than oral therapy, has been shown to reduce the number of anginal attacks per day.

Oral nitrates

The drugs considered in this section are longer acting than sub-lingual nitroglycerine (see table).

Recently the newer isosorbide mononitrate preparations have become available. Their theoretical advantage over the isosorbide dinitrate drugs is the fact that isosorbide mononitrate does not

Oral nitrates (longer acting than GTN sub-lingually)

Drug	Preparation marketed	Tablet strengths	Dose used
Glyceryl trinitrate	Nitrocontin	2.6 mg 6.4 mg	2.6–6.4 mg bd or tds with either
	Sustac	2.6 mg 6.4 mg	
Isosorbide dinitrate	Cedocard	5 mg	5–20 mg bd to tds
	Cedocard Retard	20 mg	20 mg bd with either
	Isoket Retard	20 mg	
	Isordil	5 mg 10 mg 30 mg	5–30 mg tds to 4 hrly
	Isordil Tembids	40 mg	40 mg bd or tds
	Soni-slo	20 mg	20 mg bd or tds
	Sorbid SA	40 mg	40–80 mg bd
	Sorbitrate	5 mg 10 mg 20 mg	5–20 mg bd to tds
	Vascardin	10 mg	10–20 mg bd to tds
Pentaerythritol tetranitrate	Cardiacap	30 mg	30 mg bd
	Mycardol	30 mg	30 mg bd
	Peritrate	10 mg	20–60 mg tds
	Peritrate SA	80 mg	80 mg bd
Isosorbide mononitrate	Elantan	20 mg 40 mg	20–40 mg bd or tds
	Elantan LA 50	50 mg	50 mg od
	Ismo 20	20 mg	20–40 mg bd or tds
	Monit	20 mg	20–40 mg bd or tds
	Mono-cedocard	20 mg 40 mg	20–40 mg bd or tds
	Imdur	60 mg	60 mg od

undergo first pass metabolism in the liver, and bioavailability is thus greater. Rapid hepatic metabolism of pentaerythritol tetranitrate may limit its effect, but isosorbide dinitrate has become a valuable drug in the management of angina. However, it is not clear yet whether the mononitrate preparations are really superior.

Nitrate tolerance

In many patients, tolerance to nitrate therapy develops quite rapidly. Mechanisms which have been suggested to cause this are:

- Activation of renin–angiotensin system. If this is the cause it should be blocked by captopril. Activation of the renin–angiotensin system has also been said to account for the rebound phenomenon (vasoconstriction occurring on nitrate withdrawal).
- Plasma volume expansion. This may develop during nitrate therapy. It may also be partly responsible for nitrate tolerance.
- Depletion of sulphydryl (-SH) groups in vascular smooth muscle. Administration of *N*-acetyl cysteine has been shown to reduce nitrate tolerance and may well prove to be useful in the future.

Tolerance can be avoided by arranging therapy to provide a nitrate free period during the 24 hour cycle. Oral nitrates should not be given after 6 pm in the evening and nitrate patches should be removed also. A nitrate free period at night can be achieved in this way.

Intravenous nitrates

Both preparations below are very similar in action and of similar price

- glyceryl trinitrate/nitroglycerine (Tridil); 0.5 mg/ml in 10 ml ampoules

• isosorbide dinitrate (Cedocard i.v. or Isoket), both are 1 mg/ml in 10 ml ampoules

Indications

Intravenous nitrates are used in

• crescendo or unstable angina not responding to medical treatment orally

• left ventricular failure and pulmonary oedema. This may be secondary to acute mitral regurgitation, ruptured ventricular septum, etc.

• accelerated hypertension (malignant hypertension), although nitroprusside is a better drug in this condition having more arterial vasodilator properties

• during and after coronary artery by-pass surgery. Hypertensive episodes following cardiac surgery

• during cardiac catheterisation: intra-coronary injection of nitroglycerine or isosorbide may be necessary if chest pain is associated with ST segment elevation (i.e. coronary spasm or impending myocardial infarction)

• as a prophylactic measure during PCTA (see **5.7**).

Problems and difficulties with i.v. nitrates

Direct measurement of arterial pressure may be necessary. Pulmonary artery wedge (PAW) pressure or PA pressure should also be monitored by a Swan-Ganz catheter.

Hypotension may occur with excessive dosage. The infusion should be stopped, the legs elevated, and if necessary plasma expansion/volume replacement given.

Side-effects. Palpitations, giddiness, nausea, retching, sweating headache, restlessness, muscle twitching, have all been seen.

Drug incompatibility. Both nitroglycerine and isosorbide i.v. are incompatible with PVC infusion bags or giving sets. Up to 30% potency may be lost within 1 hour.
Polyethylene or glass are not a problem, e.g.

Incompatible PVC	**Compatible polyethylene**
Viaflex (Travenol)	Polyfusor (Boots)
Steriflex (Boots)	Bottlepak/Flatpak (Dylade)

The drugs can be given either by drip infusion or by infusion pump using a glass syringe or rigid plastic syringe and polyethylene tubing.

Patient incompatibility. I.v. nitrates are best avoided in

- pregnancy
- uncorrected hypovolaemia
- patients with closed angle glaucoma
- anaemic or hypotensive patients
- patients with severe cerebrovascular disease

Dose calculation
Nitroglycerine (Tridil) 0.5 mg/ml in 10 ml ampoules
Add 5 × 10 ml ampoules (25 mg) to 450 ml 5% dextrose
Mixture = 50 mg/litre = 50 μg/ml
Start at 10 μg/min. Increase every 20–30 minute intervals by 25 μg/min until correct effect is achieved.

Nitroglycerine dose calculation
Nitroglycerine (Tridil). 10 ml ampoules contain either 0.5 mg/ml (5 mg ampoule) or 5 mg/ml (50 mg ampoule). Single-strength preparation: Add 1 × 5 mg ampoule to 40 ml 5% dextrose or 1 × 50 mg ampoule to 490 ml 5% dextrose (Concentration = 100 μg/ml).
Double-strength preparation: add 2 × 5 mg ampoules to 30 ml

5% dextrose or 2 × 50 mg ampoules to 480 ml 5% dextrose (concentration = 200 μg/ml).

Nitroglycerine

Single-strength preparation:
(concentration 100 μg/ml)

Dose (μg/min)	Paediatric microdrops/min	ml dextrose/ 24 hr
10	6	144
20	12	288
30	18	432
40	24	576
50	30	720
60	36	864
70	42	1008
80	48	1152
90	54	1296
100	60	1440
Double-strength preparation: (concentration 200 μg/ml)		
120	36	864
140	42	1008
160	48	1152
180	54	1296
200	60	1440

Start at 10 μg/min. Increase every 20–30 min by 20 μg/min until effect is achieved. To maximum 400 μg/min. Usual range needed is 10–30 μg/min.

Isosorbide dinitrate (ISDN) dose calculation

Isosorbide dinitrate (Cedocard i.v. or Isoket). Both are 1 mg/ml in 10 ml ampoules. Isoket also as 50 mg in 50 ml ampoules. Add 5 × 10 ml ampoules (50 mg) to 450 ml 5% dextrose. Mixture concentration = 1 mg in 10 ml. Start at 10 ml (1 mg)/hr—10 paediatric microdrops/min. Usual range needed is 1–7 mg/hr. In severe cases 10 mg/hr may be needed.

Isosorbide dinitrate

Using above mixture (5 × 10 ml in 450 ml 5% dextrose)

Dose ISDN mg/hr	Dose ISDN μg/min	Paediatric microdrops/min	ml dextrose/ 24 hr
1	17	10	240
2	33	20	480
3	50	30	720
4	67	40	960
5	83	50	1200
6	100	60	1440
Using double-strength mixture (10 × 10 ml ampoules in 400 ml 5% dextrose)			
7	117	35	840
8	133	40	960
9	150	45	1080
10	167	50	1200

NB

Paediatric microdrops are 60 drops/ml

Standard drops are 15 drops/ml

Paediatric microdrops make calculations easier e.g. 30 microdrops/min = 30 ml/hr.

5.5 Calcium antagonists

A group of drugs which share the property of inhibition of calcium influx during stage 2 of the cardiac action potential (the plateau phase). This phase of calcium influx is the slow calcium current in contrast to the rapid sodium influx of phase 0. The drugs may also inhibit calcium influx in vascular smooth muscle cells causing smooth muscle relaxation. In cardiac muscle cells the inward movement of calcium ions triggers the contractile proteins, and calcium antagonists may have a negative inotropic effect. The calcium channel inhibited by calcium antagonists is called the voltage dependant channel (i.e. calcium influx occurring only during depolarisation). Beta-agonists increase calcium influx via a receptor operated channel and this is not inhibited by calcium antagonists.

The increasing number of calcium antagonists have varying properties and some seem to have a predeliction for certain vascular beds. The drugs have a wide variety of chemical structures and the nature of the voltage dependant channel and how the drugs block it, are imperfectly understood. There is an overlap in drug effects but the table below outlines the more specific uses of the drugs.

Effect	**Drug**	**Condition**
Negative inotropic effect	Verapamil	HOCM Hypertension
Effect on AV node conduction	Verapamil	SVT. Fast AF or flutter
Systemic vasodilatation	Nifedipine	Hypertension Raynauds phenomenon
Coronary vasodilatation	Nifedipine Diltiazem Verapamil, etc.	Angina Coronary spasm
Cerebral vasodilatation	Nimodipine	Sub-arachnoid haemorrhage

Although the degree of negative inotropism varies, all calcium antagonists should be used with great care in patients with a history of left ventricular failure or large hearts on the CxR.

The three most commonly used calcium antagonists in the UK are verapamil, nifedipine and diltiazem.

Nifedipine

Useful in all types of angina, especially when beta-blockade is contra-indicated. It can be used synergistically with beta-blockade. It dilates both coronary and systemic vessels and is useful in systemic hypertension. It is of great value in Raynauds phenomenon but of very limited value in intermittent claudication. Not to be used in pregnancy and should be avoided in women who may wish to become pregnant. Its vasodilating properties result in a warm generalised flush half to one hour after taking the drug, and a reflex tachycardia. It is of no value in supraventricular or junctional tachycardia.

Side-effects: Flushing and tachycardia. Ankle and leg oedema gradually developing during the day. This does not respond well to diuretics and is better managed with advice about posture and support stockings if necessary. Pruritus. (Avoid in inflammatory skin disease.) Gum hyperplasia. Some patients notice a diuretic effect.

Dose: Start with 10 mg tds. A 5 mg capsule is available. The capsules can be chewed in severe angina and the drug is absorbed through the buccal mucosa. A slow release preparation is more useful in hypertension (10–20 mg bd after meals up to a maximum of 40 mg bd).

An intra-coronary preparation is available. 0.2 mg given i.c. will help prevent coronary spasm during PTCA.

Diltiazem

This drug is a potent coronary vasodilator but has less effect on dilating peripheral vascular beds. It causes less flushing and reflex tachycardia than nifedipine. Like nifedipine it can be used synergistically with beta-blockade. It increases AV nodal refractoriness and can be used for supra-ventricular tachycardia. It also appears to have an anti-platelet effect which may be shared by other calcium antagonists. It is useful in the first line treatment of angina where beta-blockade is unsuitable. Diltiazem, nifedipine and verapamil all increase coronary blood flow.

Side-effects: These are few and the drug is well tolerated. A few patients develop an irritating skin rash which resolves when the drug is stopped. Rarely a more serious exfoliative dermatitis and epidermal necrolysis have been reported.

Dose: Orally 60–120 mg tds. An i.v. preparation is not generally available yet.

Verapamil

Although introduced initially as a drug for angina, it has become very valuable in the treatment of supraventricular and junctional tachycardia because of its effect on AV nodal conduction. It can be used as an alternative to beta-blockade but should be avoided in patients on beta-blockers unless they are under close supervision, have good LV function and no conduction defect. It is useful in decubitus angina. It has a negative inotropic effect and should be used with great care in patients with a history of LVF in the past or a large heart on the CxR. Reduce the dose in liver disease.

It is of great value in the acute treatment of supraventricular (narrow complex) tachycardia. It will increase the degree of AV block in atrial fibrillation and atrial flutter with fast ventricular rates and can be used with digoxin in the chronic management of these arrhythmias. Given i.v. in atrial flutter with a fast ventricular rate it will slow the ventricular rate allowing the flutter waves to appear more clearly. Carotid sinus massage may abort an attack of supraventricular tachycardia after or during verapamil administration even if it did not do so before it.

Side-effects: Constipation is the main problem with verapamil. Haemorrhoids may be the result.

Dose: Orally. Initially 80 mg tds increasing to 120 mg tds. A slow release preparation is available (e.g. for hypertensive patients) 240 mg od as a single dose.
I.v., 5–10 mg. Repeat in 30 min if necessary. ECG monitoring is essential during verapamil administration i.v.

Verapamil should be avoided in:

- patients on beta-blocking agents unless under close supervision and LV function is good
- sino-atrial disease
- patients with AV block
- possible digoxin toxicity
- hypotensive patients
- AF and WPW syndrome (see p.302)
- wide complex tachycardias. These may be VT rather than SVT with aberrant conduction. Verapamil given to patients with VT may produce hypotension and asystole.

Other calcium antagonists

Many other calcium antagonists are shortly to appear on the market. It is unlikely they will have enormous advantages over the currently available drugs e.g.:
Bepridil
Nitrendipine
Nimodipine
Nicardipine
Niludipine
Nisoldipine
Felodipine
Falipamil
Of these Nimodipine appears to be of particular interest. It has been used in patients with sub-arachnoid haemorrhage and prevents cerebral vasospasm. The drug seems to be more selective for cerebral vessels. Early trials suggest a reduction in mortality in patients receiving nimodipine after sub-arachnoid haemorrhage, but more data is needed.

Bepridil is both calcium antagonist and an inhibitor of fast sodium influx. It dilates coronary vessels but has a definite negative inotropic effect.

Rarely used calcium antagonists

Perhexiline: Causes raised intra-cranial pressure, papilloedema, hepatitis, peripheral neuropathy, ataxia, impotence, weight loss.
Prenylamine: Negative inotrope and GI side-effects.
Lidoflazine: Long acting coronary dilator. May precipitate VT, GI side-effects.

5.6 Management of unstable angina

It is now well established that patients with unstable angina should be managed medically until the symptoms have settled. They are then investigated with coronary angiography with a view to possible angioplasty or surgery. Patients who do not settle on medical treatment require urgent investigation.

Unstable angina:

- angina occurring with increasing frequency or severity
- angina occurring at rest, or more frequently at night
- angina not relieved quickly with nitroglycerine
- associated with ST depression on the ECG

Investigation, angioplasty or surgery in the unstable phase carries only a very slightly higher risk than in stable angina.

Stage 1

Complete bed rest
Light sedation
Restricted visitors
Analgesia as required e.g. diamorphine 2.5–5 mg i.v/i.m. prn 4 hourly
Drug therapy:

- beta-blockade: e.g. propranolol 40 mg tds
- isosorbide mono or dinitrate 10–20 mg tds
- diltiazem 60 mg tds

} 'Triple therapy'

- GTN 0.5 mg/Nitrolingual spray, etc. as required
- soluble aspirin 300 mg od

Aspirin has been shown to reduce the incidence of myocardial infarction and mortality in unstable angina. The exact dose required is still unknown. It inhibits cyclo-oxygenase in platelets, reduces thromboxane A_2 synthesis, and platelet adhesiveness is reduced.

Beta-blockade is avoided if there is any suggestion that the unstable angina is due to coronary spasm (labile ST elevation during pain) as this avoids unopposed alpha effects on coronary arteries in patients with spasm.

There is evidence that anticoagulation helps in unstable angina and many physicians heparinise their patients (e.g. 1000–1500 units hourly).

One trial suggested nifedipine should not be used without a beta-blocker in unstable angina. Calcium antagonists have not been shown to reduce mortality in unstable angina when used alone but are considered safe and useful as synergistic agents with a beta-blocker.

Stage 2

If after a few hours symptoms are not settling: add isosorbide dinitrate i.v. starting at 2 mg/hr, increasing up to 10 mg/hr if necessary.

Stage 3

Coronary arteriography. This is usually performed when symptoms have settled, but may be required urgently if pain continues. Patients should be referred to a centre able to do this, preferably sedated and with i.v. isosorbide dinitrate running. Approx 7–10% patients will have left main stem stenosis, about 70% will have left anterior descending stenosis, less than 3% will have coronary spasm and a few will have normal coronary arteries ($<10\%$).

Stage 4

This depends on the coronary arteriographic findings, the facilities available and the expertise of the investigator. The options are:

- percutaneous coronary angioplasty (PTCA)
- coronary artery by-pass surgery (CABG)
- continue medical treatment
- intra-aortic balloon pumping (IABP)

PTCA is proving very valuable in unstable angina. The history is often short and the lesion if a single one is often soft: ideal for angioplasty. In unstable angina standby facilities for coronary artery by-pass surgery are necessary.

Intra-aortic balloon counterpulsation (IABP) is rarely used in unstable angina except as a holding mechanism prior to surgery or to move the patient to a surgical centre. The balloon can be inserted percutaneously without the need for x-ray screening. IABP is very useful in the short term for controlling pain. Difficult or high risk angioplasty can be performed with the balloon pump working. See **5.11**.

Medical treatment is reserved for patients with normal coronary arteries, or those with dominantly coronary spasm. A very few patients with unstable angina will have severe diffuse coronary disease which is considered inoperable. These patients must also be managed medically.

Patients with normal coronaries or spasm will continue calcium antagonists and nitrates with soluble aspirin, but their beta-blocking agent is stopped.

In spite of the enormous contribution of PTCA, it is still in the patient's best interest, initially, to manage unstable angina medically if possible. The infarction rate for medically treated patients (without PTCA) is about 14–18%. It is expected that the addition of PTCA will lower this figure.

5.7 Percutaneous transluminal coronary angioplasty (PTCA)

First performed in man in 1977, this has now become a standard technique in cardiology offering some patients a real alternative to conventional coronary artery by-pass surgery.

PTCA is performed in the catheter laboratory under local anaesthetic and sedation only. The technique is illustrated in Fig. 5.5 and can be performed via the brachial or femoral artery. Rapid advances in equipment technology have enabled cardiologists to attack more difficult and more numerous lesions. Initially the technique was restricted to single vessel disease, but multivessel dilatation is now common. Trials are now underway comparing the long term results of CABG versus PTCA.

Indications

- anyone being considered for CABG. Are their lesions suitable for PTCA?
- patients with refractory angina who are not fit for CABG for other medical reasons (e.g. renal failure, severe lung disease)
- the elderly
- patients who have already had CABG. Stenosis in a native vessel, internal mammary artery or vein graft
- severe varicose veins
- major clotting disorders
- very poor LV function
- intolerance to medical therapy

Fig. 5.5 Stages in coronary angioplasty:
a) The guiding catheter (GC) is positioned in the ostium of the left coronary artery (LCA). Angiography shows a severe stenosis in the mid anterior descending. b) A guide wire (0.014 – 0.018″) is positioned across the stenosis. The balloon catheter (dilatation catheter) remains in the shaft of the guiding catheter. c) The dilatation catheter is advanced across the stenosis. d) The balloon is inflated. e) The balloon and guide wire are withdrawn for the final angiogram.

▶

5.7 Percutaneous transluminal coronary angioplasty

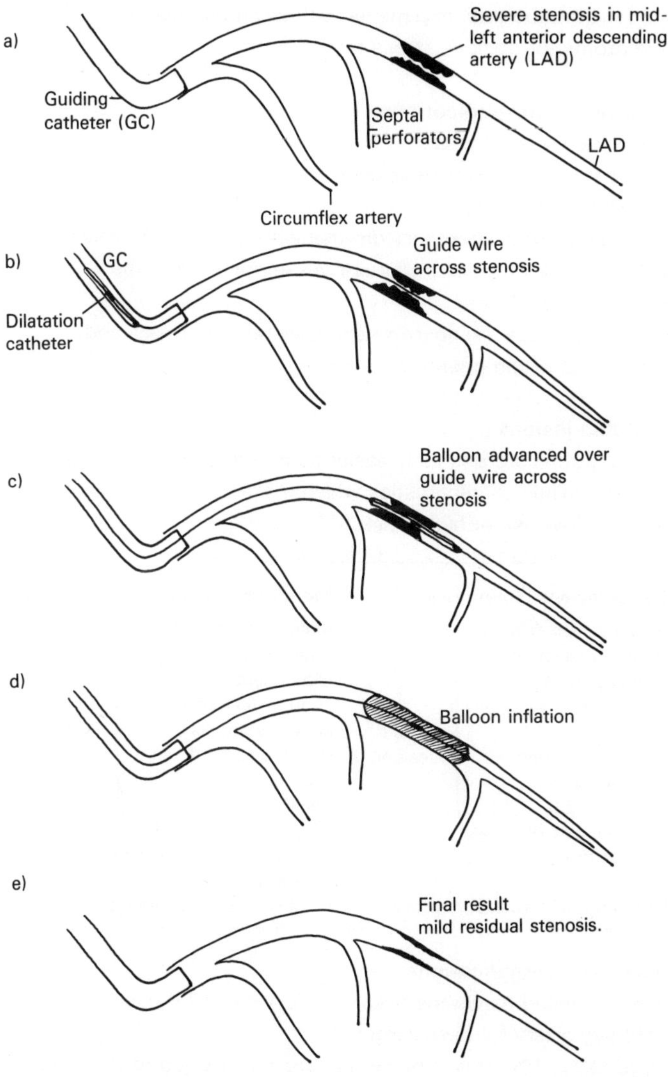

• post thrombolysis: in patients with severe stenoses, symptoms, or positive stress tests

Relative contra-indications

• left main stem disease
• very tortuous coronary vessels
• multiple restenoses
• diffuse proximal coronary disease with by-passable vessels
• total occlusion of an important vessel for >6 months
• 3 previous PTCAs

None of these are absolute and depend on the skill and experience of the operator.

Suitable lesions

Some lesions are definitely easier than others and the table below outlines characteristics which make lesions easy or difficult, low risk or higher risk.

Easier lesions. Lower risk		**More difficult lesions. Higher risk**	
Single vessel disease		Multivessel disease	
Good LV function		Poor LV function	
Young patient	Softer lesions	Old patient	Harder lesions
Short history of angina		Long history of angina	
Discrete		Longer stenosis	
Smooth concentric stenosis		Rough ulcerated eccentric	
Non calcified		Calcified	
Proximal part of vessel		Distal part of vessel	
No side branch involved		Side brances involved or bifurcation stenosis	
Left anterior descending artery		Right or circumflex vessels	

Risks and complications

In experienced hands the risks of PTCA parallel those of coronary artery by-pass surgery.

• *mortality*. 1%. This is higher in patients >65 (up to 2%) and higher still in patients who require emergency CABG (approx 6%).

• *acute coronary occlusion and myocardial infarction.* 3% or less now. This is due to acute dissection or thrombosis or both, usually at the site of dilatation. Re-dilatation or emergency CABG is necessary.
• *damage to coronary artery at site other than dilatation site* — e.g. ostial dissection with guiding catheter; perforation of the coronary artery is very rare.
• *guide wire fracture.* Distal fragment has to be removed surgically.
• *side branch occlusion.* This may reverse spontaneously. Risks of this can be reduced using a 'two wire' technique, or more rarely a pair of balloons: the kissing balloon technique.
• *distal vessel emboli.* This is probably much more common than is generally realised, involving micro-emboli into tiny distal vessels. More serious occlusion of the larger vessels can occur due to distal movement of thrombus or atheromatous material. Vigorous herparinisation during the procedure is mandatory. PTCA of acutely embolised vessels may be necessary.
• *complications of arterial catheterisation.* The guiding catheter is slightly larger than a conventional coronary catheter. Haematoma and false aneurysm formation at the femoral puncture site may occur. More serious is the possibility of systemic emboli from within the guiding catheter itself if heparinisation is inadequate.

Successful PTCA

This is judged primarily angiographically. A reduction in the stenosis by >20% was judged by Gruntzig as a primary success. Most PTCA precedures reduce the stenosis by considerably more. The vessel may look rather shaggy following PTCA, but the vessel wall quickly remodels itself, and provided there is a good lumen, with a good perfusion pressure there is usually no problem. A short and limited dissection flap may be seen and this may also remodel with a remarkably smooth artery after a period of 3 months.

Success may also be judged by a reduction of the stenosis gradient. This is usually 50–70 mmHg pre PTCA, and should fall to below 20 mmHg following successful PTCA.

Preparation of the patient

The operator must explain the entire procedure to the patient. Most patients will already be familiar with the catheter laboratory, having had previous coronary angiography. Diagrams (e.g. Fig. 5.5) help in the explanation. Important points which should be included are:

- the procedure takes a little longer than coronary angiography, but in many respects is very similar. There will be no hot flush (no need for repeat LV angiography). There is no need for a general anaesthetic. A sheath will be left in the patient's groin for a few hours after PTCA
- the patient should expect angina during balloon inflation and should tell the operator if he or she gets it
- the possible need for emergency coronary by pass surgery (<5%)
- the very small mortality risk (<1%)
- the possible need to repeat the procedure in the next 6 months (20–30% of cases)
- the patient will spend the night after the procedure in the CCU
- the operator should obtain the patient's consent on a special consent form

The house physician must help organise the drug regime, cross matching blood etc. He should have observed coronary angioplasty to answer patients questions. A standard regime is:

- stop beta-blocking agents 48 hours prior to PTCA. This is done to try and reduce any tendency to coronary spasm during PTCA
- soluble aspirin 300 mg daily
- oral nitrates and a calcium antagonist in standard doses

The morning of the procedure:
- start i.v. isosorbide dinitrate 2 mg/hour about 2 hours prior to PTCA
- starve the patient for 4 hours pre PTCA
- group and cross match 2 pints of blood
- shave the patient's chest and one leg if necessary
- premedication as in conventional cardiac catheterisation.

Additional sedation may be given i.v. in the catheter laboratory if necessary .

Management of the patient following PTCA

The patient is monitored in the coronary care unit or similar monitoring facility overnight and usually can go home within 2 days.

There is no absolute standard regime for post PTCA management, as nothing has been shown convincingly to prevent acute occlusion or restenosis.

- i.v. isosorbide dinitrate 2 mg/hour is continued overnight. Careful monitoring of the BP is necessary. It is important to avoid hypotension with excess sedation, analgesia and nitrates all causing a fall in systemic pressure and hence a drop in coronary perfusion pressure. This could potentiate the development of acute coronary occlusion. A fall in systemic pressure below 90 mmHg should be corrected by reducing the i.v. nitrates or by correcting hypovolaemia with i.v. colloid.
- i.v. heparin 1000 – 1500 units/hour is continued overnight in some centres—especially if there is an obvious dissection flap or thrombus visible in the coronary artery following PTCA.
- The arterial sheath is removed 4–6 hours after straight forward cases not on heparin. Alternatively it is removed the following morning 2 hours after stopping the heparin. Sheath removal is painful as the local anaesthetic has worn off. Patients may develop an acute vagal episode and it is sensible to predicate them: i.v. atropine 0.6 mg + i.v. Diazemuls 10–20 mg (or Omnopon 10 mg i.v.). Some patients develop oozing

around the sheath, and this may necessitate its removal earlier than planned.

- A post PTCA ECG is taken as soon as practical.
- Acute occlusion of the dilated vessel is suggested by the development of chest pain and rapidly rising ST segments over the relevant leads. This is a medical emergency and is usually managed by transferring the patient back to the catheter laboratory for a repeat PTCA procedure as soon as possible. If the first PTCA was particularly complex or difficult, the operator may opt for emergency coronary bypass surgery. Intravenous thromblysis is a third possibility, but there may be bleeding problems with the large arterial sheath *in situ*.
- Discharge home. The patients should take soluble aspirin 300 mg od, plus a calcium antagonist for 6 months. Beta-blocking agents can usually be stopped, unless PTCA has been performed in a hypertensive or post-infarct patient. Treadmill exercise testing (and possibly thallium^{201} scanning) should be performed at 1 month and 6 months post PTCA and thereafter at annual intervals.

Restenosis

It is recognised that this occurs in 20 – 30% of all cases undergoing PTCA, usually within the first 6 months. Only about 15% of patients actually require redilatation. Few centres perform routine repeat coronary angiography and restenosis is suggested by the development of angina again, or the recurrence of a positive treadmil test.

No drug regime has yet been found to prevent restenosis. However, a recent study suggests that dietary supplementation with omega-3 fatty acids (Maxepa) given 1 week prior to PTCA and continued for 6 months following dilatation may reduce restenosis. It is not prevented by either aspirin or formal anticoagulation. Factors which are thought to be associated with restenosis are:

- inadequate initial dilatation: e.g. due to balloon undersizing. An unsatisfactory initial result is the single most important factor

• high residual stenosis gradient (>18 mmHg)
• high inflation pressures needed at first PTCA (>7 atmospheres)
• male sex
• PTCA of a by-pass graft
• smokers
• variant angina
• multivessel disease
• long stenoses
• proximal lesions
• diabetics
• complex dissection at first dilatation

Restenosis is dealt with by a second PTCA. The lesion may be smoother than the first time and the procedure often easier with a lower complication rate. The cause of restenosis is unknown. Denuded endothelium stimulates platelet accretion and release of platelet derived growth factor (PDGF). This reaches the media within 24 hours and stimulates smooth muscle cell proliferation. Unfortunately antiplatelet agents have not been found to reduce the restenosis rate.

Newer technology

• coronary angioscopy has been used intra-operatively to examine the effects of PTCA. Angioscopy is now just starting in the catheter laboratory and will greatly improve our understanding of the effects of PTCA on the vessel wall
• laser technology. The problem of vessel wall perforation in the coronary tree is still limiting the advance of laser probe use. A new advance is the development of the hot balloon which may well help prevent restenosis
• coronary drill. The Kensey drill uses a high speed rotating catheter tip in a fluid vortex
• coronary atherectomy. This catheter placed across the stenosis punches out slivers of atheroma which can be removed and examined histologically

5.8 Myocardial infarction

Mortality is approximately 40% in the first 4 weeks and 50% of whom die within the first 2 hours of symptoms. The great delay in getting patients to hospital is generally due to the delay in the patient recognising the importance of his or her symptoms.

Mobile coronary care units developed in Brighton and Belfast in the UK have shown how successful they can be: possibly by

- reduction of transport deaths
- resuscitation of on site VF
- possible reduction of infarct size by early treatment of arrhythmias; although this will be impossible to prove
- reduction of the time taken to reach a coronary care unit

Education of lay people in cardiac resuscitation has proved very valuable (e.g. in Seattle) and static coronary care units (e.g. in sports stadia) are being developed.

Pathology

Approximately 90% of patients with a transmural infarct have total occlusion of the relevant coronary artery (as visualised by angiography) within 4 hours of pain onset. The incidence decreases with time (possibly due to relaxation of additional spasm or recanalisation). The majority of occlusive thrombi are associated with intimal plaque rupture and haemorrhage into the plaque.

A small proportion of patients will have normal coronary arteries. Emboli or spasm must be the prime mechanisms in these cases.

Home or hospital care

Since the original work of Mather and his colleagues in 1971 numerous publications have appeared extolling the virtures of both home and hospital care for myocardial infarction.

Since 50% of patients who are going to die do so within 2 hours of their symptoms, home care may be considered where:

• time from onset of symptoms is > 4 hours
• the patient is warm, well perfused, out of pain, and normotensive
• there are no signs of LVF
• there is no history of diabetes
• the cardiac rhythm is stable

The wishes of the patient and his/her relatives are considered, the social circumstances, the availability and proximity of a coronary care unit, and the available transport facilities.

Immediate treatment in the home

Analgesia. Diamorphine or similar opiate is the drug of choice. Diamorphine 5 mg i.m. (and 2.5 mg i.v. if the patient is in severe pain). The dose is repeated as required watching both respiratory drive and blood pressure. Diamorphine also acts as a venodilator, being of great value in acute pulmonary oedema.

Metoclopramide 10 mg i.v. or i.m. or cyclizine 50 mg i.m. or orally should be given as an anti-emetic. Both opiates and myocardial infarction cause vomiting. Cyclizine is more sedative than metoclopramide. Numerous other anti-emetics are available. Metoclopramide has the additional advantage of speeding gastric emptying and increasing the tone of the cardia (oesophagogastric junction).

Oxygen at 5 litres/min.

Bradycardia (sinus or junctional) is treated with atropine 0.6 mg i.v. repeated to a maximum of 3.0 mg.

Lignocaine. 300 mg i.m. in the absence of bradycardia, hypotension or shock may be given for frequent multifocal ventricular extrasystoles, salvos of ventricular tachycardia, etc., or prior to transfer to hospital.

Frusemide. Intravenous frusemide is given to the patient in acute pulmonary oedema (also has a venodilator effect). Dose 40–80 mg initially i.v. It should not be given for a raised JVP in the presence of an inferior infarct unless the patient is also in pulmonary oedema.

Immediate treatment in the hospital

The arrival of coronary thrombolytic agents is revolutionising the acute management of myocardial infarction in hospital and is considered separately in section **5.9**.

Diagnosis

This may pose a great problem, and there are no absolutely accepted criteria. Diagnosis is based on the following:

- typical history
- ECG changes
- cardiac enzyme elevation
- post mortem evidence

Other criteria which may help but are less reliable include:

- physical signs, e.g. new high dyskinetic apex, pericardial rub
- fever developing 48 hours after the pain
- elevated Wbc and ESR
- Myocardial scintigraphy. Not positive until 48 hours post-infarction, e.g. hot spot scanning using isotopes taken up into dead/dying cells (e.g. imido-diphosphate) or cold spot scanning using potassium analogues taken up by living cardiac cells (e.g. thallium).

The table shows the criteria modified from WHO analysis.

Summary of ECG changes (for examples see **10.1**)

1 *Pathological Q waves*. New Q waves are the hallmark of so-called transmural infarction. In standard leads pathological Q wave should be not less than 25% of the R wave and 0.04 sec in duration with negative T waves. In precordial leads pathological Q waves should be associated with QRS duration <0.1 sec (i.e.

	Definite	Probable	Possible
History	Severe, typically cardiac pain lasting 20 minutes or more and unrelieved by nitrates	As in definite category	Atypical chest pain A sense of suffocation or indigestion. General malaise. History of syncope History of acute dyspnoea or CCF
ECG	New Q waves in at least 2 ECGs ST segment elevation persisting for 24 hours, more than 2 mm in precordial leads, more than 1 mm in standard leads	Either definite ECG changes or ↓	Transient ST segment elevation T wave inversion only No new Q waves
Cardiac enzymes	Rise to more than twice normal	Definite enzyme changes	Rise to less than twice normal

not LBBB), and with negative or biphasic T waves. Q waves in V_4 or V_5 should be >0.4 mV and in V_6 >0.2 mV.

Large Q waves occur also with hypertrophy and fibrosis (e.g. HOCM), and infiltration (e.g. amyloidosis). It is most valuable to be able to establish that the Q waves are new. Q waves also occur in the chest leads in corrected transposition.

2 *Injury current/ST segment elevation.* ST segment elevation should persist preferably for 24 hours. (Transient ST segment elevation occurs with Prinzmetal angina.) It usually appears within 24 hours of a transmural infact, and returns to isoelectric baseline within 2 weeks. Persisting ST segment elevation after 1 month suggests LV aneurysm.

3 *Reciprocal ST segment depression.* This is thought to reflect a 'mirror image' of electrical activity on the opposite non-infarcted wall. It is not thought that reciprocal ST segment depression indicates additional ischaemia and coronary disease in the relevant territory.

4 *T wave inversion.* By itself it is not diagnostic of infarction. (Occurs in the normal heart in some patients with catecholamine stimulation, reversed by beta-blockade.)

Steep symmetrical T wave inversion may occur without new Q wave development either in ventricular hypertrophy or in 'subendocardial' infarction. Enzyme elevation is necessary to confirm infarction in the absence of new Q waves.

Localisation of infarcts from ECG

• anterolateral

Q waves in I aVL. V_{3-6} ST elevation with T inversion in I and AVL

• anteroseptal

Q waves in V_2 and V_3 (but often none in lateral precordial or standard leads) with ST elevation and T inversion

• anteroapical

Q wave in I with ST elevation. Apparent right axis deviation. May be Qs in V_{3-4}

- inferior (diaphragmatic)

Q waves in II. III. aVF with ST elevation and T inversion

- true posterior

Tall R waves in V_1 and V_2 (exclude RV hypertrophy type 'A' WPW, and RBBB) with negative ST depression in V_{1-3}. Can be confirmed by oesophageal lead.

Cardiac enzymes

CPK (creatine phosphokinase). MB isoenzyme. The most specific cardiac enzyme. Rises and falls within the first 72 hours. Cumulative CPK concentrations have been used to estimate infarct size. Peak concentration 24 hours post infarction. Other isoenzymes of CPK are MM (skeletal muscle) and CPK-BB (brain and kidney). Very small amounts of CPK-MB also occur in small intestine, tongue and diaphragm.

SGOT (serum glutamic oxaloacetic tranaminase, also known as aspartate aminotransferase). Less specific than CPK-MB. Rises and falls within 4–6 days. Peak concentration at 24 hours. SGOT also elevated in liver disease (+ hepatic congestion), pulmonary embolism, skeletal muscle injury, shock, or i.m. injections.

LDH (lactic dehydrogenase). Again not cardio-specific. Peaks about 4–5 days post infarction, and may take 2 weeks to return to baseline. LDH also elevated in: haemolysis, leukaemia, megaloblastic anaemia, renal disease, plus all the false positive causes of elevated SGOT.

The LDH false positives can be separated by isoenzyme electrophoretic studies. LDH_1, cardiac, red cells; LDH_4 and LDH_5, liver and skeletal muscle.

HBD (Hydroxybutyrate dehydrogenase). This is really measuring the activity of LDH_1 isoenzyme and is often used instead of LDH analysis and isoenzyme differentiation.

Myoglobin. Although not strictly an enzyme, peak levels of serum myoglobin occur before peak CPK-MB activity. It is also excreted in the urine. It is not clinically useful (due to its skeletal muscle origin).

Changes on ECG not diagnostic of infarction, but which may be ischaemic

- ST segment depression
- transient ST segment elevation (e.g. spasm)
- axis shift—left or right
- transient T wave inversion (Figs. 5.6 and 10.10)
- increase in R wave voltage (e.g. on exercise testing)
- LBBB or RBBB
- 1°, 2° or 3° AV block
- tachyarrhythmias
- transient tall peaked T waves

Non-Q wave (sub-endocardial) infarction

A total coronary occlusion usually produces a transmural Q wave infarct. Incomplete thrombosis or early lysis in a coronary artery produces a non-Q wave infarct. The diagnosis of a sub-endocardial infarct is based on a typical history of chest pain, ECG changes (ST segment elevation, ST depression or T wave inversion) plus enzyme elevation which is often mild compared with transmural Q wave infarction. See Figs 5.6 and 10.10.

Generally it is an incomplete and small infarct. It may be due to diffuse three vessel disease or a single severe stenosis in a large artery. In either case it may occur early in the course of a Q wave infarct, before the vessel is totally occluded. Frequently it progresses to a Q wave infarct within a year. Sub-endocardial infarcts account for about 20–30% of all infarcts.

Relevance of diagnosis to subsequent course and prognosis

It is very important to follow up and investigate patients with a non-Q wave infarct. The subsequent course and prognosis differs sharply from Q wave infarction:

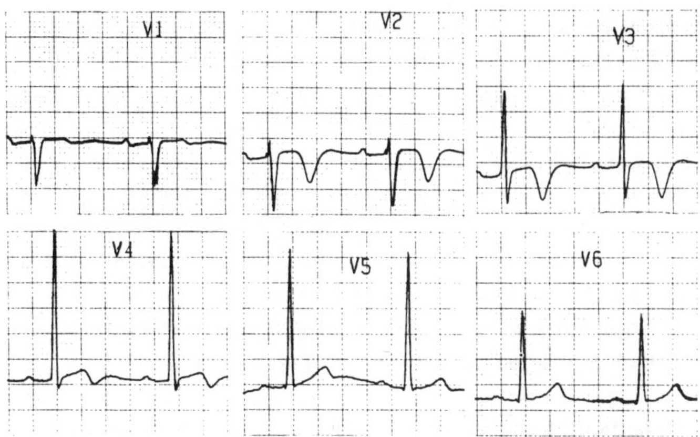

Fig. 5.6 ECG chest leads in a man with a tight LAD stenosis and history of severe chest pain lasting 30 minutes. No pathological Q waves. Enzyme elevation needed to confirm infarction. This ECG returned completely to normal following angioplasty.

- low hospital mortality: approx 2% (12–18% in Q wave infarcts)
- high late (1 year) mortality particularly with evidence of early extension: (approx 65% vs 34% Q wave infarcts)
- ST segment depression at diagnosis more dangerous than ST elevation
- high incidence of arrhythmias. 24 hour ECG monitoring needed
- more post-infarct angina than following Q wave infarction
- LV function may improve transiently following a non-Q wave infarct. If segmental wall motion can be shown to improve then that area is at high risk for a full thickness infarct subsequently

Post-infarct management

Early investigation is necessary with exercise testing and coronary angiography. PTCA is useful for suitable lesions, or coronary surgery for patients with diffuse three vessel disease.

Medical management alone is unsatisfactory, but if no other facilities are available, treatment with soluble aspirin, beta-blockade, and diltiazem is recommended.

Early hospital discharge

Selection of a low risk group of patients has allowed early discharge from hospital at about 1 week following infarction. If there have been no complications at the end of the fourth day then there are unlikely to be complications. Using an early discharge policy will very rarely release a patient who later develops problems. Early follow up is necessary.

Patients who should not be discharged early are those with:

- pulmonary oedema or evidence of LVF
- further chest pain after admission
- diabetes
- arrhythmias
- conduction defects: 2° or 3° AV block, bifascicular block
- persistent fever

Common sense and the patient's social circumstances are all important.

Early investigation

Treadmill exercise testing has been performed as little as 1 week after uncomplicated infarcts and is useful in assessing the severity of coronary artery disease, and the 1 year prognosis.

Most centres now exercise patients before returning them to work and perform coronary angiography on young patients or those with strongly positive tests and poor exercise tolerance.

Advice to the coronary patient prior to hospital discharge

Work. The patient should consider returning to work if possible 3 months after a myocardial infarct. In a few cases this time may be shortened. A return to full-time work is the single most important item in a patient's recovery. A few occupations however cannot be restarted following infarction: public service vehicle drivers, heavy goods vehicle drivers, airline pilots or air traffic control personnel, divers.

Several occupations should be considered hazardous for the post-infarct patient e.g. furniture removers, scaffolders, bricklayers, dockers, miners, steelworkers, and if possible the patient should be advised to seek a lighter job.

Exercise. Regular daily exercise is encouraged. The patient should be recommended to take initially two short walks (15–20 min) daily, with prophylactic GTN if necessary. This distance should be increased weekly. Instructions for swimming, etc. are as with angina (p. 137–8).

Weight. Weight control is important and is often difficult when giving up smoking.

Smoking. Should be stopped.

Diet. A diet which does not produce weight gain is the most important factor. A high fibre diet with vegetables and cereals should be encouraged. Reduction in saturated fats may be important in secondary prevention, but there is no evidence that reduction of serum cholesterol below 6.5 mmol/L is of any benefit in the long term.

Sex. This should be discussed. Intercourse is probably best avoided for 1 month only after myocardial infarction. GTN prophylaxis and beta-blockade will help patients with angina on intercourse, but beta-blockade may cause impotence. A relatively passive role in intercourse should be encouraged initially.

Contraception. The Pill should be discouraged and alternative methods suggested for the female patient.

Alcohol. Regular evening alcohol in moderation is perfectly satisfactory (e.g. two glasses of wine or a double whisky). Several pints of beer however should be discouraged because of its water load effect.

Travel. Travel abroad should be discouraged for the first two months, but may be unavoidable (see angina).

Secondary prevention
There is enough evidence now to recommend routine beta-blockade following myocardial infarction. It should be started as soon as possible after the infarct and certainly within 2 days. It has been shown to reduce the incidence or reinfarction and sudden death following a first infarct. Its effect on mortality is probably by reducing the incidence of cardiac rupture. Beta-blockade should be continued for at least 2 and probably 5 years after infarction. The choice of beta-blocking agent is only important in that drugs with pronounced intrinsic sympathomimetic activity are best avoided (e.g. oxprenolol); there have been positive trials with timolol, metoprolol, atenolol and propranolol.

Soluble aspirin should also be used in the long term (300 mg od) in the absence of contra-indications. There is concern about long term use of aspirin in the elderly causing an increased incidence of cerebral haemorrhage, and it should be avoided in the patient over 75 years.

There is no evidence that any of the calcium antagonists confer any benefit in secondary prevention.

Diet. There is increasing evidence that lowering plasma cholesterol into the normal range is important in lowering coronary risk. This is discussed fully in the management of hyperlipidaemias, section **5.16**.

Myocardial infarction with normal coronary arteries

Definite Q wave infarcts occasionally occur in patients who have normal coronary angiograms at subsequent investigation. It is not always possible to provide an explanation but possible considerations are:

- coronary spasm
- coronary emboli
- recanalisation following coronary thrombosis
- thyrotoxicosis
- coronary arteritis
- prothrombotic state

Spontaneous thrombus developing in a normal artery is rare but may indicate a hypercoagulable or prothrombotic state. It may occur in heavy smokers, women on the contraceptive pill and polycythaemic patients. Haematological help is needed but investigations which should be considered include:

- full blood count
- platelet count
- prothrombin time, partial thromboplastin time, and thrombin time
- platelet aggregation to ADP? Spontaneous aggregation of platelets in platelet rich plasma
- lupus anticoagulant. Check dilute Russell viper time
- antithrombin III deficiency
- protein C deficiency
- protein S deficiency

5.9 Coronary thrombolysis

It is now well established that thrombolysis has an important part to play in acute myocardial infarction. Several studies have shown a significant reduction in early (1 month) and late (1 year) mortality in those patients receiving thrombolytic agents within four hours of onset of pain.

The pre-existing high grade stenosis in the coronary artery suddenly becomes occluded by thrombus usually secondary to plaque rupture. The cause of plaque rupture remains unknown. Acute occlusion of the coronary artery results in myocardial infarction in the dependent territory. Coronary angiography at the time of acute infarction shows total occlusion of the relevant vessel in 90–100% cases. Progressive myocardial damage develops and becomes irreversible at 6 hours. The aim of thrombolysis is to produce reperfusion of the distal artery. The high grade stenosis may have to be dealt with by coronary angioplasty on a subsequent occasion.

Thrombolytic agents

Non specific thrombolytic agents:

- streptokinase
- urokinase

Fibrin specific agents:

- rt-PA (recombinant tissue plasminogen activator, single or double chain) half life 7 min (Actilyse)
- APSAC (anisoylated plasminogen streptokinase activator complex) i.v. half life 90 min

The non specific fibrinolytic agents such as streptokinase are the only agents routinely available at present in the UK. Cost of treatment is approximately £100 per patient for streptokinase (urokinase is more expensive and less easily available). It can be given either intravenously or via the coronary artery catheter. Disadvantages are that it causes a systemic lytic state and depletes fibrinogen and α_2 antiplasmin levels. It is antigenic and often causes a fever and allergic reaction (see p. 360).

The fibrin specific agents are still available on research basis in the UK; rt-PA is now available in the USA. APSAC is likely to cost >£500 per patient and rt-PA >£1000 per patient (1988 prices). They have the advantage of working only at the site of the thrombus, and deplete fibrinogen and α_2 antiplasmin levels less. Haemorrhagic complications are fewer.

Administration

Thrombolysis should be considered in any patient with an acute myocardial infarction who has had chest pain for less than 6 hours and who does not have the standard contra-indications to streptokinase:

- recent CVA (in last 6 months)
- recent gastrointestinal bleed
- haemorrhagic diathesis
- recent abdominal surgery, neurosurgery, eye surgery, liver biopsy, lumbar puncture
- pregnancy or post partum
- streptococcal infection or previous streptokinase therapy in last 6 months
- severe hypertension >200/100
- trauma
- age over 70 years (increased risk of cerebral haemorrhage)
- menstrual bleeding
- liver or renal disease
- ulcerative colitis
- i.m. injections in casualty

Prior to streptokinase administration, the patient should receive hydrocortisone 100 mg i.v. and chlorpheniramine 10 mg i.v. The need for this prophylactic anti-allergic regime is debated. It is sensible to consider it in any patient who has received streptokinase before, or in any patient with a history of a recent sore throat. Streptokinase is given intravenously 1.5 million units in 100–200 ml N saline over 30–60 min.

Intracoronary streptokinase is rarely given now, as the advantages over the intravenous route are minimal and the logistics much more difficult. The intracoronary dose is 10 000 units bolus dose followed by an infusion of 4000 units/minute for 60 min. Sometimes a second 60 min course is necessary.

APSAC is given as 30 units i.v. over 5 min; rt-PA 80 – 100 mg i.v. over 3 hours. 40 mg is given over the first hour and 40 mg over the next 2 hours.

Summary of thrombolytic agents

Agent	rt-PA	Streptokinase	APSAC
i.v. dose	80–100 mg	1.5 million units	30 mg
Infusion time	3 hours	1 hour	5 min
Half life	4 min	30 min	90 min
Storage	Room temp	Room temp	Refrigerator
Source	Recombinant human protein	Bacterial	Bacterial + human plasma
Anaphylaxis	Nil	0.1%	0.1%
Allergic reaction	Nil	2–3%	2–3%

Following the administration of streptokinase, the partial thromboplastin time and fibrinogen levels are checked and heparin is started about 12–24 hours later. Subsequent thrombin time estimations should be between 2–4 times normal. After 48 hours warfarin is started and continued for 3 months.

Recent evidence from the ISIS 2 study suggests that aspirin given in association with streptokinase confers considerable benefit in reduction of mortality. This may result in aspirin being used instead of warfarin following thrombolysis in the future. This trial also suggests that streptokinase may confer benefit in patients who have had pain up to 24 hours prior to presentation.

Reperfusion

This occurs in untreated control patients spontaneously in about 20%. Reperfusion occurs in approximately 50–70% of patients who receive thrombolysis within 4 hours of pain onset. The greatest improvement occurs in patients treated within 2 hours. It has also been shown that fibrin specific thrombolytic agents (e.g. rt-PA) are superior to streptokinase in producing reperfusion. Early reperfusion reduces infarct size and helps preserve LV function. In the large majority of patients who receive intravenous therapy, successful reperfusion is marked by a rapid fall in ST segments. Occasionally reperfusion arrhythmias occur due to wash out of toxic metabolites but these are rare. Wash out also results in a brisk rise in CPK levels. Successful reperfusion also results in rapid improvement in chest pain.

Reocclusion

Exact rates of reocclusion are unknown as coronary angiographic data is not available in large numbers. It is probable that 25% of patients reocclude within 3 months of thrombolysis unless the residual stenosis is dealt with by angioplasty.

Complications

Haemorrhage. This is by far the biggest problem. It complicates 7–10% of patients receiving streptokinase. Bleeding from drip sites and intramuscular injection sites are common and a large intramuscular haematoma can develop from simple i.m. analgesic injections. Transfusion is occasionally required. General practitioners and accident and emergency physicians should be encouraged to give analgesic injections intravenously in patients who are likely to be candidates for thrombolysis. More serious bleeding complications include haematemesis and melaena from occult peptic ulcers and cerebral haemorrhage.

Bleeding from a drip site is treated with local pressure. More severe bleeding complications require transfusion, and possible fresh frozen plasma or cryoprecipitate. Very rarely the streptokinase can be reversed by slow i.v. infusion of tranexamic acid 10 mg/kg body weight.

Allergic reactions. These are common with streptokinase. A low grade fever, and rash is common. Nausea, vomiting, headaches and flushing are also reported. A few patients who receive APSAC develop a vasculitis resembling Henoch–Schönlein purpura. This is usually self limiting after a few days. Bronchospasm has also been reported with APSAC. One of the advantages of rt-PA is that it does not cause allergic reactions and may become the agent of choice in patients who have already had a course of streptokinase in the past.

Subsequent management

Following successful thrombolysis, patients who need PTCA must be identified. This requires exercise testing in those patients who are pain free.

Patients who continue to get angina following thrombolysis or who have positive exercise tests at low work load need coronary angiography. The proportion of patients who are likely to need PTCA following thrombolysis probably exceeds 30%. The exact timing of PTCA after successful thrombolysis remains controversial. There is no evidence that very early angioplasty carries any benefit over PTCA at say 3 weeks post thrombolysis. The increase in thrombolysis will put a greater burden on cardiac catheter laboratories and facilities for performing PTCA may not be available close to the district hospital.

5.10 Complications of myocardial infarction

See separate sections for:

- Recurrent unstable angina (**5.6**, p. 157)
- Bradycardias or heart block requiring pacing (**6.1**, p. 243)
- Tachyarrhythmias; atrial or ventricular (**6.12–6.14**, pp. 286–302)
- Cardiac arrest (**5.15**, p. 225)
- Left ventricular failure (**5.11**, p. 192)

5.10 Complications of myocardial infarction

Sudden death

This can occur at any time following an infarct and is usually due to:

- acute cardiac rupture
- VF or fast prolonged VT degenarating to VF
- massive pulmonary embolism
- left main stem embolism from mural thrombus (rare)

Acute cardiac rupture occurs usually from about day 4 to 10, post-infarction. Electromechanical dissociation is typical. (Good ECG with no output all all.) Very occasionally it is contained by the pericardium (see Tamponade). Analysis of the causes of death in beta-blocking trials and myocardial infarcts suggests beta-blockers reduce mortality in infarction by reducing the incidence of cardiac rupture, but the drug has to be given early — within the first 2 days.

Massive pulmonary embolism may also show electro-mechanical dissociation on the ECG.

Right ventricular failure (RVF)

This is less common than LVF but very important as it usually is either missed or wrongly treated.

It occurs primarily following inferior infarction and is usually transient.

Persistent RVF presents with high neck veins and hepatic congestion. In the acute stage in severe cases Swan–Ganz monitoring is required and may show low left-sided filling pressures with high right-sided pressures. Cardiac output may be improved by plasma expansion in careful regulated amounts, rather than diuretic therapy, which may make the situation worse.

The differential diagnosis is pulmonary embolism (p. 354)

Pericarditis

This is often acute (within the first few days) and transient. It may occur with anterior or inferior infarcts. Pain is typically cardiac in distribution and relieved by sitting up or leaning forward. It is worse lying flat. Inferior/diaphragmatic involvement may cause shoulder-tip pain. A pericardial or pleuro-pericardial rub may be heard, but the pain is so typical in character it should be suspected with the history alone. The ECG shows transient T wave changes or 'saddle shaped' ST segment elevation (Fig. 10.9).

Treatment is with non-steroidal anti-inflammatory agents (e.g. soluble aspirin, indomethacin, ibuprofen, ketoprofen, etc.). Echocardiography should be performed frequently to check for an enlarging effusion. The ECG with an enlarging effusion shows progressive voltage reduction and sometimes electrical alternans.

Systemic embolism

From mural thrombus is more frequent following large infarctions and generally occurs 1–3 weeks post infarct. Patients with large infarctions should be heparinised until fully mobile (e.g. for first week), but the evidence that anticoagulants improve mortality figures from acute infarcts is small and only possible with pooled trials.

Peripheral limb emboli may be removed surgically (e.g. Fogarty technique). Large mesenteric emboli are generally fatal. Coronary emboli may account for a small number of reinfarctions.

Pulmonary embolism (9.2, p. 354)

This occurs due to a combination of

- low cardiac output, poor peripheral flow and venous stasis if venous pressure is high
- prolonged bed rest
- haemoconcentration with diuretic therapy
- increased platelet stickiness

Patients are thus mobilised early — within 48 hours of uncomplicated infarction to avoid pulmonary emboli — and discharged early. Patients who are likely to require several days bed rest should be heparinised parenterally until they are fully mobile.

Tamponade (**7.2**, p. 324)
This occurs following sub-acute cardiac rupture in which the pericardium acts as a barrier. A false aneurysm may follow if the patient survives (Fig. 5.7).

Examination may reveal raised neck veins filling on inspiration, with systolic 'x' descent. Small volume pulse possibly with pulsus paradoxus. Soft muffled heart sounds.

Cardiac rhythm quickly becomes slow, idionodal or ventricular bradycardia with no output (electromechanical dissociation).

Diagnosis can be confirmed by echocardiography. Needle aspiration may be of temporary benefit, but in the acute stage the condition is usually fatal unless urgent surgical repair is

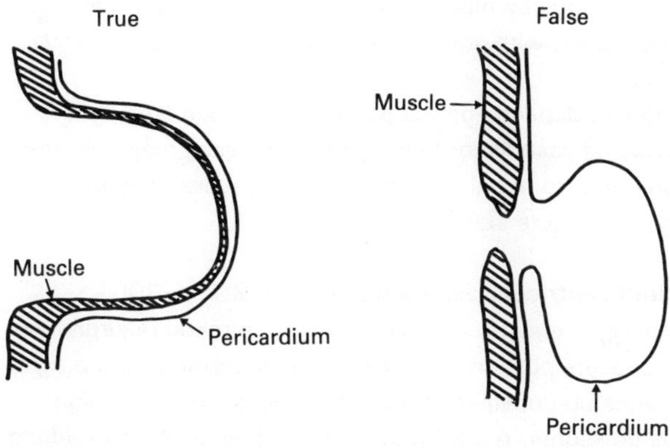

Fig. 5.7 Ventricular aneurysm. Shows the difference between a true and a false ventricular aneurysm. The true aneurysm is lined by a thin layer of a muscle/scar tissue as well as pericardium. The false aneurysm is subacute cardiac rupture with only pericardium lining the aneurysm. It tends to have a narrower neck than a true aneurysm.

possible. (The false aneurysm has a narrow neck and can be repaired occasionally in the acute stage.)

Acute cardiac rupture is a common cause of sudden death following myocardial infarction.

Mitral regurgitation (see **3.2**, p. 75)
Mild subvalvar mitral regurgitation is common following inferior or posterior infarction due to papillary muscle dysfunction. It is often transient. The murmur is ejection, in quality often midsystolic or late systolic and heard at both apex and left sternal edge.

Severe mitral regurgitation is due to chordal rupture or papillary muscle infarction and rupture. Pulmonary oedema occurs rapidly, often with a small left atrium.

Physical signs: a loud pansystolic murmur at apex or left sternal edge with possible thrill. Systolic expansion of the left atrium may be confused with a RV heave.

Echocardiography may show chaotic movement of the posterior leaflet with anterior movement during diastole and fluttering.

Treatment depends on the patient's condition (see LVF). Diuretics and vasodilator therapy (nitroprusside) may hold the situation prior to mitral valve replacement, which may be life-saving in the acute stage.

Acquired ventricular septal defect (see **2.1**, p. 20)
Physical signs may be very similar to acute mitral regurgitation, however acute pulmonary oedema is less prominent, and right-sided signs predominate in the early stages, with very high venous pressures. A VSD may occur with an anterior or inferior infarct.

Without Swan–Ganz catheterisation it may be impossible to differentiate acute VSD from mitral regurgitation. The table on p. 189 is a general guide only.

5.10 Complications of myocardial infarction

	Mitral regurgitation	**VSD**
Infarct site	Inferior/posterior	Anterior
CxR	Acute pulmonary oedema	Pulmonary plethora
Dyspnoea	Severe orthopnoea and PND	Less dyspnoeic
JVP	May be normal	Raised
But:	Both may have pansystolic murmur and thrill at left sternal edge, parasternal heave (RV or LA +). Both may be in cardiogenic shock	

Swan–Ganz catheterisation will confirm the diagnosis with a step up in saturation in the right ventricle.

Echocardiography: This is proving very valuable in diagnosis. Pulsed or continuous wave Doppler ultrasound is necessary. The sample volume is scanned up the RV border of the septum in the 4 chamber view and the Doppler signal is picked up at the site of the VSD. This technique may avoid the need for Swan–Ganz catheterisation.

Treatment: Earlier attempts to control the situation with medical treatment for as long as possible are now considered inappropriate. Surgery is recommended early now. A double patch technique either side of the septum may be needed to close the typical 'Swiss cheese' type defect. Recurrence of a small VSD post operatively is not uncommon. Postero-inferior VSDs carry a higher mortality than antero-apical VSDs. RV function is an important predictor of survival.

This is a high risk condition: 50% mortality within the first week.

LV aneurysm

Anterior

Is suspected clinically if the high paradoxical apex of an anterior infarct persists. The ECG shows persistent elevation of ST segments after 4–6 weeks.

The patient may have no symptoms. The diagnosis can be confirmed by:

- 2D echocardiography
- multiple-gated acquisition scanning (MUGA)
- LV angiography

Symptoms are commonly left ventricular failure or angina refractory to medical treatment. Occasionally patients develop recurrent ventricular tachycardia or systemic emboli.

Symptomatic patients are investigated with a view to left ventricular aneurysmectomy if the residual contractile segment function is adequate, and if medical treatment fails to control symptoms.

Inferior/posterior

This is less common than anterolateral aneurysm. It may be associated with considerable mitral regurgitation. False aneurysm may also occur infero-posteriorly.

Physical signs are less obvious, as there is no paradoxical apex. Persistent ST elevation occurs on inferior leads. Investigation and indications for surgery are as with anterior aneurysms, but additional mitral valve replacement may be necessary.

Late malignant ventricular arrhythmias

Occurring 1–3 weeks after myocardial infarction, often at about 10 days, are the cardiologist's nightmare: the patient having made an uneventful recovery, about to return home, suddenly collapses with VF,

Fortunately the problem is uncommon, even so patients with large infarcts should have 24–hour monitoring prior to discharge.

Early exercise testing may point to patients at risk. Recently signal averaging of the standard 12 lead ECG has shown that patients at risk of late ventricular arrhythmias may show late or after potentials. Signal averaging of ECGs is expensive and not generally available yet. It may prove a useful investigation for the future.

The most easily avoidable cause is hypokalaemia from excessive diuretic therapy. Digoxin should be avoided in infarcts unless the patient is in AF.

Dressler's syndrome

A syndrome of recurrent pericarditis, pleural effusions, fever, anaemia and high ESR. It occurs in about 1–5% of infarcts, usually 1–4 weeks following myocardial infarction. It is thought to be due to an autoimmune reaction to exposed myocardial antigens following infarction (and a similar illness may occur following cardiac surgery). Anti-heart antibodies have been demonstrated, but are not useful clinically.

It is a chronic condition. Treatment in the first instance is with non-steroidal anti-inflammatory agents, or steroids in more severe or refractory cases. Steroids are said to increase the likelihood of LV aneurysm development, but the evidence for this is anecdotal.

Treatment may have to be continued for several months and patients observed when treatment is stopped or weaned off as the syndrome may recur. Tamponade is rare.

Shoulder hand syndrome

This is now rare following myocardial infarction, probably due to early mobilisation. It develops 2 weeks – 2 months post infarct. It develops as stiffness and pain in the shoulder (usually left). Pain and swelling of the hand (becoming puffy and mottled).

A few cases late develop wasting of small muscles of the hand with irreversible contractures forming (like Dupuytren's).

Treatment is with mobilisation physiotherapy of hand and

shoulder with analgesia. Hydrocortisone injections into the sub-acromial bursa may help. Systemic steroids are not used.

Depression

Occurs in up to one-third of post infarct patients. It can be largely prevented by:

- a sensible encouraging approach from the doctor: worried doctors produce worried patients
- early mobilisation
- pre-discharge advice re work, driving, sex, travel, etc.
- exercise programme and follow-up to check the patient is considering returning to work
- avoidance of anti-depressant drugs if possible. If absolutely necessary mianserin, doxepin or lofepramine are said to have less cardiac effects than earlier tricyclics (amitriptyline or imipramine).
- cardiac rehabilitation course. There is renewed interest in this aspect of cardiac care. Unfortunately there is little evidence yet that it has long term physical benefits, but there is no doubt that cardiac rehabilitation provides motivation, company, reassurance and carefully graded and medically supervised exercise.

Depression following infarction may result in denial of symptoms, with the patient too frightened to admit to any problems.

5.11 Left ventricular failure (LVF)

The concept of treating LVF with afterload reduction is now firmly established. In heart failure there is an inappropriately raised systemic vascular resistance due to sympathetic overdrive and activation of the renin-angiotensin system. The use of inotropes on top of this vasoconstriction may increase afterload still further.

Flogging a failing heart in this way has other problems:

- no oral agent available other than digoxin
- increased myocardial oxygen consumption

- possible increase in infarct size
- arrhythmias with increased myocardial excitability (β_1 effect)
- increased heart rate with shorter diastolic coronary flow
- possible vasoconstrictor effect on coronary arterioles (α-effect)
- central line administration with most drugs

In view of these heart failure is managed with bed rest, diuretics and vasodilating agents. Vasodilators are divided into:

1 *Venodilators.* Reduce preload by dilating venous capacitance vessels, e.g. nitrates, some diuretics. They lower filling pressures without initially much improvement in stroke volume. At higher doses they also become arterial dilators.

2 *Arterial dilators.* Reduce afterload. Dilate arterial resistance vessels, e.g. hydralazine. They improve stroke volume without much reduction in filling pressure or pulmonary venous pressure.

3 *Combined arterial and venous dilators.* Drugs such as nitroprusside and α-blocking agents. These improve stroke volume and reduce filling pressure. They are very useful in LVF.

A wide variety of vasodilating drugs is now available (see next table).

Choice of vasodilators

Left ventricular failure (acute) with pulmonary oedema with normotension, e.g. acute mitral regurgitation, septal infarction with VSD. Acute infarction in normotensive patient:

- Nitroprusside: if full haemodynamic monitoring available, with
- frusemide i.v.

If no monitoring facilities available other than ECG:

- frusemide i.v. + isosorbide dinitrate i.v., then:
- oral isosorbide dinitrate plus ACE inhibitor + oral diuretic as the patient improves

The great majority of patients with LVF can be managed with this regime without the need for arterial pressure monitoring.

Low output states: hypotensive, cool, oligaemic patients (so-called 'forward failure')

• dopamine (see inotropes section), monitoring haemodynamics. Once normotension is restored addition of nitroprusside may be beneficial. Alternatively dobutamine if urine output satisfactory

Chronic congestive cardiac failure (oral therapy only)

- frusemide (+ amiloride if hypokalaemic)
- ACE inhibitor, especially if history of hypertension
- long acting nitrate
- avoid adding salt to food. Allow salt for cooking in most cases

} In combination

Prazosin has not been included because of its tachyphylactic problem and hypotensive first dose effect. Hydralazine is less used now, as tachyphylaxis also is thought to be a problem and it produces the lupus syndrome in high doses (>150 mg/day). Nifedipine and other calcium antagonists are usually used in patients with angina as the dominant symptom, rather than as first choice in LVF (see **5.5**). The ACE inhibitors have already revolutionised the treatment of chronic cardiac failure and have been shown to reduce mortality in the long term (The Consensus Study).

Drugs in acute LVF

I.v. nitrates. See **5.4**

I.v. sodium nitroprusside (SNP)

Controlled infusion of nitroprusside is of great value in the treatment of acute LVF (e.g. ruptured chordae), the management of hypertensive crises and the post-cardirac surgical control of hypertension. It can be used to lower blood pressure in aortic dissection prior to surgery.

Its great advantage is its rapid onset and equally rapid

cessation of action on switching the infusion off. A computerised feed-back technique is available in which automatic control of the SNP infusion rate is governed by the arterial pressure.

It is a potent dilator of arteries and veins by acting locally on vascular smooth muscle.

Infusion preparation:

1 Weak solution. Dissolve 50 mg sodium nitroprusside (Nipride) in 2 ml 5% dextrose; add this to 500 ml 5% dextrose. Infusion strength 100 mg/L (100 μg/ml). Start at 1 μg/kg/min (40–70 μg/min usually). Maximum infusion rate 400 μg/min.

Wrap infusion bottle/paediatric giving set/infusion line in aluminium foil to protect from light.

Renew infusion every 4 hours. Must be in a separate line from bicarbonate.

2 Strong solution. This is often easier to manage clinically and involves smaller volume load. Add 50 mg sodium nitroprusside to 100 ml 5% dextrose solution (in paediatric giving set) = 500 μg/ml. Then 6 dpm (paediatric microdrops) = 50 μg/min; 12 dpm = 100 μg/min, 30 dpm = 250 μg/min, etc.

Cyanide toxicity

Over 90% cyanide released from nitroprusside is bound by erythrocytes. Cyanide free in plasma is freely diffusible and causes a cytotoxic hypoxia by inhibition of cytochromic oxidase. Cyanide is slowly metabolised to thiocyanate.

- toxicity is related more to the rate of infusion than to total dose, but care must be taken once a total dose of 50 mg is exceeded
- plasma cyanide or thiocyanate levels are not necessarily a reliable guide to toxicity
- a metabolic acidosis (arterial lactate from anaerobic metabolism) occurs with cyanide toxicity, but may not necessarily be due to it. However it is the easiest guide to nitroprusside dose and usually reverses quickly when the infusion is stopped.

Vasodilating drugs

Drug	Arterial dilator	Venous dilator	Oral dose	I.v. dose (adult)	Side-effects other than hypotension
Isosorbide dinitrate	(+)	+++	10 mg 6 hrly to 30 mg 4 hrly	1–7 mg/hour	Headaches. Nausea
Hydralazine	+++	—	25 mg tds to 150 mg qds	20 mg over 5 mins (0.3 mg/kg)	Lupoid reaction (> 200 mg/day) Fluid retention. Tachyphylaxis
Minoxidil	++	+	2.5 mg bd to 10 mg tds	—	Hirsutism. Gut disturbances Fluid retention. Breast tenderness
Diazoxide	++	+	100 mg tds	150 mg at 5–10 min intervals	Diabetes mellitus. Action i.v not sustained. Fluid retention
Salbutamol	+	(+)	4–8 mg tds	10–40 µg/min	Tremor. Hyperglycaemia. Apparent hypokalaemia
Nifedipine	++	++	10 mg qds	—	Flushing. Headaches. Ankle swelling

Nitroprusside	+++	+++	—	1–6 µg/kg/min	Cyanide toxicity. Metabolic acidosis. Hypothyroidism
Prazosin	++	++	0.5 mg test dose 1 mg tds to 10 mg tds	—	First dose syncope. Drowsiness. Impotence Tachyphylaxis
Phentolamine	+++	+	50 mg qds	5–10 mg i.v. stat 10–20 µg/kg/min	Diarrhoea. Flushing. Tachycardia
Phenoxybenzamine	+++	+	10 mg nocte to 30 mg bd	10–40 mg slowly i.v.	Paralytic ileus — dry mouth. Impotence
Trimetaphan	++	+	—	3mg/min	Tachycardia
Captopril	++	+	25 mg tds to 150 mg tds	—	Stomatitis. Rashes. Proteinuria. Leucopenia. Agranyulocytosis. Loss of taste

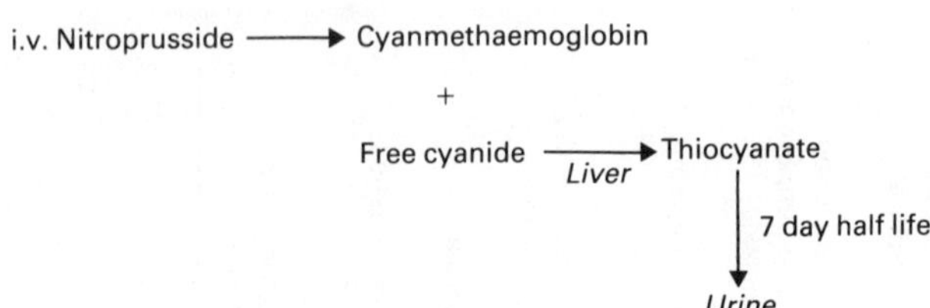

Summary of nitroprusside infusion

- monitor arterial and preferably PAW pressure
- frequent measurement of acid-base balance
- keep levels as below (if assays available)
  plasma cyanide <3 μmol/l
  plasma thiocyanate <100 μg/ml
  red cell cyanide <75 μg/100 ml
- maximum infusion rate <400 μg/min (approx 5–6 μg/kg/min in adults)

Toxic levels of thiocyanate may cause hypothyroidism. If possible nitroprusside infusion should not be used for more than 48 hours. Hydroxycobalamin infusion given at the same time as SNP infusion reduces plasma cyanide levels (forming cyanocobalamin). This infusion also has to be protected from light. Dose of B12 = 25 mg/hour (mixture of 100 mg B12 in 100 ml 5% dextrose).

Emergency treatment of cyanide toxicity

- amyl nitrite inhalation or isosorbide dinitrate i.v. (increase methaemoglobin)
- sodium thiosulphate injections
- bicarbonate for lactic acidosis
- hydroxycobalamin infusion

Hydralazine

This drug causes arteriolar vasodilatation and a rise in stroke volume. Its inotropic effect may be primary or secondary to vasodilatation. It does not reduce pulmonary capillary wedge pressure or systemic venous pressure to any great extent. In heart failure a compensatory reflex tachycardia does not necessarily occur.

Starting oral dose is 25 mg tds (half life 2–8 hours). It is acetylated in the liver, and excreted in the urine.

The lupus syndrome

Is more likely to develop in patients who:

- receive >200 mg daily (check ANF and LE cells)
- are slow acetylators
- have histocompatibility locus DR4.

However the lupus syndrome may occur on doses less than 200 mg daily. Positive ANF is not an indication to stop the drug, as it occurs in 30–60% patients receiving hydralazine for 3 years or more, but lupus occurs in only 1–3%. The lupus syndrome is less common in black patients. It is fully but slowly reversible on stopping the drug.

Tachyphylaxis

Unfortunately recent reports suggest that long-term tolerance to the drug occurs, possibly due to reduction in the number of receptor sites in the arterial wall, or to a change in the receptor itself.

Benefit from acute administration may not persist and a change of drug may be necessary. The drug may cause fluid retention and should be used with a diuretic.

Parenteral administration

Is possible in emergency situations (e.g. severe hypertension, pre-eclampsia). The drug can be given i.m. (20 mg) or slowly i.v. (20 mg slowly over 5 min).

Drugs in chronic congestive cardiac failure

Angiotensin coverting enzyme inhibitors (ACE inhibitors)

A group of drugs which inhibit the conversion of inactive angiotensin I to the powerful vasoconstrictor angiotensin II. At present there are three ACE inhibitors available in the UK, but there will be many more in the next few years. The profound vasoconstrictor effect of angiotensin II is reduced and the reduction in congestive cardiac failure where other drugs have failed and have a sustained action. They may be useful even when plasma renin activity is low. This may by mediated by reduction of bradykinin degradation and activation of prostaglandin production.

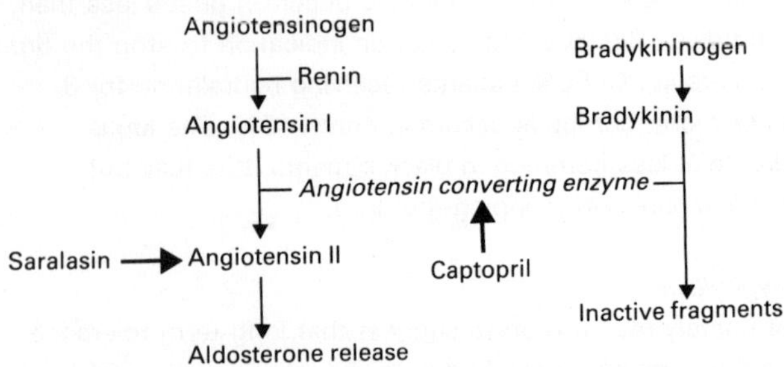

ACE inhibitors

Drug	Starting dose	Doses/day	Maximum dose
Captopril (Capoten) (Acepril)	6.25 mg bd	3	50 mg tds
Enalapril (Innovace)	2.5 mg od	1	40 mg od
Lisinopril (Zestril) (Carace)	2.5 mg od	1	40 mg od

Starting therapy with ACE inhibitors
Hypertensive patients can safely be started on ACE inhibitors on an out-patient basis. Patients with congestive cardiac failure however are best admitted to a hospital bed if possible before starting therapy. The first dose should be given at night. The starting doses above are the lowest possible and should be used in the elderly. In younger fitter patients with good renal function the starting dose could be doubled. Many physicians start their patients on captopril and then switch to a longer acting ACE inhibitor when the patient is established on it.

Problems and side-effects with ACE inhibitors
• *Hypotension.* This is the commonest problem especially with the first dose. Severe hypotension can result in a neurological deficit or renal failure. It is important to make sure patients are not hypovolaemic or severely hyponatraemic (excess diuretics) before starting treatment. May need i.v. N saline.
• *Chronic cough.* Responds to a reduction in dose. May be due to bradykinin.
• *Loss of taste.* Apthous ulcers may develop. Dysgeusia.
• *Hyperkalaemia.* Due to a reduction in aldosterone. Care needed with postassium retaining diuretics.
• *Deteriorating renal function.* This may be due to hypotension and 'pre-renal failure'. In hypertensive patients with pre-treatment normal renal function who suddenly deteriorate on ACE inhibitors consider renal artery stenosis. Deteriorating renal function is the commonest long term reason for restricting or reducing the dose. Careful monitoring of blood urea and creatinine needed.
• *Urticaria and angioneurotic oedema.*
• *Rarely: proteinuria, leucopenia, fatigue, exhaustion.*
• *False positive urine test for ketones (captopril).*

There is little evidence to suggest that ACE inhibitors without the -SH group (e.g. Enalapril and Lisinopril) may have less side-effects, e.g. with taste problems than Captopril. There is no rebound hypertension on stopping ACE inhibitors.

Contra-indications to ACE inhibitors treatment

- severe renal failure. Serum creatinine >300 umol/l
- hyperkalaemia
- hypovolaemia
- hyponatraemia
- pregnancy or lactating mothers
- LV outflow obstruction
- hypotension. Peak systolic pressures <90 mmHg
- cor pulmonale

Use with other drugs

ACE inhibitors can be safely used with digoxin and diuretics (care with volume and sodium depletion). Potassium retaining diuretics are reduced or stopped. The drugs may be used with other hypotensive agents if necessary e.g. nitrates and beta-blockers. The effect is synergistic.

Drugs of second choice in heart failure

Prazosin

Acts on the α_1-receptors in the vessel wall and causes arterial and venous dilatation. Unfortunately tachyphylaxis is a problem.

Initial dose is 0.5 mg taken on going to bed. In spite of this a few patients develop first dose syncope which limits its use. If the test dose is taken satisfactorily then the patient is started on 1 mg tds.

The drug is well absorbed following oral administration (half life 3–4 hours). It is probably more useful in hypertension than chronic heart failure.

Care should be taken in using nitrites with prazosin, as both are powerful venodilators and may cause syncope together. Although prazosin reduces systemic vascular resistance, renal plasma flow is reduced and fluid retention may result.

Salbutamol
This β_2-agonist causes arterial dilatation, an increase in stroke index, but also an increase in heart rate. It does not restore normotension in the hypotensive patient with LVF. It is not suitable for the patient in acute pulmonary oedema.

It causes tremor. It shifts potassium into the cells and causes an apparent hypokalaemia. It causes restlessness and insomnia.

α-blocking agents
Phenoxybenzamine, Phentolamine. These drugs can be used in the management of acute LVF, but nitroprusside is better with its more pronounced venodilating properties.

They are more useful in hypertensive crises or management of phaeochromocytoma. Phenoxybenzamine may be of some use in coping with severe Raynaud's phenomenon.

Of these two drugs phentolamine may be the most useful in heart failure by having a weak inotropic effect (noradrenaline release) as well as α-blocking properties.

Diazoxide. Is rarely used now in hypertension or LVF. Acute intravenous administration (150–300 mg) causes a sudden fall in BP, but the fall is not sustained and the dose needs to be repeated in 10–15 min. Chronic use causes diabetes mellitus. It also causes fluid retention. Infusion of diazoxide is not as hypotensive as bolus administration.

Minoxidil. This drug causes salt and water retention and is not suitable for chronic heart failure. It is more useful in hypertension and must be given with a diuretic. Hirsutism limits its use to men. Reflex tachycardia requires additional beta-blockade. The drug has a long half life (1–4 days) and can be given as a single oral dose daily (starting 5 mg od) initially.

5.12 Digoxin

The controversy regarding the use of digoxin in sinus rhythm continues, but controlled crossover studies with placebo are making the situation clearer, especially regarding its long-term use in heart failure.

Action

Digoxin is thought to inhibit the action of sarcolemmal membrane Na^+/K^+ ATPase; inhibiting the sodium pump. This allows greater influx of sodium and displacement of bound intracellular calcium. The increase in calcium availability exerts the inotropic effect. Other effects of digoxin are:

- AV node refractory period prolonged
- AV node conduction slowed
- mild peripheral vasoconstriction (arteries and veins)
- vagotonic effect
- automaticity increased (myocardial excitability)
- possible acceleration of bypass conduction in WPW syndrome

It is the only oral inotrope commercially available apart from xamoterol. Its inotropic effect is much weaker than sympathomimetic inotropes.

Indications

Congestive cardiac failure with atrial fibrillation

This is the classic situation for digoxin. Its effect on the AV node slows ventricular response to fast AF, and its positive inotropic effect helps the dilated failing left ventricle increase its stroke volume.

Control of chronic atrial fibrillation (e.g. mitral valve disease)

The drug is used for its effect on the AV node although additional therapy with a beta-blocker or verapamil may be needed.

Management of paroxysmal atrial fibrillation
Digoxin does not prevent paroxysmal AF, merely controls the ventricular response when its occurs. More recent drugs (e.g. amiodarone) may prevent AF relapsing, as quinidine has been shown to in the past. Amiodarone may replace digoxin in paroxysmal AF, if its side-effects do not prove too troublesome.

Heart failure in children
Digoxin is still the mainstay of therapy.

Congestive cardiac failure and sinus rhythm
Several studies have shown that digoxin is of benefit in this situation and that the effect is sustained. The presence of a third sound is a strong correlate of a good response to digoxin. However not all patients benefit from digoxin and in a group of patients already on digoxin about one-third deteriorate when digoxin is withdrawn.

Thus digoxin is not the first drug of choice in CCF with sinus rhythm. If bed rest, diuretics and vasodilators do not achieve or maintain an improvement digoxin should be tried. It is likely to help in patients who:

- have a third sound with a large heart
- do not have valvar obstruction

Once heart failure has been controlled and the heart is smaller digoxin may be withdrawn under supervision.

Digoxin is no longer the drug choice in:

- supraventricular tachycardia. This is better managed with intravenous verapamil or adenosine
- sino-atrial disease. This is probably better managed with beta-blockade, amiodarone and/or pacing
- cor pulmonale. There are no studies to show it helps. The side-effects of digoxin could be dangerous. It can be used only if the patient is in AF

- myocardial infarction, unless the patient is in AF
- valvar or subvalvar aortic stenosis, unless the patient is in uncontrolled AF. Digoxin will increase the gradient in muscular subaortic obstruction (HOCM)
- hypertensive heart failure. This is better managed with afterload reduction

Digoxin should be avoided in:

- WPW syndrome
- HOCM
- second or third degree AV block. Chronic first degree AV block is not a contraindication to digoxin although acute prolongation of the PR interval (e.g. myocardial infarction, infective endocarditis) is more dangerous and patients should be monitored carefully
- severe renal failure (creatinine clearace <10 ml/min)
- patients with recurrent ventricular arrhythmias
- prior to DC cardioversion
- cardiac amyloidosis

Digitalisation

Acute intravenous

This is not often necessary and the patient should be normokalaemic. Use digoxin 0.25 mg i.v. 2 hourly until effect is achieved, usually 0.75–1 mg is required. Following control of the fast AF then the patient is maintained on 0.125 mg i.v. as required 4 hourly.

Using intermittent doses of 0.25 mg i.v. is safer than a bolus dose of 0.75–1 mg over 30 min.

Oral

The loading dose depends on lean body mass as skeletal muscle binds digoxin. It is only necessary if a rapid result is required. Often patients can be started on the maintenance dose. Loading dose is 1.0–1.5 mg orally for 70 kg adult;

maintenance dose depends on renal function and is 0.25 mg. Larger doses (up to 0.5 mg daily) may be required, but care must be taken and, with larger doses, plasma levels are helpful.

A useful compromise in the absence of an emergency is to use: digoxin 0.25 mg bd for 2 days then 0.25 mg od. Digoxin can be given intramuscularly if necessary, but not subcutaneously (very irritant).

Plasma levels
Normal level for satisfactory therapeutic effect is 0.8–2 ng/ml (1–2.5 nmol/l). Blood is taken 6–8 hours after an oral dose. Serum half life is 30 hours. However the level should never be used as more than a guide and the clinical effect must be taken into consideration, i.e. levels > 2 ng/ml do not necessarily mean digoxin toxicity unless the patient's condition or ECG are consistent with this.

Very high plasma levels are associated with acute i.v. administration (e.g. up to 100 ng/ml), but these levels are transient and not toxic.

If the required effect is not achieved with plasma levels of 3–4 ng/ml then additional therapy with beta-blockade or verapamil should be used.

Approximately 20–40% of digoxin is bound to plasma proteins. Most digoxin is excreted unchanged by the kidney both by filtration and active tubular secretion. About 10% is excreted in the stools, and a smaller percentage metabolised in the liver.

Reduction in digoxin dose
This is required in the following situations.
• Symptoms of digoxin toxicity: anorexia, nausea, vomiting, xanthopsia (very rare), neurological symptoms (paraesthesiae, fits, mental confusion), gynaecomastia, etc.
• ECG changes: junctional bradycardia, ventricular bigeminy, salvos of ventricular ectopics or paroxysmal VT. 2° or 3° AV

block. Paroxysmal atrial tachycardia with varying block (PATB) may be a sign of digoxin toxicity in patients who are fully digitalised. The digoxin effect on the ECG is not an indication to reduce the dose.

• Other drug therapy. Several drugs increase plasma digoxin levels, possibly by protein displacement, reduced renal clearance or diminished distribution to the tissues. In several cases the cause is unknown.

Drugs increasing plasma digoxin are: quinidine (probably reduced renal clearance); verapamil; amiodarone (probably protein displacement); nifedipine. In patients taking additional quinidine or amiodarone the dose of digoxin should be halved.

• Development of renal failure. Plasma digoxin levels may help. Digitoxin does not need dose reduction in renal failure. If the creatinine clearance is < 10 ml/min it is probably better to avoid digoxin altogether. 10–25 ml/min, 0.0625–0.125 mg daily; 25–50 ml/min, 0.125 mg/0.25 mg alt. days; 50 ml/min, 0.25 mg daily. Cardiac glycosides are not removed by dialysis.

• The elderly require a smaller dose of digoxin. The paediatric 0.0625 mg tablets are small and blue and easily recognisable. If digoxin is necessary they can usually be managed on 0.0625–0.125 mg/day.

• Increased sensitivity to digoxin occurs in the following conditions and dose reduction may be necessary: hypokalaemia; hypercalcaemia; hypoxia, chronic pulmonary disease; hypomagnesaemia (e.g. chronic diarrhoea or prolonged diuresis); hypothyroidism.

Increase in digoxin dose

May be needed in:

• other drug therapy, i.e. cholestyramine (reduces absorption), barbiturates and phenytoin

• malabsorption

Children

Paediatric digoxin elixir (lime flavour) contains 0.05 mg/ml. Children tend to need more digoxin than their small weight would suggest. Digitalising dose is 0.01 mg/kg 6 hourly until therapeutic effect obtained; maintenance dose is 0.01 mg/kg/day. Toxicity in children: sinus bradycardia, vomiting, drowsiness. AV block is not as common as in adults.

Other digitalis glycosides

These are rarely if ever needed now. Careful dose regulation of standard digoxin will cope with almost all situations.

Digoxin overdose

The development of digoxin antibodies has made a great difference to the therapy of digoxin overdose. Infusion of the antibody fragment Fab (raised in sheep) rapidly reverses the toxic effects of digoxin. The dose is calculated from the plasma digoxin concentration assuming an interval of >6 hours from ingestion.

Digoxin load (mg) = plasma concentration (ng/ml) × body weight (kg) × 0.0056. Antibody load needed (mg) = 60 × digoxin body load. If digitoxin has been ingested the factor 0.00056 is used not 0.0056.

The Fab fragments are excreted in the urine (half life 16 hours). With reduction in serum digoxin hypokalaemia may result as potassium goes back into the cells. Hypersensitivity and anaphylactic reaction are a theoretical possibility as this is a sheep protein.

Drug trade name: Digibind; 40 mg of Fab fragments/vial.

5.13 Inotropic sympathomimetic drugs

Most inotropic drugs work by increasing the level of intracellular cyclic AMP which with intracellular calcium promotes contractility. The increase in cyclic AMP may be achieved by:

- stimulation of beta-receptors:

Digitalis glycosides

Drug (trade name)	Tablet/elixir strength	Injection strength	Advantages/disadvantages
Digoxin (Lanoxin) (Lanoxin PG) (Diganox Nativelle)	0.25 mg 0.125mg 0.0625 mg 0.05 mg/ml	0.25 mg/ml	Standard digoxin for all routine therapy. Maximum effect after i.v. dose in 2–3 hours. Serum half life 1½ days. Has largely replaced all other digitalis glycosides
Digitoxin (Digitaline Nativelle)	0.1 mg 1 mg/ml	0.2 mg/ml	Cumulative. Serum half life 4–6 days. Hepatic metabolism and gut excretion, so may be used with renal impairment. Oral dose 0.1 mg daily (range 0.05 mg–0.3 mg/day)

Medigoxin (Lanitop)	0.1 mg	0.1 mg/ml	β-methyl digoxin. Better gastrointestinal absorption. oral dose 0.2 mg bd for two days, then 0.2 mg od. Same dose i.v.
Lanatoside C (Cedilanid)	0.25 mg	0.2 mg/ml	Similar to digoxin, but said to cause less vomiting. Rarely used except with intolerance of other digitalis glycosides
Ouabain (Ouabaine Arnaud)	—	0.25 mg/ml	Most rapid action i.v. (1 hour). Not used orally. 0.25 mg i.v. initially. repeated 2–4 hourly. Switch to oral digoxin when possible

5.13 Inotropic sympathomimetic drugs

Beta 1: isoprenaline, dobutamine, dopamine, xamoterol.
Beta 2: salbutamol, terbutaline, pirbuterol, prenalterol dopexamine.

- stimulation of glucagon receptor: glucagon
- stimulation of H_2 receptor; histamine
- inhibition of phosphodiesterase, the enzyme which converts cyclic AMP to inactive 5′ AMP. There are many drugs in this group:

bipyridines: amrinone, milrinone.
imidazoles: enoximone, piroximone.
imidazopyridine; sulmazole.
xanthine derivatives: caffeine, aminophylline
Other inotropes:

- digitalis glycosides (see **5.12**)
- alpha agonists: Stimulate post-synaptic α receptors in the myocardium without increasing cyclic AMP: noradrenaline, adrenaline, high dose dopamine (via noradrenaline)

Many of these drugs are still under development, and in time some may be available as an oral agent (see section on newer inotropes).

Down regulation of beta receptors
The normal myocardium contains both beta 1 and beta 2 receptors in a ratio of about 4 : 1. In heart failure this ratio is reduced or reversed as the number of beta 1 receptors falls. This may be due to chronic high levels of circulating noradrenaline. Beta 1 agonists will therefore have less effect, and treatment with beta 2 agonists in heart failure assumes more importance. Newer drugs like xamoterol which partially block the beta 1 receptor may help prevent this down regulation.

Dopamine
The precursor of noradrenaline dopamine has become a standard drug in the management of cardiogenic shock, and low output left ventricular failure secondary to myocardial infarction.

It is also used in septic shock, and post-cardiac surgery.

It acts on several different receptors with activity changing with increasing dose.

1–5.0 μg/kg/min. Dopaminergic receptors activated. Dilatation of renal, coronary, splanchnic and cerebral arteries. Sometimes called the 'renal dose' of dopamine. Other sympathomimetics only increase renal blood flow by increasing cardiac output. Dopamine has this unique action on renal vascular bed.

5.0–10.0 μg/kg/min. β-receptors activated. The inotropic dose. It does increase heart rate, probably more than dobutamine. Doses > 10.0 μg/kg/min are likely to cause arrhythmias.

> 15.0 μg/kg/min. α-receptors activated. The drug also releases noradrenaline from myocardial adrenergic nerve terminals. Vasoconstrictive doses of dopamine are not beneficial. Renal blood flow falls.

Addition of nitroprusside or an α-blocking agent helps prevent this.

Precautions:

- As with all sympathomimetic agents except dobutamine, the drug must be given by a central line. Peripheral administration causes vasoconstriction and skin necrosis. This can be reversed by injections of subcutaneous phentolamine (5–10 mg phentolamine in 10–15 ml saline).
- The drug is inactivated by bicarbonate or other alkaline solutions.
- Dopamine is metabolised by β-hydroxylase and monoamine oxidase. It is contra-indicated in patients on MAOIs.
- It is contra-indicated in phaeochromocytoma, ventricular arrhythmias.

Dopamine infusion preparation

Four ampoules of dopamine (Intropin) each of 200 mg are added to 500 ml 5% dextrose. Using paediatric giving set (60 microdrops = 1 ml) infusion strength: 1 microdrop = 26.7 μg dopamine.

Infusion rate chart (microdrops/min)

Weight of patient (kg)	Dopamine dose (μg/kg/min)					
	2	5	10	15	20	25
30	2	6	12	18	23	29
40	3	8	16	23	31	39
50	4	10	20	29	39	49
60	5	12	23	35	47	58
70	5	14	27	41	55	68
80	6	16	31	47	62	78
90	7	18	35	53	70	88
100	8	20	39	58	78	97

Dobutamine

This synthetic inotrope is structurally similar to dopamine, but differs from it in several respects (see table of inotropes). It does not activate dopaminergic receptors, and does not cause local release of noradrenaline from myocardial stores. Its advantage over dopamine is its lack of chronotropic effect at low doses, where it seems to be an exclusive inotrope. Also dobutamine can be given via a peripheral line if there is no central line available. Dopamine must never be given via a peripheral line.

Dobutamine is a racemic mixture of *l*- and *d*-dobutamine. *d*-dobutamine is a potent beta 1 agonist, and *l*-dobutamine a potent alpha agonist with weak beta 1 and beta 2 action. As with all beta 1 agonists dobutamine may be liable to down regulation.

Both dopamine and dobutamine have their advocates. Cross-over studies have suggested:

- heart rate lower with dobutamine for same increase in cardiac output
- pulmonary wedge pressure lower with dobutamine
- fewer ventricular ectopics
- more sustained action over 24 hours

Its α-effects are less than noradrenaline, and its β_2-effects less than isoprenaline.

Precautions are the same as for dopamine. Both drugs have very short half lives (e.g. dobutamine approx 2½ min). Of the two drugs dobutamine and dopamine, the former is probably the superior inotrope.

Second line sympathomimetic drugs

Isoprenaline

Is rarely used as an inotrope now unless an increase in heart rate is required. Junctional bradycardia, transient second degree AV block, or sinus bradycardia unresponsive to atropine following myocardial infarction or cardiac surgery will be helped by isoprenaline, and may obviate the need for temporary pacing. However the risk of increased myocardial excitability must be considered. It reduces systemic vascular resistance and dilates skeletal and splanchnic vessels (β_2-effect) which is not where the flow is needed.

Dose and infusion preparation

(Various ampoule strengths available, e.g. 0.1 mg/ml, 1 mg/ml.) Add 2 mg isoprenaline to 500 ml 5% dextrose: mixture strength = 4 µg/ml. Start infusion at 1 µg/min = 15 microdrops/min. Increase dose as required, generally up to 10 μg/min.

Adrenaline

Very occasionally there is still a place for adrenaline infusion when other inotropes have failed. It has a mixed β- and α-receptor activity.

Inotropic sympathomimetic drugs

Drug and receptor affected	Increase heart rate β_1-effect	Myocardial release of noradrenaline	Peripheral vasoconstriction α-effect	Peripheral vasodilatation β_2-effect	Renal blood flow Dopaminergic	Dose i.v.
Dopamine Dopaminergic, β, α at high dose	++	+ +	− to ++	+ + Low doses	++	*Renal dose:* 1–5.0 μg/kg/min Inotropic dose: 5.0–10 μg/kg/min Constricting dose > 15 μg/kg/min
Dobutamine β_1 (β_2 small)	+	−	− to +	++	−	2.5–15.0 μg/kg/min. Low dose — inotropic High dose — inotropic + chronotropic
Salbutamol β_2 (β_1 small)	+ +	−	−	++	−	10–40 μg/min (up to 0.5 μg/kg/min)
Isoprenaline β_1 and β_2	+++	−	−	+++	−	1–10 μg/min
Adrenaline $\beta_1 > \beta_2$ (α small)	+++	+	+	−	−	1–12 μg/min
Noradrenaline α (β small)	− or +	++	+++	−	−	1–12 μg/min

Infusion preparation. 5 ml of 1:1000 adrenaline (= 5 mg) in 500 ml 5% dextrose; mixture = 10 μg/ml. Start at 1–2 μg/min (6–12 paediatric microdrops/min).

Glucagon

This activates adenylcyclase by a mechanism separate from the β_1 myocardial receptor. It can be used in beta-blocked patients. It is not a powerful inotrope, does not have a sustained effect and causes hyperglycaemia, hypokalaemia and nausea. It is expensive and of little value in left ventricular failure or cardiogenic shock. It is of more use in treating hypoglycaemia.

Dose 1–5 mg slowly i.v. repeated after 30 min. Infusion rate is 1–7.5 mg/hour.

Choice of parenteral inotrope

In low output states with oliguria (<30 ml/hour) low dose dopamine is the drug of choice. If urine output is > 30 ml/hour then dobutamine is preferable. In hypotensive states with pulmonary oedema a combination of dopamine or dobutamine with nitroprusside should be tried. Dopamine and dobutamine may be used together using the 'renal' dose of dopamine and dobutamine as the inotrope.

Newer inotropes

1 *Dopexamine*. An alternative to dopamine. Only available as an i.v. preparation. Stimulates DA1 dopamine receptors (e.g. renal vessels dilate), potent beta 2 agonist, weak beta 1 agonist. Also inhibits noradrenaline re-uptake. It is thus a potent vasodilator plus the effects of dopamine.

2 *Ibopamine*. The only oral inotrope available related to dopamine. Converted to active metabolite epinine. Appears to activate alpha, beta and dopaminergic receptors.

3 *Xamoterol*. (Corwin). This is the only inotrope other than digoxin available in the UK which can be given orally on prescription. It is a partial beta 1 agonist increasing contractility. At the same time it blocks the effects of high endogenous catecholamines on the beta 1 receptor. It is said to lower LV diastolic pressure by improving relaxation. It has been shown to be superior to digoxin in a single controlled trial.

Xamoterol should be avoided in severe acute LVF or severe chronic CCF until more is known about its effects. It is compatible with other drugs in heart failure; digoxin, diuretics, ACE inhibitors, vasodilators etc.

Dose: 200 mg bd. Reduce dose in renal failure.

Avoid Xamoterol in: Patients with chronic obstructive airways disease, LV outflow obstruction, pregnancy and lactating women. Severe acute LVF.

4 *Enoximone.* Phosphodiesterase inhibitor. Will be available as both oral and i.v. preparation. Preliminary trials show a sustained benefit in LV ejection fraction exercise tolerance and symptoms. Can be used as an i.v. preparation with dobutamine.

5.14 Cardiogenic shock

A syndrome of inadequate blood supply to vital organs with failure of elimination of metabolites resulting in their functional and structural disturbance. Clinically this amounts to a hypotensive patient with cool pale moist skin, low volume rapid pulse, oliguria (<30 ml/hour), and obtunded consciousness.

Causes

It usually results from massive myocardial infarction with more than 40% of the myocardium involved. Mortality is approximately 80%. It may result from arrhythmias or valve lesions.

Pathophysiology

Reduction in cardiac output following myocardial infarction results in sympathetic-adrenal discharge and vasoconstriction. Shunting may occur as a result (e.g. lungs) and decreased tissue flow causes tissue hypoxia, anaerobic metabolism and lactic acidosis. Precapillary dilatation and post-capillary

5.14 Cardiogenic shock

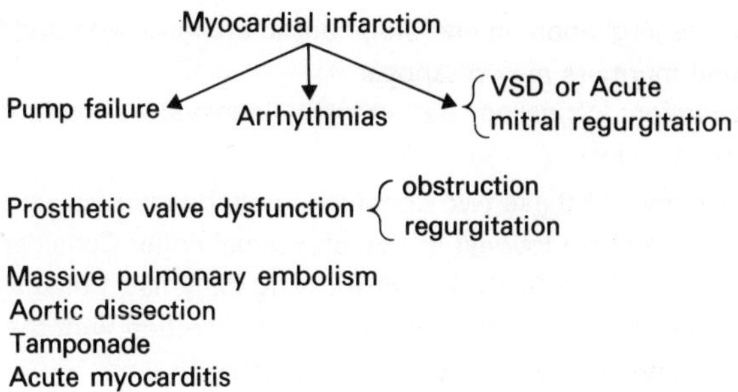

constriction may cause fluid extravasation. Stasis, sludging of red cells further reduces flow. Mitochondrial damage, lysosome release and cell death result. Shunting may result in the wrong organs getting the small output (e.g. splanchnic bed) at the expense of renal, coronary and cerebral vascular beds.

Examination

Should be quick and thorough. Examples of signs to note are:

• general condition: state of consciousness, dyspnoea. peripheral cyanosis, xanthomata. Flows are more important than blood pressure

• blood pressure in both arms

• pulse: volume, rhythm, ?anacrotic, ?pulsus paradoxus, ?pulsus alternans. Check all peripheral pulses. Auscultate carotids and subclavian arteries

• venous pressure: is no guide to LV filling pressure. May be normal in anterior infarction. High in RV infarction or pulmonary embolism. Systolic ('x') descent in tamponade rising with inspiration

• apex heat: position and quality, ?high apex beat of anterior infarction, paradoxical of LV aneurysm. ?Hyperdynamic of acute MR. ?Double apex of high LVEDP (prominent 'a' wave). Absent in tamponade. ?RV heave of acute pulmonary embolism

• thrills: ?Apical with ruptured chordae. retrosternal with VSD or mitral regurgitation, in end-stage aortic stenosis with low flows thrills and murmurs may disappear

• auscultation: ?S_3 gallop, ?left or right, ?pansystolic murmur of acute VSD or MR

The murmur of these two conditions may be identical, and both may be heard loudest at the left sternal edge. Consider VSD in anterior infarction with the patient lying fairly flat. Consider mitral regurgitation in inferior or posterior infarction with the patient sitting up in acute pulmonary oedema.

Management

The most important factor in cardiogenic shock is time. If more than 2 hours have elapsed from the onset of shock then it is unlikely any intervention will make any difference. Several medical personnel will probably be needed to perform the necessary monitoring requirements:

Stage 1. General measures

Analgesia; oxygen via MC mask or ventilation if necessary; ECG monitoring; 12 lead ECG; urinary catheter; skin (toe) and core (rectal) temperature measurement; bloods for FBC, U + E, LFTs; cardiac enzymes; blood gases.

Insertion of monitoring lines

Swan–Ganz to PA/PAW via subclavian vein; radial artery pressure (acid – base status and arterial gases also); CVP lines × 2 (may be used for drug administration).

Initial CxR

Is performed after insertion of Swan–Ganz catheter to check its position and to exclude a pneumothorax. It is also used to check: heart size, lung fields, size of aortic root and upper mediastinum, position of endotracheal tube if patient is ventilated.

Echocardiogram

As soon as possible to exclude pericardial effusion. It provides information about LV size and function, and on 2D machine may show an LV aneurysm. Ruptured chordae will be seen on M-mode as chaotic mitral valve (anterior or posterior leaflet) movement. VSD due to septal perforation can be diagnosed reliably by Doppler echocardiography. A double aortic wall suggestive of dissection may be visualised, but once again echocardiography cannot be relied on, unless trans-oesophageal echocardiography is available which is much better at visualising dissection.

Swan–Ganz monitoring

The measurement of left ventricular filling pressure can be performed by right heart catheterisation using a balloon flotation catheter introduced by subclavian vein puncture. It can be shown that in the absence of mitral valve stenosis or pulmonary vascular disease then LVEDP = mean PAW pressure.

If a good wedge pressure cannot be obtained, then PAEDP = LVEDP. The catheter can be safely left in PA for more than 24–48 hours if necessary. Serial measurements can be made following drug intervention (or exercise testing in fitter patients). Thermodilution cardiac outputs can be performed. The catheter can be used for:

- cardiac output
- LVFP/PAW/PAEDP measurement
- PA: O_2 content (e.g. for Fick cardiac output)
- right heart saturations (to check for septal perforation in acute myocardial infarction)
- central core temperature (thermistor in PA)
- PA systolic pressure: a useful monitor of ventilation

Technique

The balloon is tested prior to insertion (usually via subclavian route). Once in RA the balloon is inflated and the catheter gradually advanced until a sudden rise in pressure indicates arrival in RV. The catheter usually easily floats into PA. The balloon is deflated in PA and the pressure recorded. The catheter is advanced until a wedge pressure is achieved. The catheter should not be left in the PAW position for any length of time. The catheter is marked with 10 cm graduation marks to indicate how much catheter has been inserted.

In experienced hands the technique is safe. However numerous complications have been reported:
- all complications of subclavian puncture (see **6.2**)
- ruptured pulmonary artery (by the balloon)
- damage to pulmonary or tricuspid valves
- catheter knotting
- pulmonary infarction
- septicaemia
- infective endocarditis
- arrhythmias, often from RV outflow tract

Stage 2. Correction of filling pressure

As soon as the Swan-Ganz catheter is *in situ* attempts are made to get the filling pressure of the left ventricle (mean PAW or PAEDP) to 16–18 mmHg. This is the optimum filling pressure with a normal serum albumin to achieve maximum stroke volume without pulmonary oedema.

Filling pressure too high

- with normotension (mean aortic pressure > 90 mmHg) use vasodilators (e.g. nitroprusside), keeping mean aortic pressure > 70 mmHg
- with hypotension use dopamine 5–10 μg/kg/min

Filling pressure too low (rare)

Give 200 ml plasma and repeat measurement. Vasodilators can always be used if too much plasma is given, and small amounts of plasma may be enough.

Stage 3. Improvement of stroke volume

Inotropes are usually required. The choice lies between dobutamine or dopamine (see inotrope section). Note that the skin temperature gradually warms up as peripheral flows improve.

Although set out in stages the management of cardiogenic shock depends on many of these procedures being performed quickly and more or less simultaneously.

Stage 4. Further measures

Percutaneous transluminal coronary angioplasty (see **5.7**)
This should be considered in patients with acute myocardial infarction who are going into cardiogenic shock, whether or not streptokinase has been given (see Thrombolysis, **5.9**). It may still be possible to salvage some myocardium if PTCA is performed early enough and there is little to lose in a condition like this with such high mortality. This can be performed with intra-aortic balloon pumping via the other femoral artery or brachial artery.

Intra-aortic balloon pumping (IABP) (Fig. 5.8)
The intra-aortic balloon can now be inserted percutaneously without arterial cut down procedure and without x-ray screening. The R wave of the ECG triggers balloon deflation. The sudden 'sump' effect of balloon deflation acts as afterload reduction, reducing systolic work (Fig. 5.9).

The balloon is timed to inflate just after the dicrotic notch of aortic valve closure. Inflation increases coronary and cerebral blood flow. Helium is used as inflation gas.

Patients are fully heparinised while on the balloon. The balloon can be removed percutaneously after deflation and firm pressure over the femoral artery entry site will secure haemostasis. Surgical removal is advised after prolonged use.

IABP quickly settles unstable angina but is rarely necessary now with drug treatment, followed by coronary angiography and

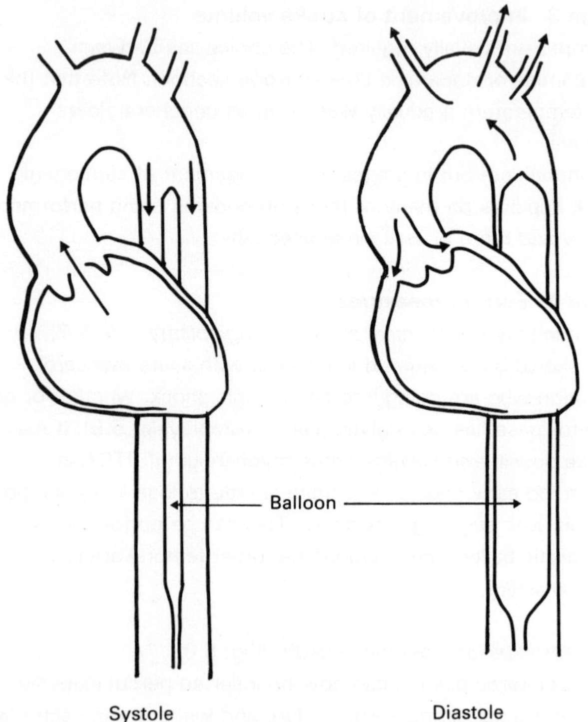

Fig. 5.8 Intra-aortic balloon pumping. Inflation of intra-aortic balloon in diastole increases cerebral and coronary blood flow.

possible PTCA or coronary by-pass surgery. Nevertheless it remains a useful tool in severe unstable angina and conventional coronary angiography can be performed with the balloon *in situ* via the other leg. The main indication for IABP remains the low output state in the pre-operative or post-operative cardiac surgical patient. It is also a useful back-up in patients who are at higher risk for coronary angioplasty.

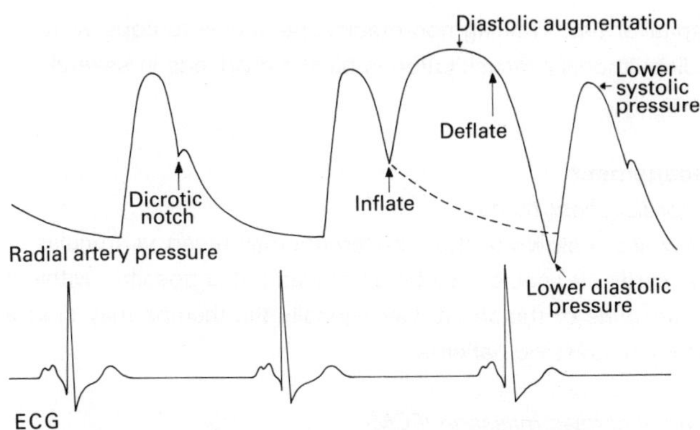

Fig. 5.9 Effect of balloon pumping on arterial pressure. Shows schematic representation of EGG and radial artery pressure during intra-aortic balloon pumping. The balloon is inflated during the second EGG cycle only to show diastolic augmentation of pressure. The balloon is timed to inflate just after the dicrotic notch, and deflation is triggered by the R wave of the EGG. Note also the lower pressure at end-diastole prior to the 3rd cycle and the lower systolic pressure of the 3rd cycle. This represents successful afterload reduction by the balloon.

Surgery

In cardiogenic shock this is really reserved for urgent mitral valve replacement (e.g. ruptured papillary muscle), for repair of acquired VSD, or for repair of aortic dissection (p. 368). Very occasionally repair of sub-acute cardiac rupture is possible (p. 187).

5.15 Cardiac arrest

The recognition of cardiac arrest is based on absent arterial pulsation and an unconscious patient. Spontaneous respiration may continue sporadically for up to a minute following an arrest and the state of the pupils is merely a guide to the time from an arrest.

Ideally an arrest team containing at least three medical personnel (one an anaesthetist) are trained to be called to any hospital arrest. Training non-medical personnel to cope with cardiopulmonary resuscitation is paying dividends in several cities.

Management

Precordial chest thump
A few sharp blows to the midsternum may revert ventricular tachycardia. It should only be employed if it is possible within a few seconds of the arrest. Occasionally the thumps may start a rhythm in asystolic patients.

External cardiac massage (ECM)
70/min as minimal rate in adults, 100/min in infants. When artificial ventilation is underway pause every 5–6 beats for respiratory cycle. With good cardiac massage pressure similar to native pressure can be achieved.

With infants the chest is encircled with both hands and the chest compressed with the thumbs. With children ECM is performed with one hand only.

A hard surface beneath the patient is necessary for effective massage. Correct ECM should not fracture ribs although this occasionally occurs in the elderly. Massage too near the xiphisternum will not be effective and may damage the liver.

Airway and artificial ventilation
The airway should be cleared, false teeth removed and vomit aspirated with a sucker. Pillows are removed and the head extended. Initially the patient is ventilated using an oral airway (Guedel) a mask and self inflating bag connected to an oxygen cylinder. If these are not available a Brooke airway or mouth-to-mouth ventilation is used.

Intubation should be performed as soon as possible if equipment is available. It should not be attempted by inexperienced personnel and ventilation using a mask and self inflating bag should be continued until experienced help arrives.

Whatever type of ventilation is established the chest should be auscultated to check the lungs are being inflated effectively.

When help arrives:

Establish ECG monitoring

Pass a nasogastric tube and aspirate the stomach

Insert a central venous line or preferably two. The internal jugular is the safest in an emergency. Subclavian vein is an alternative but a pneumothorax will make resuscitation unlikely to succeed. A peripheral vein may be of temporary help only, but several drugs given through a peripheral line will cause skin necrosis (e.g. dopamine, adrenaline).

Venous blood sample for serum K^+ or preferably:

Arterial blood sample for blood gases, acid–base status and serum K^+

If the arrest has been longer than 2 minutes give 50 mmol sodium bicarbonate i.v. before blood gas results return.

Check the clock

Subsequent action depends on the ECG

If the monitor shows ventricular fibrillation:

• Immediate DC shock 200 watt seconds (Joules) in an adult. This energy should cardiovert 95% adults. If the patient is very heavy or if the first shock is delayed greater energy may be needed. The electrodes should be widely separated. Neither should be directly over the sternum (bone has high impedance to electric current). An electrode paste 'bridge' will short circuit the shock and prove useless.

• If this shock fails repeat the DC shock immediately with 400 watt seconds.

• If this fails and blood gas results are not available give a further 50 mmol sodium bicarbonate i.v. (50 ml of 8.4% sodium bicarbonate).

• If VF is 'coarse' (large amplitude): give lignocaine 100–200 mg i.v. and repeat the shock.

10 ml 1% lignocaine contains 100 mg
10 ml 2% lignocaine contains 200 mg
Continue massage and ventilation between shocks. The value of good massage and ventilation over a long period cannot be overemphasised and may 'ride out' arrhythmias (other than VF) which are not being successfully managed with drugs.

- If this fails: give bretylium tosylate 100 mg i.v. (2 ml) and repeat the shock. Then continue lignocaine infusion at 2 mg/min.
- If the VF is 'fine' (low amplitude) give adrenaline 0.5 mg (0.5 ml of 1:1000) i.v. to increase amplitude before cardioversion. Coarse VF is much more likely to be cardioverted successfully than fine VF. Catecholamines should not be added to a line containing bicarbonate as they are inactivated.

If the monitor shows asystole or a severe bradycardia:

- Give atropine 1.2 mg i.v. There is little to be gained by giving more than 3 mg in total.
- Calcium chloride 10 ml 10% solution. Calcium gluconate provides fewer calcium ions. This must obviously be given separately from the bicarbonate line.
- Then isoprenaline infusion. Start with bolus dose of 1 mg then continue at 1–5 μg/min: up to 10 μg/min e.g. 5 mg in 500 ml 5% dextrose
  = 10μg/ml. Starting at 12 paediatric microdrops/min
  = 2μg/min.
- Consider blind endocardial pacing. This is occasionally successful until screening is established.

Correction of acidosis
If the arrest was for less than two minutes before successful cardioversion, do nothing re base deficit. If longer:

$$\frac{\text{Base deficit} \times \text{Body wt (kg)}}{6}$$

gives an approximation of mmol sodium bicarbonate required. 8.4% sodium bicarbonate = 1 mmol/ml.

- it is always safer to give less than this and repeat the blood gases
- an isolated figure gives no idea of the rate of acid production
- excess sodium bicarbonate is a sodium load, and may cause hyperosmolality
- if no blood gases are available 50–100 mmol sodium bicarbonate should be given for every ten minutes of an arrest procedure
- one central line should be reserved for sodium bicarbonate only. It inactivates dopamine, adrenaline, etc., and it precipitates out with calcium chloride or gluconate solutions.

Correction of hypotension
If the rhythm is reasonably stable but pulse of low volume:

- check CVP. This is particularly important in inferior (right ventricular) infarctions where a fluid load may improve the cardiac output. Fluid load should not be attempted without Swan–Ganz monitoring (see cardiogenic shock). Generally the CVP should be 5–10 cm H_2O from the mid-axillary line
- start dopamine 5 μg/kg/min increasing to 10 μg/kg/min. (For dose regime see **5.13**, p. 214) via a central line not used for bicarbonate, administration

Correction of potassium status
Hyperkalaemia ($K^+ > 5.0$ mmol/litre). Give calcium chloride 10 ml 10% and check for possible metabolic acidosis. Correction of metabolic acidosis should reduce serum K^+.

Hypokalaemia. Give 20 mmol KCl through central line over ten minutes if K^+ is < 3.0 mmol/litre.

Further measures which may be necessary

- insertion of radial artery and Swan–Ganz catheter in

pulmonary artery
- insertion of urinary catheter
- intermittent positive pressure ventilation continued. In the presence of pulmonary oedema and a reasonable arterial pressure ($>$100 mmHg) positive end expiratory pressure (PEEP) may help
- insertion of temporary pacing with screening facilities available
- echocardiography to exclude pericardial effusion, check LV function, mitral and aortic valve movement and aortic root
- aspiration of a pericardial effusion if documented

Procedures which are not recommended
Dexamethasone i.v. This does not reduce cerebral oedema if given after the event. It should only be used if the arrest was secondary to an anaphylactic reaction.

Intra-cardiac injections. With a good central line this is unnecessary. It may damage the anterior or inferior surface of the heart.

Attempts to assess neurology during resuscitation. This is very unreliable. Pupils are affected by a wide variety of drugs used in resuscitation. It is preferable to wait and concentrate on resuscitation.

When to discontinue resuscitation attempts
This is difficult and depends on so many factors, e.g. age and condition of patient, precipitating cause for the arrest if known, other medical conditions, results of resuscitation measures.

Usually resuscitation attempts continue for half an hour and longer in the younger patient if there is no electrical activity.

Electromechanical dissociation (no pulse or arterial pressure, but stable ECG rhythm in spite of inotropic support) usually means extensive myocardial damage or cardiac rupture and pericardial tamponade. It also occurs in massive pulmonary embolism. In this situation attempts at resuscitation are usually continued a little longer (e.g. up to 1 hour).

5.16 Management of hyperlipidaemias

There is at last good evidence that active reduction of plasma cholesterol reduces coronary risk, particularly in patients with very high cholesterol levels. Reduction of triglycerides is important in reducing episodes of pancreatitis and peripheral neuropathy in relevant cases, but has not yet been shown to reduce coronary risk.

Motivation of patients is important. The diet is unpleasant and rigid. The drugs have unpleasant side effects and patients rarely feel better on medication. In addition the doctor rarely sees any immediate benefit and therapy is expensive. Patient compliance will be a problem.

Screening

Fasting blood is only needed for estimation of triglycerides. Patients should also avoid alcohol for 24 hours prior to the test. A random test is sufficient for cholesterol alone. The following groups of patients should be screened:

- family history of coronary disease, especially if presenting < 50 years
- family history of hyperlipidaemia
- xanthomas
- xanthelasma or corneal arcus <40 years (as less specific signs than xanthomas except in younger age groups)
- obesity
- hypertension
- history of myocardial infarct, CVA or intermittent claudication <60 years

Finger prick testing kit is now available. It can be used in outpatients with results available immediately. The reagent strips are not cheap (approx 60p each, 1988 prices)

If a random test is performed and a total cholesterol level of

>6.5 mmol/l is found, the test is repeated fasting with estimation of both LDL and HDL cholesterol and triglycerides. The ratio of HDL to LDL cholesterol is often calculated. A ratio of <0.2 is considered a risk factor for coronary disease.

Secondary hyperlipidaemia

Dietary
- excess dietary fat or calories
- excess alcohol
- anorexia nervosa

Renal
- nephrotic syndrome
- chronic renal failure
- long term dialysis

Endocrine
- hypothyroidism
- poorly controlled diabetes

Intestinal
- biliary obstruction
- acute pancreatitis

Drugs
- steroids
- oestrogens (norgestrel)
- thiazides
- non selective beta-blockers
- isotretinoin (acne)

The drugs listed cause a rise in plasma triglycerides and a fall in plasma HDL. Women with a history of hyperlipidaemia, coronary or cerebrovascular disease should not take the oestrogen containing pill. Otherwise drug effects on lipids are not important.

Types of lipid measured (in decreasing order of size)

Chylomicrons: The largest lipid particle. Size >800 Å. Formed in the small bowel mucosal cells and carried in the lymphatics and plasma. Consist mainly of triglyceride. This is removed in the peripheral tissue by the action of lipoprotein lipase. The remnant particles are reabsorbed by the liver.

VLDL. Very low density lipoproteins. Size 300–800 Å. Synthesised in the liver. Endogenously synthesised triglyceride. Broken down by lipoprotein lipase to smaller LDL particles.

LDL. Low density lipoproteins. Size 200 Å. Major carrier of cholesterol in the plasma. Derived from intravascular breakdown of VLDL particles. LDL is primarily removed by the liver from the circulation. Its removal depends on the available number of LDL receptors on the liver and peripheral cells. The receptors available partly depend on the need for intracellular cholesterol and on a genetic factor. Thus a reduction in the intrahepatic cholesterol pool (e.g. by bile acid depletion with cholestyramine) increases the number of LDL receptors on the hepatocyte membrane, resulting in an increased uptake of LDL by liver and peripheral cells and a fall in plasma LDL cholesterol. High levels of LDL cholesterol are associated with coronary disease. (e.g. LDL >5 mmol/l).

HDL. High density lipoproteins. Size 100 Å. The smallest lipoprotein, rich in phospholipid and carries about 1/4 total cholesterol. Secreted by the liver and also produced from chylomicron metabolism. Low levels of HDL are associated with coronary disease (e.g. <1 mmol/l). Regular exercise increases HDL levels.

Apoproteins. There are at least ten different apoproteins which form an essential part of the lipoprotein particle. Each is specific for a type of lipoprotein or involved in lipid transport, enzyme activation or cellular uptake and receptor recognition.

Normal lipid levels

Plasma lipid levels rise with age. These figures are a guide to patients under the age of 70.

- Total cholesterol: 4.0–6.5 mmol/l (150–250 mg/100 ml)
- HDL cholesterol: 0.8–2.0 mmol/l
- LDL cholesterol: <4.9 mmol/l
- triglycerides: 0.8–2.0 mmol/l (70–170 mg/100 ml)

The aim of treatment is to reduce the cholesterol level to <6.0 mmol/l. Maximum reduction in saturated fat intake will only reduce the plasma cholesterol by a maximum of 15%. Patients with cholesterol levels > 6.5 mmol/l who are already on a low cholesterol diet and who are under the age of 70 should be considered for additional drug therapy.

Treatment

Diet

Weight reduction, cutting back on alcohol intake, and low fat diet are the first stage in treatment. This means avoiding: egg yolks, butter, cream, lard and fatty meats. Reduce cheese intake, cottage cheese allowed.

Substitute margarine for butter, vegetable oils for lard, chicken and turkey for red meat.

Encourage fish intake (avoid fish roe), vegetables and fibre.

Reduce red meat intake to 3 oz per day.

This diet will reduce both cholesterol and triglycerides. If still high on diet then drug treatment is needed.

Drug therapy for hypercholesterolaemia (e.g. Type IIa).

Several of the drugs below may be needed in combination.

First choice: Anion exchange resins.

cholestyramine 4 gms tds–8 gm tds.

colestipol 5 gms tds–10 gm tds.

These bind the bile acids in the small bowel preventing their reabsorption in distal 200 cm of the terminal ileum. The intrahepatic bile salt pool is reduced, there is an increase in LDL receptors on the hepatocyte and more cholesterol is absorbed from the plasma to synthesise more bile salts.

Side-effects:
- constipation, bloating, flatulence, haemorrhoids, even intestinal obstruction
- fat soluble vitamin supplementation may be needed (ADEK)
- drug absorption reduced; e.g. digoxin, thyroxine, warfarin. Dose may need increasing

Second choice: Nicotinic acid.
100 mg tds. Gradually increasing to 1 gm tds.
Reduces hepatic VLDL synthesis. Inhibits release of FFA from fat cells. Reduces LDL synthesis by reducing synthesis of apoprotein B in the liver.

Side-effects:
- limit its use
- flushing soon after taking the drug (reduced by adding small dose of Aspirin)
- nausea, abdominal discomfort, diarrhoea
- rarely; itching, hyperpigmentation, acanthosis nigricans, macular oedema
- rise in serum alkaline phosphatase, liver enzymes, uric acid and glucose
- avoid in; liver disease, gout, history of recent peptic ulcer

Third choice: Fibrates.
bezafibrate; 600 mg od (200 mg tds or monopreparation od).
gemfibrozil; 600 mg bd
clofibrate; 500 mg tds after meals. Less used now.

Frederickson classification of primary hyperlipidaemia types

Type	Frequency	Lipoprotein abnormality	TG and cholesterol	Clinical features
I	Rare	Chylomicrons+++ Plasma lipaemic LDL↓ VLDL→	Triglyceride+++ Cholesterol+	Abdominal pain Hepatosplenomegaly Pancreatitis Eruptive xanthomata
IIa	Common	LDL+++ VLDL →	Cholesterol+++	Premature atheroma Tendon xanthomata
IIb	Common	LDL++ VLDL+	Cholesterol++ Triglyceride+	As in Type IIa
III	Uncommon	VLDL+ Remnants+ Abnormal apolipoprotein E	Cholesterol++ Triglyceride++	Diabetes gout Premature atheroma Orange palmar crease Eruptive xanthomata

IV	Common	VLDL+ LDL→	Triglyceride++	May have diabetes, gout obesity, premature vascular disease
V	Uncommon	VLDL++ Chylomicrons++ Plasma lipaemic LDL↓	Triglyceride++ Cholesterol+	Pancreatitis Hepatosplenomegaly Diabetes gout Eruptive xanthomas

Other terms commonly used to descirbe sub-types:

- Type I: Familial hypertriglyceridaemia or chylomicronaemia. Lipoprotein lipase deficiency.
- Type IIa: Familial or primary hypercholesterolaemia. This may be homozygous presenting in childhood with angina, myocardial infarction, or aortic stenosis. More commonly it is heterozygous (1 in 500 of the population) presenting in early adult life.
- Type IIb or IV: Familial combined hyperlipidaemia.
- Type III: Broad *B* hyperlipoproteinaemia.
- Type IV: Endogenous hypertriglyceridaemia.

Primarily drugs for lowering triglyceride. They activate lipoprotein lipase and increase the number of LDL receptors. They may partly inhibit HMG CoA reductase also.

Side-effects:
• nausea, abdominal discomfort, rarely a myositis like syndrome
• gallstones, possible neoplasms of GI tract (clofibrate). Clofibrate is best avoided

Fourth choice: HMG CoA reductase inhibitors:
mevinolin and synvinolin. 10–40 mg bd.
Direct inhibitors of intrahepatic cholesterol synthesis. Increase in liver LDL receptors.
Once these drugs have a product licence in the UK they will probably rapidly become a drug of first or second choice.

Side-effects:
• headaches, nausea, fatigue, insomnia, rashes myalgia
• cataracts in high doses in animals

Drugs rarely used now: D-thyroxine, probucol, neomycin.

Drug therapy for hypertriglyceridaemia (e.g. Types I, V)
First choice: Fibrates.
See above. The best single drug type for high triglycerides

Second choice: Nicotonic acid.
See above.

Third choice: Marine oil supplementation.
Inhibit hepatic VLDL synthesis. Fish oils providing 5–20 g omega-3 fatty acids daily lower triglycerides. They are expensive, (approx £40.00 per month on low dosage).

Fourth choice: Consider low fat diet with MCT (medium chain triglyceride) supplementation.

Other forms of treatment for hypercholesterolaemia
In patients with homozygous hypercholesterolaemia high levels of cholesterol (15–30 mmol/l) may not be reduced satisfactorily on diet and combination drug therapy. These patients are usually children and further options to be considered are:

- plasma exchanges every 2–3 weeks
- plasma exchange using an LDL immunoabsorber column
- surgery:

resection of distal 200 cm of ileum: preventing reabsorbtion of bile acids
portacaval shunt
liver transplantation; providing new LDL receptors

These are obviously highly specialised procedures requiring referral to a centre with particular experience in this condition.

6 Disturbances of cardiac rhythm

6 Disturbances of cardiac rhythm

For examples of all the ECGs discussed see **10**.

6.1 Indications for temporary pacing

AV block in acute myocardial infarction

Complete AV block
In inferior infarction complete AV block usually results from right coronary artery occlusion. The AV nodal artery is a branch of the right coronary artery. Second degree AV block (Wenckebach type) does not always represent AV nodal artery occlusion, as vagal hyperactivity may play a part. A localised small inferior infarct may thus cause complete AV block.

In anterior infarction complete AV block usually represents massive septal necrosis with additional circumflex artery territory damage. The prognosis in complete AV block is dependent on infarct size and site rather than the block itself.

Complete AV block in either type of infarction should be temporarily paced.

Second degree AV block (Fig. 10.3)
1 *Wenckebach (Mobitz type 1).* Incremental increases in PR interval with intermittent complete blocking of the P wave. This is decremental conduction at AV node level. In inferior infarction it does not necessarily require pacing unless the bradycardia is poorly tolerated by the patient. It may respond to atropine. In anterior infarction Wenckebach AV block should be temporarily paced.
2 *Mobitz type II AV block.* Fixed PR interval with sudden failure of conduction of atrial impulse (blocking of the P wave). Often occurs in the presence of a wide QRS as this type of block is usually associated with distal fascicular disease. It carries a high risk of developing complete AV block. It usually occurs in association with anterior infarction, but should be prophylactically paced with either type of infarct.

6 Disturbances of cardiac rhythm

6.1 Indications for temporary pacing

First degree AV block

Does not require temporary pacing, but approximately 40% will develop higher degrees of AV block, and observation is necessary.

Bundle branch block (Figs. 10.5, 10.6)

This is a more complex group with conflicting evidence from various series. Patients with evidence of trifascicular disease or non-adjacent bifascicular disease complicating myocardial infarctions should be prophylactically paced, i.e.

Trifascicular disease:
- Alternating RBBB/LBBB
- Long PR interval +
  - new RBBB + LAHB
  - or new RBBB + LPHB
- Long PR + LBBB:

Non-adjacent bifascicular disease; RBBB + new LPHB (Fig. 10.6).

There is no proof that LBBB with a long PR interval is genuine trifascicular disease without measurements from His-bundle studies, but if it develops in the presence of septal infarction, LBBB is assumed to be LAHB + LPHB. One of the commonest bundle branch blocks complicating anterior infarction is RBBB and LAHB (usually manifest by RBBB + left axis deviation), as these two fascicles are in the anterior septum. In anterior infarction this combination should only be paced if a long PR interval develops. Measurement of the H–V interval is theoretically useful in acute infarction, but involves insertion of an electrode under fluoroscopy and is not generally practical.

Sino-atrial disease

Profound sinus bradycardia or sinus arrest may occur in acute infarction (typically inferior infarction and right coronary occlusion). The sinus node arterial supply is usually from the right coronary artery. Vagal hyperactivity may contribute and be partially reversed by atropine. However sinus bradycardia or sinus arrest may need temporary pacing if not reversed by atropine and poorly tolerated by the patient.

Temporary pacing for general anaesthesia

The same principles apply as those in acute infarction. 24-hour monitoring for those thought to be at risk may provide useful information. Notice should be taken of recent ECG deterioration (e.g. lengthening of PR interval, additional LAHB).

Asymptomatic patients with bifascicular block and a normal PR interval do not need temporary pacing. Patients with sino-atrial disease should have 24-hour ECG monitoring prior to surgery, as vagal influences may produce prolonged sinus arrest.

Temporary pacing during cardiac surgery

Temporary epicardial pacing may be necessary in surgery adjacent to the AV node and bundle of His, e.g.

- aortic valve replacement for calcific aortic stenosis (with calcium extending into the septum)
- tricuspid valve surgery, and Ebstein's anomaly
- AV canal defects and ostium primum ASD
- corrected transposition and lesions with AV discordance

A knowledge of the exact site of the AV node and His bundle can be obtained by endocardial mapping at the time of surgery. Closure of a VSD in corrected transposition, or of the ventricular component of a complete AV canal defect may damage the His bundle and permanent epicardial electrodes may be required.

Other indications for temporary pacing

Indications include termination of refractory tachyarrhythmias, during electrophysiological studies, drug overdose (e.g. digoxin, beta-blocking agents, verapamil).

6.2 Pacing difficulties

Failure to pace or sense

Wire displacement
This is the commonest reason for failure to pace and is a common problem with temporary wires which have no tines or screw-in mechanisms. To some extent it can be avoided by stability manoeuvres during wire insertion. Positions just across the tricuspid valve tend not to be very stable.
Positions in the RV apex are usually more stable but sometimes threshold measurements are not ideal here. Wire displacement requires repositioning in either temporary or permanent systems.

Microdisplacement
If not appreciated on a chest x-ray this may be overcome by increasing pacing output voltage or pulse width. Otherwise repositioning is necessary.

Exit block
This may develop in the first two weeks due to a rise in threshold. As the electrode becomes fibrosed into the endocardium the threshold levels off. With temporary units the threshold is checked daily and the voltage increased if necessary. With programmable permanent pacing units the programmer may be used to increase the output.

During temporary wire insertion a threshold of <1.0 volt at 1 msec pulse width is preferable. With permanent pacing the pulse width of the unit to be implanted is used. An acute threshold of <1.0 volt is again preferable, If the wire has been implanted for a few months then a chronic threshold of <2.0 volts is satisfactory as it is unlikely to rise further. Exit block tends to be more of a problem now with epicardial electrodes. Newer endocardial lead design (e.g. carbon porous tip) may reduce the incidence of exit block.

Wire fracture
This may occur due to kinking of the wire or too severe looping after implantation. Tight silk ligatures may damage the insulation. Complete fracture may be detected on the CxR.

Partial fracture results in intermittent pacing, and analysis of the stimulus shows reduced amplitude. A rate drop is not essential with partial wire fracture.

Perforation
This is a rare complication of permanent pacing. It sometimes occurs in patients who are temporarily paced for heart block complicating myocardial infarction. There may be loss of pacing plus signs and symptoms of pericarditis.

The diagnosis can be confirmed by measuring the intra-cardiac electrogram from the temporary wire. The temporary wire is connected to the V lead of a standard ECG machine. With impaction against the RV wall there should be an endocardial potential of 1.5–8 mV. This is lost with perforation and ST depression and T wave inversion are recorded (Fig. 6.1). Repositioning is necessary.

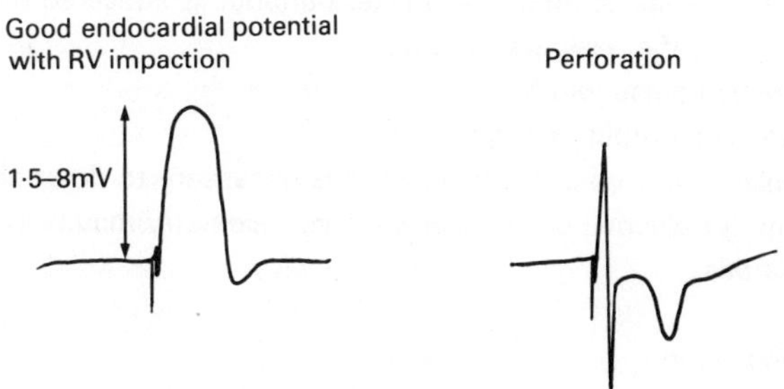

Fig. 6.1 Change in ECG on perforation by pacing wire.

Battery failure

Each permanent pacemaker has its own end-of-life characteristics. Premature battery failure has been a problem with some lithium cell designs. Several other factors than cell design may lead to early battery failure, some of which may be avoided, e.g.

- low lead impedance with large electrode tip
- wide pulse width
- constant pacemaker use, or fast pacing rate
- complex circuitry in automatic pacemakers with two sensing and two pacing circuits (DDD units). Recent units have incorporated microprocessors which drain current

Thus the choice of electrode is important. If a pacemaker with hysteresis mode is available, the take over rate may be set lower than the basic pacing rate, conserving battery life. Generally the more complex the pacemaker the shorter the expected battery life.

A pacemaker which is programmable for rate, pulse width and output may have its battery life prolonged by reducing these.

However reducing pulse width or output voltage should not be performed until enough time has elapsed from implantation to allow for the establishment of the chronic threshold (e.g. 3 months).

The end of life of most pacemaker batteries is indicated by:

- slowing of the basic pacing rate
- increasing pulse width
- decreasing output voltage

Regular follow-up at a pacing clinic is necessary to determine the time for elective pacemaker change. Telemetry may help in some areas.

EMG inhibition

Electromyographic voltage (e.g. from use of the pectoral muscles) may be of sufficient strength to be sensed by the permanent pacemaker cause it to be inhibited and hence fail to pace the ventricle. It may cause syncope when it is obviously self-limiting. For this reason, in right-handed people it is preferable to insert the permanent unit on the left side. The problem may be overcome by (in order):

- waiting until any effusion round the unit has been resolved
- if a programmable unit has been used, reduce sensitivity or reprogramme to VOO mode
- placing a non-conducting 'boot' around the pacemaker unit
- converting the permanent system to a bipolar system

Sensing failure

The pacemaker fails to notice an intrinsic cardiac impulse and is not inhibited. This may be because the R wave of the intrinsic ECG is too small, the slew rate too slow, or because the pacing unit too insensitive. In temporary pacing this may be a problem in myocardial infarction (with reduction in or loss of R waves) resulting in stimulus on T phenomenon. The use of a subcutaneous indifferent electrode as the second pole may help avoid this.

In permanent pacing the sensitivity of the unit may be changed in some programmable units (e.g. R wave sensitivity increased from 2.0 mV to 10 mV). A porous tip electrode may offer better sensing capabilities.

False inhibition (oversensing) (Fig. 6.2)

Inhibition of the pacemaker by an electrical signal other than by the R wave. EMG inhibition is an example. It may also occur with spurious signals from electrode fracture, or inadequate contacts or bad connections to the internal or external unit. Occasionally large T wave voltage may inhibit the unit. Electromagnetic interference (e.g. leak from microwave ovens) is another possibility. This used to cause false inhibition of early permanent pacing units, but is not a problem now.

6.2 Pacing difficulties

Ventricular inhibited pacing

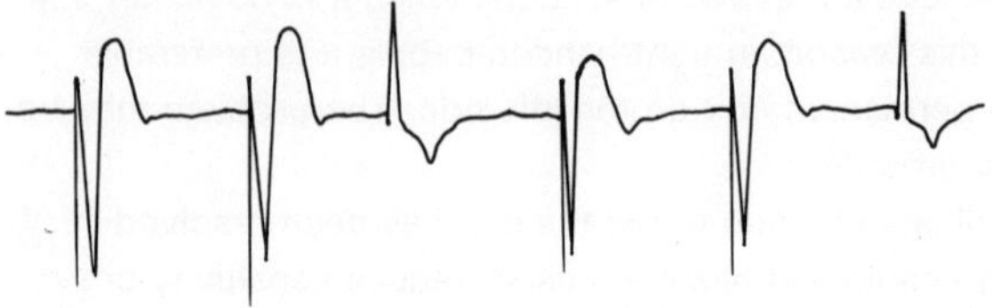

Missing

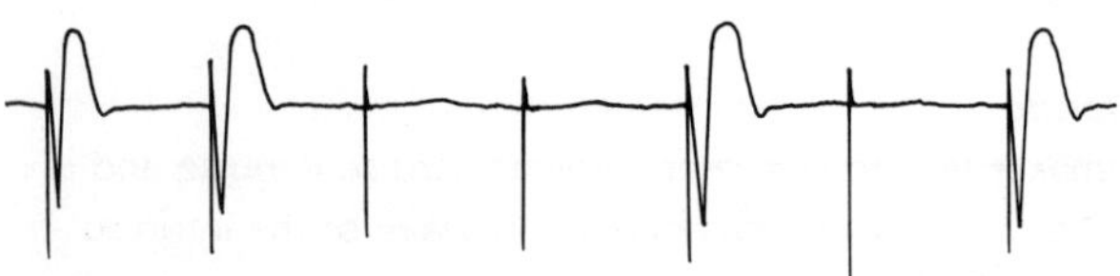

False inhibition

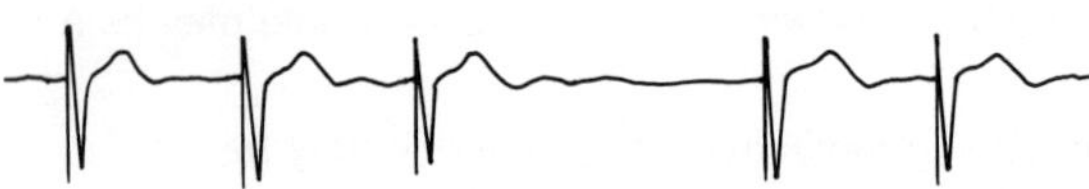

Ventricular triggered pacing

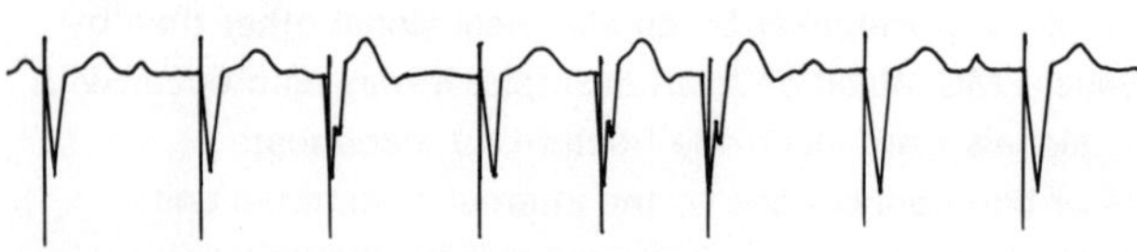

Fig. 6.2 Examples of pacing ECGs.

Complications of wire insertion

Pneumothorax

Following insertion of a pacing wire the patient should have a chest x-ray to check the wire position and to exclude a pneumothorax.

Infection

Antibiotic prophylaxis is not required for temporary pacing and is only indicated for clinical reasons. Blood cultures should be taken first, and the wire entry site should be covered with a sterile dressing. It has been shown by a prospective trial that antibiotic prophylaxis is useful for insertion of permanent pacemakers. Amoxycillin 500 mg and flucloxacillin 500 mg i.m. may be given with the premedication 1 hour prior to implantation and continued for five days orally.

Once a permanent unit is infected (e.g. extrusion of a corner of a box through ulcerated skin) it should be removed together with the wire (if possible). There is no point in trying to rescue the situation with antibiotics and resuturing. A new system should be implanted on the other side.

Haemorrhage

This uncommon complication may result from puncture of the subclavian artery with a haemothorax or widening mediastinum features appearing on the chest x-ray. The subclavian artery lies posterior to the vein and arterial puncture occurs if the entry site is too posterior (supraclavicular approach) or if the needle is directed too posteriorly (supra and infra-clavicular approach). Usually needle puncture of the subclavian artery does not result in complications if the clotting screen is normal. In elective permanent pacing, if the patient is on anticoagulants, these should be discontinued where possible to allow the BCR/prothrombin time ratio to fall to 1.5:1 or less.

Thrombophlebitis
This is usually only a problem with cubital vein entry site which should be avoided where at all possible. Temporary pacing from the femoral vein (other than at formal cardiac catheterisation) should be avoided because of the risk of infection and deep vein thrombosis.

Brachial plexus injury
This is rare and also occurs with entry site being too posterior. If the needle track is kept strictly sub-clavicular this will be avoided.

Thoracic duct injury
This is rare. The main thoracic duct drains into the junction of the left subclavian and left internal jugular vein. Temporary pacing via the right subclavian vein should therefore be attempted first.

Arrhythmias
Manipulation of the wire in the RA may produce atrial ectopics, atrial tachycardia or atrial fibrillation. Manipulation in the RV (especially post-infarction) may produce ventricular tachycardia or VF. If the RV is very irritable a lignocaine infusion should be set up (starting with 100 mg i.v. stat and 4 mg/min). Atrial arrhythmias are usually transient and of less serious consequence, especially if the wire is being inserted for complete AV block.

6.3 Glossary of some pacing terms in common use

Automatic interval (basic interval)
The stimulus–stimulus interval during regular pacing.

Bipolar pacing system
Most temporary wires use a bipolar pacing wire with two ring electrodes. The proximal ring electrode (approx 1 cm from

electrode tip) is the anode, and the distal (tip) electrode the cathode. Sometimes the position of the anode may be higher up the wire (e.g. in the SVC). The pacing spike is small on the surface ECG. Bipolar wires are also available for permanent pacing. A permanent bipolar system is immune to external signals. See **6.9**.

Demand pacing (inhibited)
Unlike the fixed-rate mode, spontaneous cardiac activity is sensed and inhibits the pacemaker, which fixes a stimulus only after a preset interval if no further impulse is sensed. Thus pacing is inhibited by sensed impulses (atrial or ventricular, see codes).

Epicardial system
Pacing wires attached to the epicardium either at thoracotomy or by subxiphoid route. The permanent unit is usually intra-abdominal (beneath the rectus muscle and extraperitoneal). It is used in

- recurrent failure of endocardial systems (infection, exit block, etc.)
- small children where rapid growth makes transvenous pacing difficult
- heart block developing during cardiac surgery
- tricuspid mechanical valve prosthesis

Epicardial systems tend to be less reliable in the long term. Wire displacement and fracture may occur due to kinking and vigorous movement.

Escape interval
The interval between a spontaneous cardiac impulse which is sensed and the next pacing stimulus. This is usually the same as the automatic pacing interval unless the pacemaker is programmed to hysteresis mode, in which case the escape interval is longer than the automatic interval.

6.3 Glossary of pacing terms in common use

Fixed rate pacing
Constant stimulation of the heart at a fixed rate not influenced by spontaneous cardiac activity.

Hysteresis
The take-over rate of the pacemaker is lower than the pacing rate, e.g. a pacemaker with a pacing rate of 72 bpm and hysteresis mode set at 60 bpm will not start pacing until the patient's heart rate falls below 60 bpm, then the pacing rate jumps to 72 bpm. Patients may notice the abrupt change in rate, but it conserves battery life.

Lead impedance
This is a vital factor in battery life. It includes the electrical resistance of the electrode itself plus the impedance of the electrode tip-tissue interface. The size of the electrode tip influences impedance of the wire. (The larger the tip the lower the impedance.) Low impedance wires result in early battery depletion. Average lead impedance is 510 Ω. Development of newer electrodes has resulted in smaller electrode tips (from standard 12 or 14 mm^2 down to 6 mm^2).

Magnet rate
Application of a magnet over some VVI units converts them to a faster (fixed) pacing rate. This is used to test battery life and satisfactory pacing if there is competition at a slower demand rate.

Missing
The term used to denote failure of a pacing stimulus to capture and depolarise atrial or ventricular myocardium. It may be due to incorrect lead positioning, too low an output voltage, or too high a myocardial threshold. Initial management is to increase pacing voltage if a temporary system, and then reposition the wire if this is not successful. Missing with a permanent system

cannot be ignored. The unit must be removed, the wire threshold tested and either repositioned or changed.

Paired pacing
A double impulse fired in rapid succession to the ventricle results in an increased force of contraction, but a much greater MVO_2 and a risk of inducing VT. It is not used in clinical pacing.

Pulse width/pulse duration
The duration of the pacing stimulus (usually between 0.5 msec and 1.0 msec). The broader pulse width may capture the ventricle and pace it when narrower pulse widths fail. but this will drain more current and shorten battery life of permanent units. The same applies to atrial pacing.

Relative threshold
Some pacing units have an analysable threshold once implanted permanently. The relative threshold is the minumum percentage of total available voltage required to pace the heart. Thus a relative threshold of 25% with maximum unit voltage of say 5.2 volts is 1.3 volts.

Sequential pacing
Pacing of the atrium followed at a preset interval by pacing of the ventricle. This allows physiological atrial transport (see physiological pacing).

Slew rate
The rate of rise of the endocardial potential (dV/dt). Potentials with a slew rate may not be sensed.

Triggered pacing (Fig. 6.2)
A sensed spontaneous R wave results in immediate pacing stimulus fired into the R wave (the heart obviously refractory and not paced). Triggered pacing units have a built in refractory

period to protect against fast electrical interference inducing ventricular tachycardia. Ventricular triggered pacing may be used:

- To avoid EMG inhibition.
- When a temporary wire is inserted to cover a failing permanent unit. Stimuli from the failing implanted unit trigger the external unit to fire an impulse. This falls in the absolute refractory period (if the internal unit's impulse depolarised the heart) or alternatively paces the heart if the internal/permanent unit impulse fails to depolarise the heart. It is thus a fail-safe mechanism.

Unipolar pacing system
Most permanent units are unipolar: using the pacing box as the anode (+) and the pacing wire as the cathode (–). The pacing spike is large on the surface ECG.

Voltage threshold
Minimum voltage which will pace the heart.

6.4 Permanent pacing for bradyarrhythmias

There has been an enormous increase in pacemaker technology since the first pacemaker was implanted by the Karolinska Hospital team in 1958. Permanent pacing is one of the most cost effective forms of treatment in the whole of medicine. Numbers of implants are increasing, but the implant rate in the UK is amongst the lowest in Europe, due in part, to the lack of pacing centres and in part to the low referral rate for pacing.

Indications for permanent pacing

These vary from country to country, but certain definite categories are recognised.

6.4 Permanent pacing for bradyarrhythmias

World survey of cardiac pacing 1986

Country	Population (millions)	No of pacing centres	No of first implants /million population
USA	239	3000	359
West Germany	61	650	421
France	55	400	413
Switzerland	6	36	230
Holland	14	111	227
Italy	57	188	200
UK	56	92	148
Greece	10	17	136

Chronic complete AV block with Stokes–Adams episodes
This is usually due to central bundle branch fibrosis (Lenegre's disease), often with normal coronary arteries In the older group. QRS complex is wide. Pacing should abolish symptoms and prolong life (1 year mortality: 35–50% unpaced, 5% paced). Symptoms other than frank syncope, which may be due to AV block, include giddiness, transient amnesia and misdiagnosed epilepsy.

In the younger age group coronary artery disease may be an additional prognostic factor.

Chronic complete AV block with no symptoms
This is a smaller group of patients who should also be paced as life expectancy is increased, and the first Stokes–Adams episode may be fatal. 24-hour ECG monitoring usually reveals very slow idioventricular rhythm at night (e.g. <20 bpm)

Congenital complete AV block
In this condition the level of block is higher up in the His bundle or AV node. The QRS complex is narrow, the idioventricular rhythm faster and it may respond slightly to exercise or to other autonomic stimuli. Asymtomatic children may survive into adult life, when a permanent transvenous system is easier to

insert. Indications for pacing in congenital complete AV block are:
• development of any rate-related symptoms
• wide QRS
• other cardiac lesions and cardiac surgery
• early presentation
• failure of AV node to respond to exercise, etc. ('lazy junction')
• 24-hour monitoring evidence of junctional exit block or paroxysmal tachyarrhythmias
• a daytime mean junctional rate <50/min: as this carries a higher long term risk of syncope and sudden death.

Mobitz type II AV block (Fig. 10.3)
This type of AV block is characterised by a constant PR interval and the sudden failure of conduction of an atrial impulse through the AV node. There is a high incidence of complete AV block developing and patients with this type of AV block should be paced permanently.

It should be noted that Wenckebach type II AV block is not an indication for permanent pacing. It may be due to high vagal tone in athletes or children, and may be a transient phenomenon in acute inferior infarction (involving the AV nodal artery). It may result from drug toxicity (digoxin, beta-blockade, verapamil). Generally it is a benign, transient rhythm disturbance.

Post-myocardial infarction

Following inferior infarction second or third degree AV block is normally transient, and permanent pacing does not need to be considered for 2–3 weeks post infarct.

Following anterior infarction complete AV block usually represents massive septal necrosis and mortality from LV failure is high. Persistent complete AV block is permanently paced. More difficult is an AV block which regresses during hospital stay. This is still a subject for debate, but 24-hour Holter monitoring may help identify subjects at risk who need permanent pacing. The ventricular myocardium is often very irritable in the post-infarct period and if possible permanent pacing should be avoided in the first 3–4 weeks.

Chronic bundle branch block

Early work which suggested that His bundle electrograms would identify patients at risk has not been substantiated. Theoretically a prolonged H–V interval in the presence of bifascicular block would indicate the third fascicle at risk. However this does not seem to be prognostically useful. The incidence of chronic asymptomatic patients with bifascicular block developing complete AV block is low. It does not seem to be precipitated by general anaesthesia. Again 24-hour Holter monitoring may be helpful. Generally asymptomatic patients with bifasicular block do not merit permanent pacing. Pacing is indicated for patients with symptoms plus bifascicular block, e.g. symptoms plus:

• RBBB + LAHB • RBBB + LPHB	Bifascicular disease (Fig. 10.6)
• RBBB with alternating LAHB/LPHB • LBBB with alternating RBBB • LBBB + Long PR interval	'Trifascicular' disease

Sick sinus syndrome (SSS)

SSS is also known as sino-atrial disease, tachycardia-bradycardia syndrome, or generalised conduction system disease. Although primarily involving the sinus node and atrial myocardium it may develop into a condition including AV node disease, or even be associated with a cardiomyopathy. Systemic emboli are a recognised complication (possibly related to prolonged periods of sinus arrest).

Common ECG abnormalities include (often switching from one to another) (Fig. 6.3).

• sinus arrest. Chronic or paroxysmal

6.4 Permanent pacing for bradyarrhythmias

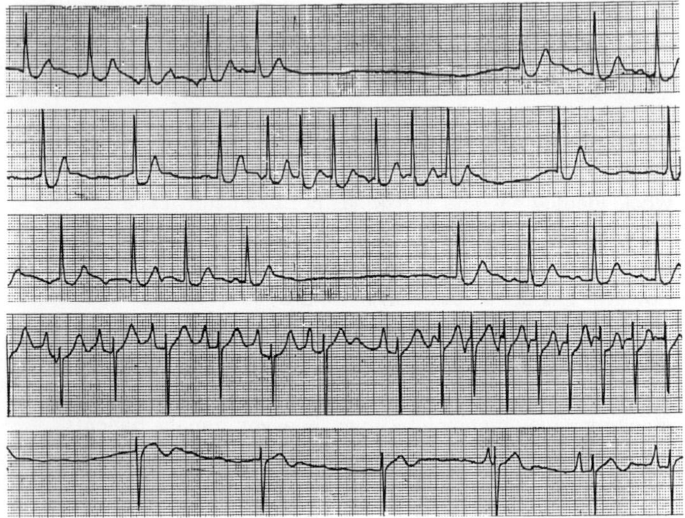

Fig. 6.3 Sino-atrial disease. Segments of a single 24-hour monitored ECG in a patient with this condition (also known as sick sinus syndrome). The ECG shows episodes of wandering atrial pacemaker and sinus arrest (1st line), junctional escape rhythm and AF (2nd line), sinus arrest (3rd line), sinus rhythm and supraventricular tachycardia (4th line), and junctional bradycardia moving into sinus rhythm (5th line).

- sinus bradycardia: not necessarily responding to effort or atropine
- sinus exit block
- paroxysmal { atrial tachycardia / atrial flutter / atrial fibrillation }
- carotid sinus hypersensitivity
- AV block—usually in the older age group who may have AF with complete AV block and a slow idioventricular rhythm

Permanent pacing in SSS does not prolong life. The indications for permanent pacing are:

- symptoms with a documented bradycardia

• symptoms due to drug-induced bradycardia (used to control the tachyarrhythmias). AAI pacing will maintain atrial transport while AV nodal conduction is still normal. However the development of AV block may require a change to VVI pacing or even DDD units in the younger age group.

6.5 Pacing for tachyarrhythmias

Antitachycardia pacing has several advantages over drug therapy for arrhythmias:

• no drug side-effects
• automatic. No patient co-operation required
• possible method of arrhythmia control in pregnancy
• no negative inotropic effect on LV function
• may work when drugs fail
• rapid termination preventing hypotension or cerebral hypoperfusion
• patient normal between attacks
• easily reversible (explantation or reprogramming)

Implantation of a permanent pacemaker for tachyarrhythmias should be considered when drug treatment is unsatisfactory or producing side-effects, and where bursts of tachycardia are infrequent. It should also be considered in patients with poor LV function, and in women who may wish to become pregnant.

Generally the technique should be avoided in

• frequent arrhythmias
• easily inducible AF or atrial flutter
• patients whose tachycardias easily degenerate (e.g. atrial ectopics → SVT → VT)
• WPW syndrome

Methods of antitachycardia pacing

Prevention/suppression

1 Permanent overdrive pacing: Single chamber.
Suppression of ectopics by overdrive pacing may prevent SVT or VT. Prevention of bradycardia may abolish episodes of

bradycardia dependant VT although this is not very effective in the long term.

2 Permanent overdrive pacing: Dual chamber.

AV pacing with a short preset AV delay (e.g. 50–150 msec) prevents recurrent re-entry tachycardia using the AV node as part of the circuit.

Tachycardia termination/version

Bursts of tachycardia can be terminated using overdrive, underdrive or bursts of extrastimuli. The pacemaker must detect an increase or sudden change in heart rate. Alternatively the patient may activate the pacemaker during tachycardia using radio frequency activation.

Underdrive pacing: termination by interference; VOO mode. Random competition of paced beats at a slower rate than the tachycardia. At some point an extrastimulus is timed appropriately to terminate the tachycardia. Problems with this technique are:

- it is usually ineffective at tachycardia rates >160/min
- the tachycardia rate may vary with variable cycle lengths
- the tachycardia must be terminated by a single extrastimulus only
- dual demand pacemakers may not be activated by slower tachycardias
- scanning time may be a problem so that the tachycardia is not terminated immediately, and may take several seconds
- the termination window (the interval in the cardiac cycle when the tachycardia can be terminated) varies in length with physiological position. It is shorter on standing, and still shorter on exercise

Overdrive burst stimulation. Rapid stimulation of the atrium in junctional re-entry tachycardia may revert the patient to sinus rhythm, but there is a risk of inducing AF. Similarly rapid ventricular stimulation in VT may accelerate the tachycardia or induce VF. Careful electrophysiological studies are needed prior to pacemaker implantation.

Additional drug therapy may be needed.

Extrastimuli. Multiple extrastimuli can now be delivered by a programmable pacemaker during tachycardia. They are more commonly used for re-entrant superventricular arrhythmias than ventricular.

A variety of programmable scanning devices is now available which automatically change the R wave–first stimulus interval if the first premature stimulus is unsuccessful. Additional stimuli can then be added so that up to seven may be delivered. Autodecremental, self-searching, geometric scanning and concertina pacing are all different algorithms designed to terminate the tachycardia as swiftly as possible by automatic alteration of the timing and number of extrastimuli.

Automatic implantable cardioverter defibrillator (AICD)

An implantable cardioverter was initially tried in 1980 for ventricular tachycardia. It was implanted exactly as a permanent pacemaker with a single venous wire under local anaesthetic. Since 1982 a larger device has been developed with defibrillating capacity.

Indications for considering an AICD:

- recurrent sustained (>30 sec) symptomatic ventricular tachycardia which is monomorphic
- refractory to drug therapy
- history of several DC cardioversions
- general condition and operability as a thoracotomy is required

The AICD weighs 290 gm and with its lithium battery is capable of delivering about 100 shocks. It is implanted in a pocket in the abdominal wall and attached to the heart by pairs of electrodes for sensing (RV bipolar lead) and two epicardial patches and an SVC electrode for defibrillating. Advances will soon obviate the need for an open thoracotomy using only transvenous wires.

The device takes about 10–20 seconds to recognise the ventricular arrhythmia and a further 5–15 seconds to charge its capacitors. The first shock delivered is usually 25 joules with a further three possible shocks of 30 joules if the arrhythmia continues.

The AICD should be avoided if:

- the ventricular arrhythmia is secondary to drugs or a metabolic upset
- the ventricular tachycardia is not sustained
- very frequent ventricular arrhythmias
- the arrhythmia is supraventricular
- there is already a permanent pacemaker *in situ*

Over 300 devices have been implanted with a significant reduction in mortality in this high risk group of patients. The cost of the unit is high (£10 000). The AICD is being developed with more sophisticated circuitry. This will allow:

- pacing back up for bradycardia
- better sensing of ECG morphology: e.g. to avoid false triggering by AF
- full telemetry and programming facilities
- antitachycardia pacing

In time an overall antiarrhythmic device will be available capable of pacing for bradycardia or tachycardia on a dual-demand basis, plus the ability to cardiovert or defibrillate for unresponsive malignant ventricular arrhythmias.

Catheter ablation

The administration of high energy electrical current down a suitably positioned intra-cardiac electrode will result in localised tissue destruction. This is used to treat arrhythmias refractory to drug treatment.

Since 1982 catheter ablation has become an established technique in cardiology. The commonest site for ablation is the

AV node, but various other sites have been ablated including sinus node, accessory pathways in WPW syndrome, and sites in the ventricle for refractory VT. Successful AV node ablation should produce permanent AV block. The heart rate is then maintained by permanent pacing.

AV node ablation

This is very useful for very fast, frequent supra-ventricular arrhythmias which are resistant to drug treatment and in this group is probably superior to antitachycardia pacing. It should be considered in:

- fast AF
- fast atrial flutter
- AV nodal re-entrant tachycardia (AVNRT)

} no extra-nodal pathway involved

Generally it should not be considered in tachycardias where the AV node forms only part of the re-entry circuit, and there is an additional atrioventricular pathway: e.g.

- WPW syndrome
- atrioventricular re-entrant tachycardia (AVRT)

} extra-nodal pathway involved

In these conditions drug treatment or surgical ablation is preferable. Careful electrophysiological studies are essential prior to ablation. The procedure is performed percutaneously, usually via the right femoral vein, as in electrophysiological studies, but under general anaesthesia. It is usually totally effective in 70% patients, ineffective in 10% and of transient or partial effect in the rest. Complete heart block may be produced for a few days with the patient then reverting to normal condition. It is performed under temporary pacing cover and the temporary wire is left in situ for 2 or 3 days in case the ablation has to be repeated if normal conduction returns. Once it is felt complete heart block has been achieved permanently, then a permanent pacemaker is implanted (preferably a rate responsive VVIR unit).

Problems and complications of the procedure are few. There may be:

- ventricular arrhythmias. 24-hour Holter monitoring may be considered in follow up of these patients
- hypotension: requiring volume loading +/− inotropes
- permanent RV dysfunction: some patients are troubled with dyspnoea post ablation
- electromechanical dissociation: usually transient
- permanent pacing is essential for life. This is a major undertaking in the young patient

Newer techniques include the use of low energy shocks with higher peak voltage. Initially the energy delivered for AV node ablation was 300–3000 joules. With the newer low energy equipment 3–20 joules may suffice.

Surgical techniques for the management of arrhythmias

The management of arrhythmias which are refractory to drug treatment may include:

- antitachycardia pacing (temporary or permanent) (p. 261)
- catheter ablation of AV node, by-pass tract or arrhythmogenic focus (p. 264)
- implantation of automatic cardioverter/defibrillator (p. 263)
- other surgical procedures

Direct division or ablation of an accessory pathway or arrhythmogenic focus can be performed during open heart surgery. Careful epicardial and occasionally endocardial electrographic mapping is required to detect the activation sequence over the atrial and ventricular myocardium. Detection of the earliest activation site on the myocardium helps establish the site of the accessory pathway (e.g. in WPW syndrome) or the arrhythmogenic focus (e.g. in ventricular tachycardia).

Surgical techniques may involve:

- cryotherapy: A cryoprobe can produce temporary ablation at −10°C, or permanent at −65° C: e.g. of accessory pathway or His Bundle.

- ventriculotomy. Encircling ventriculotomy is performed during VT
- endocardial resection: performed during cardiopulmonary by-pass
- ventricular aneurysmectomy. Performed alone may miss the site of origin of the VT, as this is often at the junction of scar tissue and more normal myocardium
- mitral valve replacement (for arrhythmias with mitral valve prolapse)
- cardiac transplantation. For the extreme case where drugs and other ablative techniques have failed

Combinations of these techniques may be necessary: e.g. mapping-directed endocardial resection plus the implantation of an automatic cardioverter defibrillator.

6.6 Pacemaker codes

With increasing complexity of permanent pacemakers, codes have been developed to enable operators to identify the capabilities of individual units.

The initial three letter code was introduced by Parsonnet in 1974 and is currently in use on the European Pacemaker card. This has been agreed by the International Association of Pacemaker Manufacturers. The three letter code is now in general use, but already likely to be superseded by a five letter code, to cope with facilities available on newer programmable units. A sixth letter may one day be included to cope with telemetric capabilities.

As will be seen in the pacemaker code table the first letter of the code always relates to the chamber paced, the second to the chamber sensed. The third letter indicates the pacemaker response to the sensed impulse. Formerly this third letter was replaced by a 'fraction', e.g. T/I or TI/I, since the more complex pacemaker responded in different ways to stimuli from atrium and ventricle.

The most frequently used pacemaker in the UK has the code VVI (94% of UK implants in 1979–80 survey).

Individual pacing codes explained

These are shown diagrammatically with a schematic ECG along side each.

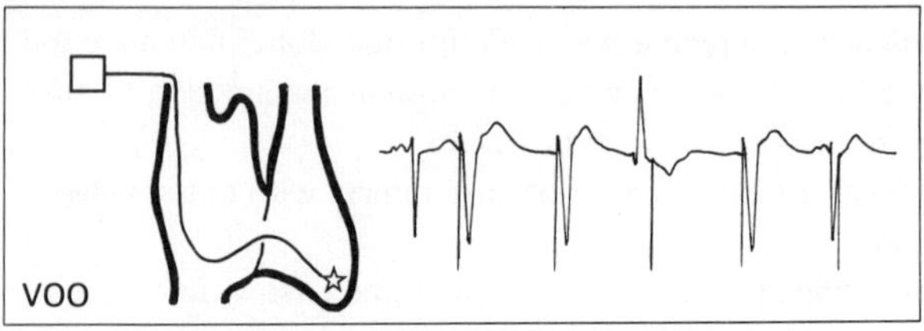

VOO

VOO This is fixed rate ventricular pacing only, and is now rarely used, i.e. ventricular pacing, no sensing and no response. The pacemaker is not inhibited by spontaneous ventricular impulses, and there is a risk of stimulus on T phenomenon causing ventricular tachycardia.

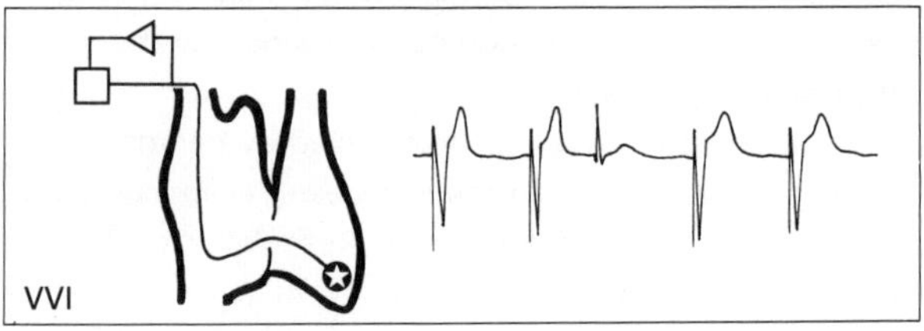

VVI

VVI Ventricular pacing which is inhibited by sensed ventricular impulses. It is the unit of choice in patients with AV block and atrial fibrillation, or sick sinus syndrome with intermittent AF, or atrial paralysis.

However patients with AV block and persistent sinus node function will lose atrial contribution to ventricular filling as often the atria contract against closed AV valves. There will be cannon waves in the JVP, and intermittent reversal of atrial flow. Retrograde AV conduction compounds the problem.

Programmable VVI units may partly overcome this by being programmed to a lower rate, or with hysteresis.

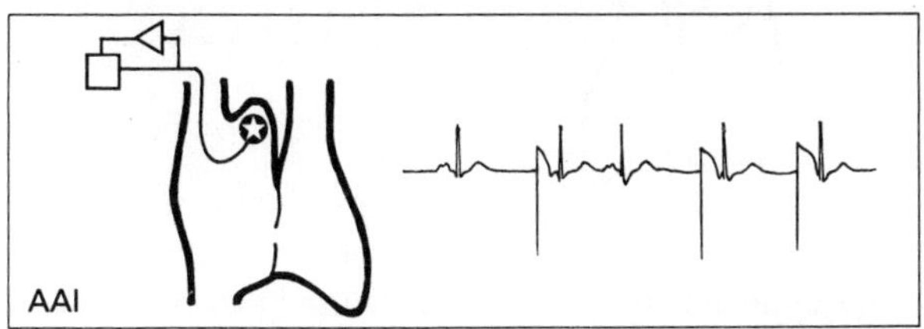

AAI This is atrial pacing only which is inhibited by sensed P waves. This type of pacemaker is used in patients with sick sinus syndrome who have normal AV node function. (It does not matter if they have retrograde AV conduction.) It may be used in patients with profound sinus bradycardia or in drug-induced sinus bradycardia (in the sick sinus syndrome) (Fig. 10.4). Atrial transport is preserved.

However this pacing relies on normal AV node function, and patients with SSS may develop abnormalities in AV conduction after the unit has been implanted (up to 30% in one series). Also it is obviously unsuitable for patients with SSS and intermittent AF, which may also develop after the unit was implanted.

Contraindications to AAI pacing are:

- AV block, or Wenckebach block with atrial pacing up to 150/min
- bifascicular block on 12-lead ECG
- atrial flutter, fibrillation or atrial paralysis
- carotid sinus syndrome
- H–V interval > 55 msec or prolonging with high atrial rates

Thus His bundle electrograms and atrial pacing studies are necessary before choosing to implant an AAI unit.

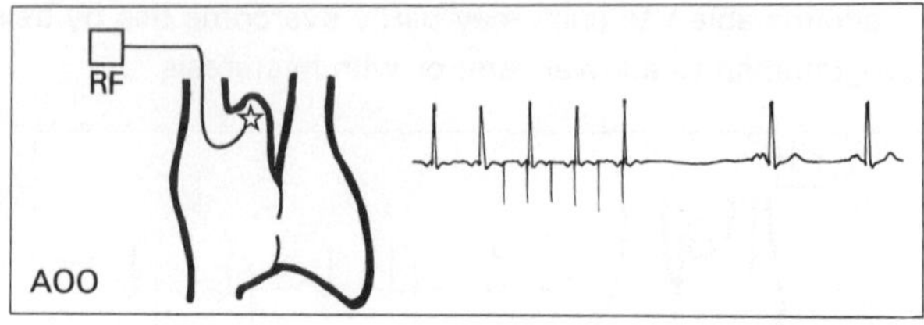

AOO Asynchronous atrial pacing. Rarely used except in patient-activated bursts to overdrive atrial tachycardias. In using rapid atrial stimulation bursts it is Important to be certain there is no pre-excitation pathway to the ventricle.

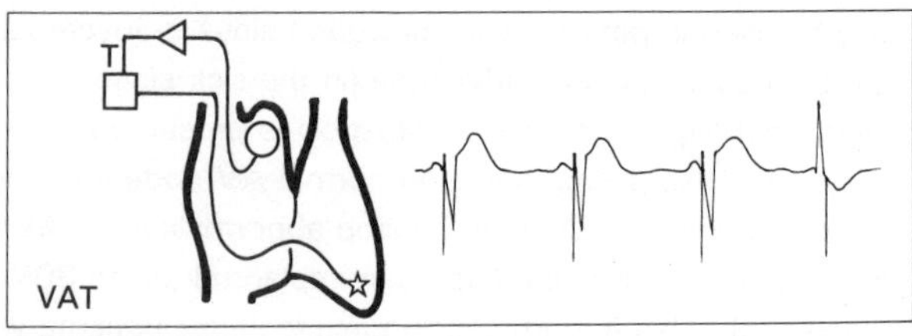

VAT Ventricular pacing triggered by a sensed atrial impulse. Two leads are required. This is P wave synchronous pacing and preserved atrial transport. It is appropriate in AV block with preserves sinus node function. It cannot be used in patients with atrial dysrythmias, AF or atrial flutter.

Its major disadvantage is that it does not sense ventricular impulses, and hence will compete with spontaneous ventricular activity. If the patient has frequent ventricular ectopics there is the risk of stimulus on T phenomenon.

It is the simplest and cheapest way of preserving atrial transport in patients with AV block (Fig. 10.4).

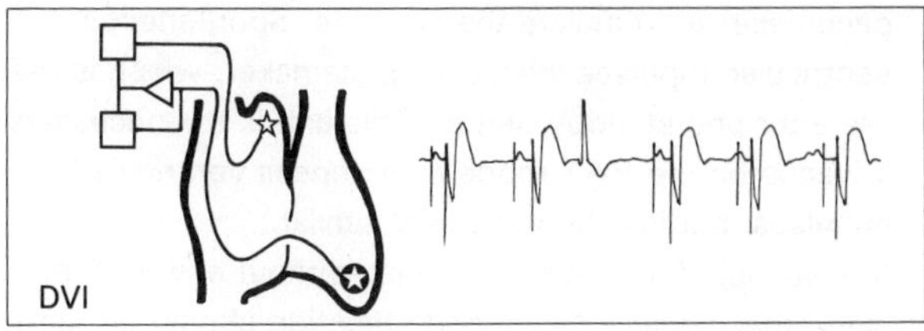

DVI Atrial and ventricular pacing, but only spontaneous ventricular activity is sensed. Spontaneous atrial activity is ignored. Two leads are required. After a spontaneous ventricular impulse is sensed the pacemaker resets to one V–A interval and fires an atrial impulse followed by a ventricular impulse. Spontaneous P waves occurring within this V–A interval are not sensed.

It can he used in complete AV block or sinus bradycardia. It cannot be used in AF. Although atrial synchrony is maintained at a basal rate it will not follow an increase in sinus rate with exercise, and competes with atrial rates faster than the pacemaker rate. It is useful in patients with retrograde AV conduction.

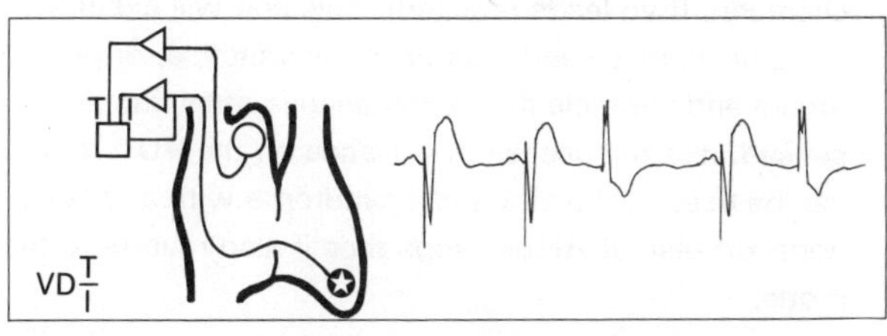

$VD\frac{T}{I}$ (also known as VDD and ASVIP) Atrially sensed ventricular inhibited pacing. Both chambers are sensed (two leads required) and the spontaneous atrial impulse triggers the pacemaker to stimulate the ventricle. Spontaneous ventricular impulses inhibit the pacemaker, which is reset to fire after one standby period. This unit is the necessary advance on the VAT mode as it senses ventricular impulses, but is otherwise very similar.

It is suitable for simple AV block without any evidence of sino-atrial disease. Sinus node function should be normal. If AF develops the pacemaker reverts to VVI mode. This also occurs if the spontaneous atrial rate falls below the escape rate of the pacemaker.

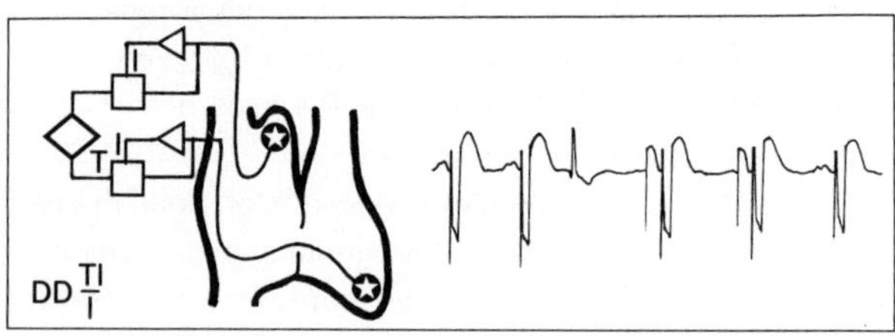

$DD\frac{TI}{I}$ (also known as DDD)

This is the fully automatic unit which paces and senses both chambers (two leads required). This unit will either sense the atrial impulse and then pace the ventricle, or pace the atrium and ventricle if no spontaneous atrial impulse is sensed. It is the necessary advance on the VD T/I unit as it can be used in the sick sinus syndrome with additional AV nodal disease. If AF develops then if also reverts to the VVI mode.

KEY TO SYMBOLS

☆ Pacing only ◯ Sensing only

✪ Pacing and Sensing

□ Pacing output circuit

◁ Sensing circuit

◇ Logic function

I Inhibited

T Triggered

RF Radio frequency signal

6.6 Pacemaker codes

Pacemaker code table

Code letter position	**1st**	**2nd**	**3rd**	**4th**	**5th**
Category	Chamber(s) paced	Chamber(s) sensed	Mode of pacemaker response	Programmable functions	Tachyarrhythmia functions
Letters used	V = ventricle A = atrium	V = ventricle A = atrium	T = triggered I = inhibited	P = Programmable (Rate and/or output only)	B = Burst N = Normal rate competition
	D = dual	D = dual 0 = none	D = dual R = reverse	M = multi-programmable	S = Scanning
			$\frac{T}{I}$ = atrially triggered and ventricular inhibited	O = none R = rate responsive	E = Controlled external (magnet or RF)
			$\frac{TI}{I}$ = Fully automatic		

6.7 Physiological pacing

The VVI unit involves a single ventricular pacing lead only, and ignores atrial contribution to cardiac output. Atrial systole may contribute up to 25% of cardiac output in some patients by increasing LVEDV and stroke volume. Utilisation of atrial systole by either sensing and/or pacing in synchrony with ventricular pacing has been called 'physiological pacing'. It has many limitations and cannot be strictly physiological at high heart rates. Nevertheless it may improve cardiac output in patients with borderline left ventricular function. It may prove also to avoid systemic emboli in patients with sick sinus syndrome by avoiding stagnation in a flaccid left atrium.

A few patients with AV block may actually do worse with VVI pacing. The AV node may still conduct retrogradely and atrial stimulation may cause atrial contraction against closed AV valves. This has been shown to put up pulmonary wedge pressure: the pacemaker syndrome.

Thus the choice of a physiological pacing unit requires a knowledge of certain facts:

- The cardiac output should be measured with ventricular pacing and AV synchronous pacing to ensure that the more expensive and sophisticated physiological unit will confer extra benefit to the patient.
- A knowledge of sinus node function. 24-hour ECG monitoring will provide some information. Tests of sinus node function (sinus node recovery time, sino-atrial conduction time) unfortunately do not reliably predict sinus node function if normal.
- A knowledge of AV conduction, both antegrade and retrograde.
- Does the patient develop SVT or other atrial tachyarrhythmias? If so this would rule out VAT pacing. 24-hour ECG monitoring, and provocation with atrial extrastimulus testing may help here.

With normal sinus node function

VAT or VDD pacing with AV block and no retrograde AV conduction. DVI or DDD pacing with AV block with retrograde AV conduction.

With normal or abnormal sinus node function

AAI pacing if AV conduction normal. VVI pacing if AV block, no retrograde AV conduction, and little improvement with AV synchronous pacing. DVI or DDD pacing with AV block and retrograde AV conduction.

Generally most elderly patients with syncope from Stokes–Adams syndrome are cured by VVI pacing. Physiological pacing is increasingly used in the younger patient with AV block and those with borderline LV function. The expense of the physiological units may prove the major limiting factor in their taking over from VVI units in the UK.

Problems with physiological pacing units

Against the obvious advantages of greater cardiac output and higher BP with physiological pacing there are several disadvantages compared with VVI pacing:

- Two leads required (except in AAI pacing). Single pass leads (with both atrial and ventricular electrodes) are being developed.
- Units more expensive.
- Shorter battery life.
- Problems with reliability of complex units and their programming equipment.
- Angina (e.g. SVT developing in VDD pacing causing high ventricular rate).
- Uncertainty at high atrial rates (e.g. SVT developing in VAT pacing causing ventricular tachycardia).
- Self-inhibition of earlier units. (A sensed P wave inhibiting the ventricular pacing circuit in DDD units. This resulted in a P wave with no subsequent ventricular complex.) This dangerous situation has been ironed out by blanking (switching off) the

ventricular amplifier during atrial sensing.

• Retrograde AV conduction with reciprocating tachycardia. Retrograde conduction of a P wave can be sensed by the atrial lead which results in a paced ventricular impulse and a re-entry tachycardla using the pacemaker. This can be prevented by increasing the atrial refractory period after a paced ventricular impulse. This limits the maximum physiological pacing rate, but 150 bpm is usually considered fast enough.

• Disease progression which limits the pacemaker's potential, e.g. development of AV block in AAI pacing, development of sick sinus syndrome in VDD pacing, development of AF in any physiological pacing system.

Most physiological pacing systems are vulnerable to progression of conduction system disease. DDD units are vulnerable to the development of AF and have to be programmed to VVI mode.

Rate responsive pacing (adaptive rate pacing): VVIR

This is a form of physiological pacing which is a useful alternative to dual chamber pacing. Only one chamber (the ventricle) is paced (as in VVI units), but the pacemaker increases its pacing rate during exercise and slows down physiologically to its basal rate at rest.

A variety of biological sensors have been developed which detect a physiological change and signal for an increased (or decreased) heart rate. These must imitate the atrium in physiological terms, and many sensors are still in development. The three most commonly used are:

1 *QT interval.* This shortens during exercise due to catecholamine release, the pacemaker senses the stimulus to T interval (the evoked QT interval). This is the most physiological of all forms of rate responsive pacing. Early problems resulted from a misconception that the QT interval and heart rate were linearly related. This produced a slow rise in heart rate with effort. The new algorithms have solved this problem.

2 *Body activity.* A piezo-electric crystal is mounted inside the pacemaker can. Vibrations from increased body activity are sensed. However on some occasions there is little increase in heart rate: e.g. mental activity, isometric exercise, and swimming as there is little body vibration.

3 *Respiratory activity.* A short second wire is implanted across the upper thorax which measures impedance changes during exercise. The second wire can be a problem under the skin on the front of the chest and erosion has been reported.

Other sensors detect changes in:

- mixed venous oxygen saturation.
- RV dP/dt
- stroke volume
- temperature
- pH of right atrial blood
- changes in thoracic impedance
- minute volume

Rate responsive pacemakers are rapidly increasing in popularity. They allow an increased cardiac output on exercise denied to the patient with a single VVI unit. Their advantages over DDD pacing and their drawbacks are summarised below.

Advantages of VVIR rate responsive pacing compared with DDD pacing:

Single ventricular wire only. Easier and quicker to implant. No problem with unstable atrial wire.

Units cheaper than DDD units.

Possible use in sino-atrial disease or AF.

Advantages of DDD pacing compared with VVIR:

The only system to incorporate atrial contribution to cardiac output.

Avoids the pacemaker syndrome.

Of greater benefit in patients with poor LV function and high LVEDP.

6.7 Physiological pacing

Units are now being developed which incorporate the best of both systems. This is a dual chamber system with rate responsive back-up should the patient develop sino-atrial disease or atrial fibrillation (i.e. DDDR).

6.8 Electrophysiological measurements and pacing

Sinus node recovery time (SNRT)

The right atrium is paced at a rate faster than the intrinsic sinus rate for up to 5 min and then pacing is switched off. Rates up to 160 bpm are used. The SNRT is the longest interval between the last paced beat and first sinus beat. Maximum SNRT is <1.4 sec. Corrected SNRT = SNRT − (spontaneous cycle length) before pacing <400 msec.

Sino-atrial conduction time (SACT)

This is calculated by firing an atrial premature stimulus late in the spontaneous cycle. The atrial premature beat collides with and extinguishes the next sinus impulse. A pause follows as the sinus node is reset. The atrial premature stimulus has to enter the sinus node and the subsequent reset sinus impulse has to leave it to the atrium. Thus:

$$\text{SACT} = \frac{(A_2 - A_3) - (A_1 - A_1)}{2} \text{ (see Fig. 6.4)}$$

$$= <100 \text{ msec}$$

Where $(A_1 - A_1)$ = Spontaneous cycle length

$(A_2 - A_3)$ = Premature atrial stimulus to next spontaneous cycle

The distance of the catheter from the sinus node is important. The SNRT and SACT are only useful if abnormal. Normal results are unhelpful and cannot be relied upon to predict normal sinus node function.

6.8 Electrophysiological measurements and pacing

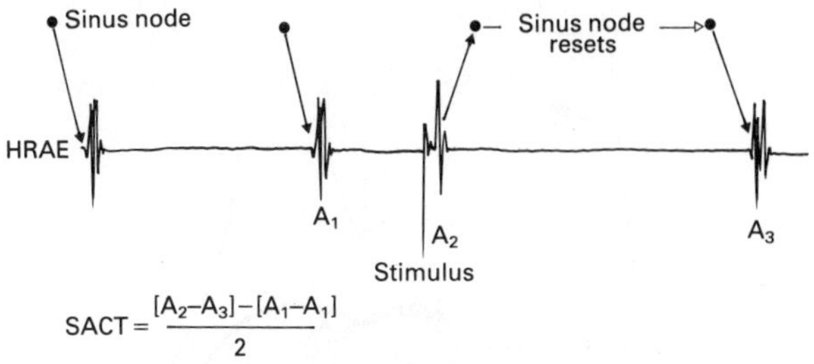

Fig. 6.4 Calculation of sino-atrial conduction time.

His bundle intervals (Fig. 6.5)
Prolongation of the PR interval may be due to electrical delay in any part of the atrioventricular conducting system. His bundle studies divide the PR interval into A–H interval (AV node conduction) and H–V interval (His-Purkinje conduction) (Fig. 6.5).

PA interval (20–40 msec)
Lengthening of this is uncommon, usually associated with atrial dilatation or large atrial septal defects. The delay is prior to the P wave.

A–H interval (50–120 msec)
This represents AV node conduction time. The AV node normally shows decremental conduction (increasing delay in conduction with increased frequency of impulses), With graded atrial pacing the AH time is gradually prolonged to the 'Wenckebach point'. This depends on vagal tone and may be altered by drugs.

Long A-H time is intra-AV-nodal delay. It occurs in:

- first degree heart block; vagal overactivity; athletes
- Wenckebach second degree AV block
- Interior infarction
- congenital heart block

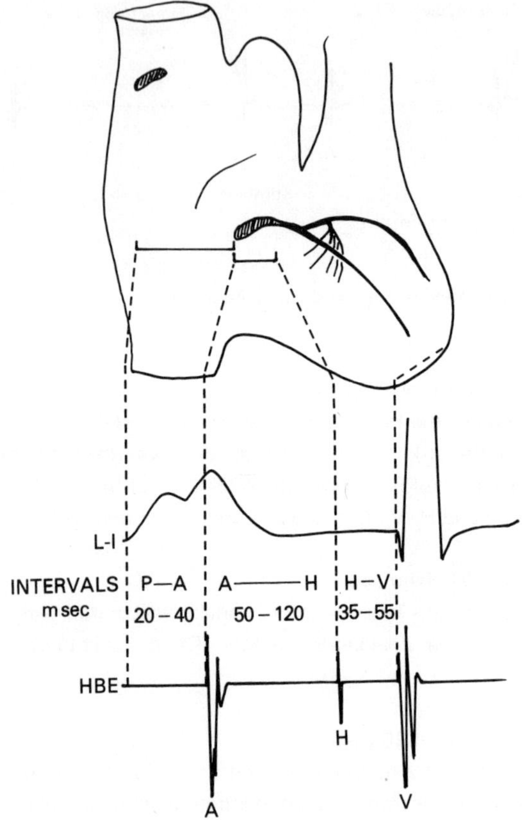

Fig. 6.5 Normal HBE intervals. L–I standard lead I of ECG. HBE = His bundle electrogram.

• drugs, i.e. digoxin, verapamil, beta-blocking agents, amiodarone

Shortening of the AH time is usually due to accessory pathways or sympathetic overactivity. It occurs in:

• sympathetic overactivity
• drugs: atropine, catecholamines

- accessory atrio-nodal or atrio-His pathways (James pathways)
- junctional ectopics

In Wolff–Parkinson–White syndrome the accessory pathway (Kent pathway) is not part of the AV node and does not affect the A–H time.

H–V interval (35–55 msec)

This represents His–Purkinje system conduction. Rarely two His spikes may be seen (split His potential) suggesting conduction delay within the His bundle. Lengthening of the H–V time indicates delay in conduction within the His bundle or intraventricular conduction system. It occurs in:

- acquired heart block in the elderly (Lenegre's disease)
- Mobitz type II AV block
- anterior infarction
- surgical trauma
- drugs (quinidine, disopyramide, ajmaline, flecainide)

Measurement of the H–V interval in patients with bifascicular block will not predict the small number of patients who will develop complete AV block (approx 6% patients with RBBB and LAHB).

Shortening of the H–V interval usually is due to accessory pathways arising from the normal AV node or His bundle (Mahaim pathways) or direct atrioventricular pathways (Kent pathway). Shortening occurs in:

- sympathetic overactivity
- drugs; catecholamines
- nodoventricular or His ventricular pathways (Mahaim)
- atrioventricular pathways (Kent)
- idioventricular rhythm arising from one of the fascicles

Spurious short H–V intervals may be produced by recording right bundle branch activity. Delivery of increasingly premature atrial stimuli until RBBB develops should help differentiate this. If the so-called His spike disappears with the development of RBBB the spike was not a true His spike, but arose from the right bundle branch.

6.9 Advice to the pacemaker patient before going home

Pacemaker interference from environmental factors

Before a patient with a permanent pacemaker goes home he or she should be warned that external signals may rarely interfere with the pacemaker and alter its function. The pacemaker wire acts as an aerial for the signal and it usually only is a problem with a unipolar system. The typical response of the pacemaker to an external signal is to switch to fixed rate pacing (magnet rate, p. 254). This increase in heart rate is noticed by the patient, who can then walk away from the source of interference.

Bursts of interference may cause inhibition of the pacemaker and pulsed electromagnetic fields are particular culprits (e.g. airport weapon detectors). The inhibition is quickly noticed by the patient.

As long as the patient is aware of the possibility of pacemaker interference he can check his own pulse if he is near a possible signal source. He should be particularly warned about getting too close to the following:

- mains driven electric motors, especially if sparking or with faulty suppression (e.g. old car engines, electrical kitchen equipment, Vacuum cleaners, electric razors, electric power drills, motor cycles, lawn mowers, outboard motors)
- airport weapon detectors. Hand-held detectors are safe
- microwave ovens if faulty with inadequate door seal
- high power radar stations. Hand-held police radar guns are safe
- CB radio transmitting systems
- some dental drills (e.g. ultrasonic cleaner)
- some equipment used by physiotherapists (e.g. shortwave heat therapy, faradism, etc.)
- shop anti-theft equipment. The pacemaker may trigger the alarm system as the patient walks out of the shop, and he should warn the shopkeeper
- public libraries have a system which can inhibit the pacemaker

• vibration. Hovercraft, helicopters and other sources of vibration may increase the rate of activity sensing pacemakers (e.g. Activitrax). Patients should be warned that this effect may occur.

If a patient is at frequent risk from external interference he can use a magnet to switch his pacemaker to fixed rate mode, during which it is immune to external signals. If this is inconvenient the unipolar system may have to be explanted and changed to a bipolar system (as in EMG inhibition, p. 248). Generally the risks are very small and are chiefly related to faulty electric motors.

Pacemakers and sport

Vigorous contact sports are best avoided in patients with permanent pacemakers, to avoid injury to the unit (e.g. rugby football, soccer, boxing, judo or karate). Squash should be discouraged if possible. A full golf swing may be uncomfortable with a pacemaker in the supramammary pouch, often more so if it is implanted on the left side.

Pacemakers and radiotherapy

Ionising radiation may damage pacemaker circuitry. If possible the pacemaker should be shielded during courses of irradiation. Close monitoring of pacemaker function is necessary after each dose of irradiation. A typical sign of pacemaker damage is a noticeable drift in the automatic pacing interval to a slower rate.

Pacemakers and surgery

Should a patient with permanent pacemaker require surgery there is usually no problem provided the anaesthetist is aware of the hazards. A common problem is prostatic surgery with permanent pacemakers *in situ* and a few precautions are necessary:

• the patient should have ECG monitoring throughout

• full DC cardioverting equipment should be available
• the diathermy plate should be as far from the pacemaker as possible (i.e. not on the chest or back). Diathermy should not be performed near the pacemaker box
• short bursts of diathermy may inhibit the pacemaker temporarily. This can be avoided by placing a magnet over the unit converting it to fixed rate mode (VOO)
• there is a remote risk of VT or VF induced by diathermy with the pacing electrode acting as an aerial. This will not be prevented by magnet override

Pacemakers and driving
Patients with permanent pacemakers may not hold HGV or PSV licences. They should not drive a car for three months after the unit's implantation. Provided they are under regular pacemaker follow-up they may hold a driving licence and should not have to pay an extra insurance premium.

6.10 Principles of paroxysmal tachycardia diagnosis

In patients with intermittent (paroxysmal) tachycardias diagnosis may be difficult. It is useful to know if the arrhythmia starts and stops suddenly, if it is regular or irregular, and if there are any factors which start it or stop it. 'Catching' the arrhythmia may not always be possible with the limited services of 24-hour ECG monitoring, and the patient may not be able to get to a hospital to have his arrhythmia recorded when it occurs. A patient-activated recorder may help.

Diagnosis of paroxysmal tachycardia involves:

• Recognition of likely associated cardiac lesions. AF: alcohol, mitral valve disease, thyrotoxicosis, coronary artery disease, pericarditis, post-cardiac surgery, etc. VT: LV aneurysm. Recent myocardial infarct.
• Recognition of resting 12-lead ECG abnormalities, e.g.

6.10 Principles of paroxysmal tachycardia diagnosis

Short PR interval:	Lown–Ganong–Levine syndrome	Pre-excitation
Short PR interval + delta wave:	WPW syndrome	
Long QT interval:	Hypocalcaemia Hypokalaemia (prominent 'u' wave) Romano–Ward syndrome (familial) Jervell–Lange Nielson syndrome (familial with deafness)	Increased risk of VT

• Recognition of cardiotoxic drugs taken by the patient, e.g. tricyclic antidepressants (VT, or AV block), digoxin (paroxysmal SVT with varying block, VT), L-dopa (VT), sympathomimetics, B_2 agonists (SVT or VT), quinidine (VT, Torsades de pointes).

• Recognition of other precipitating factors: caffeine (tea or coffee excess), smoking, alcohol, emotional stress, fatigue.

• Metabolic upsets: K^+ or Ca^{2+} high or low, hypoxia, hypercapnia, metabolic acidosis, hypomagnesaemia, phaeochromocytoma, febrile illnesses, pneumonia, etc.

• 24-hour ECG monitoring. Several recordings are often needed in a single patient. Telemetry is an alternative, and is useful for ambulant patients during hospital admission.

• Provocation of the arrhythmia. This is sometimes necessary to establish a diagnosis, to assess provocation factors and to assess treatment. The commonest provocation test is the exercise test. Unifocal ectopic beats in the normal heart are common, and usually decrease in number during exercise, recurring with rest. The abnormal heart may develop multifocal and frequent ectopics, or even ventricular tachycardia on effort. A few patients with WPW syndrome may develop tachycardia on effort, but this is not common.

Other provocative tests in patients with paroxysmal tachycardia include the use of the tilt table (orthostatic tachycardia), isoprenaline infusion (WPW syndrome), electrophysiological stimulation or cardiac catheterisation with LV and coronary angiography.

Most intermittent tachycardias can usually be diagnosed without provocation tests. Electrophysiologcal studies may be needed to assess the effect of drug therapy.

6.11 Classification of anti-arryhthmic drugs

The table on pp. 288–9 shows the Vaughan–Williams classification. Some drugs fit into more than one class and some drugs fit into none of them. The table also shows a classification based on the clinical effects of the drugs and their sites of action. It does not contain any electrophysiological data but is probably more useful at the bedside.

6.12 Management of specific tachyarrhythmias

Atrial fibrillation (AF)

Established AF

In established AF drug therapy is used to control the rate of ventricular response by increasing AV node refractoriness. Vagal manoeuvres will do this temporarily and may be useful in the diagnosis of fast AF.

Digoxin is still the drug of choice in AF (see inotropes section). If the ventricular response is still too fast in a well digitalised patient a small dose of a beta-blocking agent is added (e.g. metoprolol 50 mg tds) and the dose gradually increased if necessary. Before adding a beta-blocking agent it is important to be sure that LV function is adequate and the patient is not thyrotoxic. If the LV function is poor verapamil is added to digoxin, starting at 40 mg tds and increasing the dose if necessary up to 120 mg tds. If this fails to control the response amiodarone can be tried. Usually however digoxin plus beta-blockade controls the ventricular response.

Very occasionally in AF the conduction pathway to the

ventricles is via an anomalous pathway (e.g. Kent accessory pathway in WPW). In this situation digoxin, beta-blockade and verapamil are not effective. Digoxin and verapamil may even increase anterograde conduction in the accessory pathway and is contraindicated. If an ECG in AF shows intermittent or constant delta waves or if the ventricular response in AF is very fast (e.g. RR intervals 200–250 msec) then WPW is a strong possibility. Intravenous disopyramide 50–150 mg is the drug of choice. Other agents which can be effective are quinidine, procainamide, amiodarone or aprindine. The first three can be dangerous i.v. and DC cardioversion retains an early phase in this situation.

Paroxysmal AF

In paroxysmal AF therapy is aimed at reducing the number of bursts of AF. No treatment is ideal for this. The four drugs which have the greatest chance of maintaining sinus rhythm are amiodarone, disopyramide, flecainide and quinidine.

Digoxin is not in this list and merely controls ventricular response if AF occurs. Amiodarone is very useful, but photosensitivity is its most limiting side-effect.

Drug cardioversion

Intravenous disopyramide may chemically cardiovert AF into sinus rhythm. 50–150 mg are given i.v. Fibrillatory waves may coarsen and the ventricular response increase before sinus rhythm is achieved. Amiodarone given orally (200 mg tds up to 400 mg tds for 1 week) may also result in version to sinus rhythm. The dose is reduced after 1 week. Amiodarone is also very useful given intravenously: 5 mg/kg over 4 hours. The maximum i.v. dose over 24 hours in an adult is 1200 mg. An immediate result should not be expected: it may take 24–48 hours to convert the patient back to sinus rhythm. The patient can be converted to oral amiodarone when practical.

Classification of anti-arrhythmic drugs (Vaughan–Williams)

CLASS	CLASS 1			CLASS 2	CLASS 3	CLASS 4
Method of action	Block fast sodium channel			Beta sympathetic blockade	Hypothyroid effect	Slow calcium channel blockade
Effect on cardiac action potential	Slow phase 0 rate of rise Depress phase 4 rate of rise Also effect on APD varies: Ia ↑ APD	1b ↓ APD	Ic No effect APD	Depress phase 4 rate of rise	Increase APD	Depress phase 2 and 3
Primary site of action	Atrium Ventricle Bypass	Ventricle	His–Purkinje Ventricle Bypass	Sinus and AV nodes	Atrium AV node His–Purkinje Ventricle Accessory pathway	AV node

Examples of drugs	Quinidine Procainamide Disopyramide Ajmaline	Lignocaine Phenytoin Mexiletine Aprindine	Flecainide Encainide Lorcainide	Beta-blocking agents Bretylium Guanethidine	Amiodarone Disopyramide Sotalol Several other beta-blocking agents. Bethanidine. Bretylium	Verapamil Diltiazem
Effect on AV node and His–Purkinje system	Variable on AV node ↑His–Purkinje refractory period	Variable on AV node ↓His–Purkinje refractory period	↑ A–H↑ H–V times ↑His–Purkinje refractory period	↑ A–H time ↑AV node refractory period No effect on His–Purkinje refractory periods	↑ A–H time Little effect On H–V time ↑ Refractory periods of both AV node and His–Purkinje system	↑ A–H time ↑ AV node refractory period

DC cardioversion
This is not used for established or paroxysmal AF. Its role is chiefly in two types of situation:
1 As an elective procedure following a first attack of AF with an identifiable cause, e.g. attack of pneumonia, a thoractomy, pulmonary embolus, controlled thyrotoxicosis following thyroidectomy, following coronary artery surgery, ASD closure, mitral valve surgery, etc. If there is no known cause the patient is labelled as 'lone AF' and one attempt at cardioversion is certainly worth trying.
2 As an emergency procedure where atrial transport is vital to the maintenance of a reasonable cardiac output. The patient is usually very sick and the chances of success are not great. Examples are in HOGM, aortic valve stenosis and acute myocardial infarction.

Prior to DC cardioversion in the elective patient digoxin may be stopped for 24 hours. If there is any suggestion of digoxin toxicity the patient is not cardioverted (DC shock may produce refractory VT or VF in this situation).

If the left atrium is small, and AF has been present only for a few days, prior anticoagulation is unnecessary. If the left atrium is dilated, or there is mitral valve disease, or AF has been prolonged, then the patient is anticoagulated prior to cardioversion. This means a minimum of 3 days heparin, and preferably a week's oral anticoagulation. The factors mentioned above (dilated LA, prolonged AF) make it less likely that cardioversion will succeed. The risk of systemic emboli is small (0.5–3%). Anticoagulation following successful cardioversion should be continued for one month. Reversion to AF is common and approximately 30% stay in sinus rhythm.

Atrial flutter (Fig. 10.1)
The atrial rate in atrial flutter is 280–320/min and two to one ventricular response results in a ventricular rate of 150/min. With a four to one response the ventricular rate is 75/min, however

Drugs available for specific tachycardias

	Sinus tachycardia	Atrial fibrillation Atrial flutter Supra-ventricular tachycardia	Junctional tachycardia	WPW bypass tachycardia	Ventricular tachycardia
Drugs	None initially Look for cause: Pain Anxiety Fever, sepsis Hypovolaemia Low output state Shock Thyrotoxicosis	*Version to SR* Disopyramide Amiodarone *Rate control at AV node* Digoxin Verapamil Beta–blockade *Prevention* Quinidine Disopyramide Amiodarone (Procainamide)	(Vagal manoeuvres) Verapamil Beta-blockade Digoxin Flecainide	*At AV node* Beta-blockade At accessory *pathway* Disopyramide Quinidine Amiodarone (Procainamide) Ajmaline Flecainide	*Prevention and termination* Lignocaine Mexiletine Tocainide Procainamide Quinidine Phenytoin Beta-blockade Amiodarone Disopyramide Aprindine *Version only* Bretylium tosylate Ajmaline

it is unusual to be able to keep the response at a regular four to one.

Carotid sinus massage will increase the degree of AV block temporarily and this can be useful in diagnosis of the rhythm, as the typical saw-tooth pattern of flutter becomes obvious (especially in leads II and V_1 in the ECG). An isolated event of atrial flutter is best treated by DC cardioversion. It is the most likely arrhythmia to convert to SR and only small energy shocks are needed (25–50 Joules in the adult). If AF is produced the patient is shocked again into sinus rhythm.

Paroxysmal atrial flutter has to be controlled by drug therapy. Digoxin may produce atrial fibrillation which tends to be easier to manage. In difficult cases of paroxysmal atrial flutter the atrium can be fibrillated using a right atrial endocardial pacing lead.

Amiodarone is also useful as it reduces the atrial flutter rate, making even two to one ventricular response more acceptable (e.g. down to 130–140/min). It probably also reduces the number of bursts of flutter.

Atrial tachycardia (Fig. 10.1)
This is usually divided into two types:

- Primary atrial tachycardia (supraventricular tachycardia. SVT, PAT). Atrial rate is 150–250/min, usually about 160/min, and ventricular response is frequently 1:1. P waves may be not visible on the ECG at a ventricular response rate of 1:1, but appear with carotid sinus massage.
- Paroxysmal atrial tachycardia with varying block secondary to digoxin toxicity (PATB). Ventricular response is less likely to be a 1:1 response: P waves are usually visible.

Verapamil is the drug of choice in an acute episode of atrial tachycardia. It is given i.v. 1–10 mg over 5 min. The dose can be repeated in 20 min if still necessary. It is more effective than beta-blockade intravenously. It is more hazardous in patients already on beta-blockade, but can still be used with careful monitoring (risk of complete AV block) in an emergency. DC shock may be needed.

Paroxysmal atrial tachycardia in the long term can be managed on oral verapamil, or beta-blockade or even digoxin. Disopyramide or amiodarone are also very useful. Long acting quinidine preparations are still used, but gastrointestinal side-effects may prove a problem.

In atrial tachycardia with block (digoxin toxicity) the drug is stopped, and the K^+ checked. The potassium should be >4.5 mmol/l and oral or i.v. KCl may be necessary. Verapamil or beta-blockade is used to slow ventricular response if necessary. DC cardioversion is avoided if possible and if used low-energy shock is given (25–50 Joules) under lignocaine cover. Rapid atrial pacing can be used to extinguish the atrial focus.

The use of disopyramide in atrial tachycardia may slow the atrial rate, but quicken the ventricular response before version to sinus rhythm. Disopyramide prolongs atrial effective refractory period slowing atrial rate, but its anticholinergic effect on the AV node may increase ventricular response. The net effect depends on vagal tone. It is a more useful drug for long term prophylaxis than for acute i.v. administration in atrial tachycardia.

Junctional tachycardia (Fig. 10.1)
This is usually due to re-entry within the AV node. Accessory extra-nodal pathways may be involved in the circuit.

Vagal manœuvres are useful in junctional tachycardia and the patient may be taught these (eyeball massage is dangerous and so is excluded).

- ice cold water splashed on the face. Ice-cubes in a polythene bag placed on the face. The 'duck-diving' reflex
- carotid sinus massage. One side at a time with the patient flat
- stimulation of the soft palate (gag reflex)
- Valsalva or Müller manœuvres
- straining, lifting heavy weights, changes in posture

If the AV node is involved in one or more limbs of the re-entry pathway antegrade AV conduction will be blocked by verapamil or beta-blocking agents. If verapamil fails to block the tachycardia it is unlikely that the AV node is involved in the circuit. Amiodarone is very useful in long-term management, as is Flecainide.

Wolff–Parkinson–White syndrome is discussed separately although the AV node is involved in the circuit (p. 302).

Differentiation of SVT with aberrancy from VT

The table on p. 295 provides a general guide. Also see Figs. 10.1, 10.2.

In spite of this guide it may be impossible to decide on the source of the tachycardia. The finding of capture or fusion beats is diagnostic of VT, and a diligent search for P waves may help differentiate the two. Vagal manœuvres are always worth trying. Electrophysiological studies with provocation may be necessary to decide between the two, especially in cases of paroxysmal tachycardia documented on 24-hour ECG monitoring associated with symptoms.

6.13 Ventricular premature beats (VPBs)

Ventricular ectopics on routine 24-hour monitoring

Routine 24-hour ECG monitoring in an apparently healthy population will reveal ectopic beats in more than half, and in about 10% these will be multifocal. They do not necessarily imply underlying heart disease. They probably occur with increasing frequency in the older population. Important points in the decision to treat them are:

- are the ectopics producing troublesome symptoms?
- is there an excessive consumption of alcohol, tea, coffee, coca-cola, tobacco?
- any recent febrile or influenzal-type illness?
- any associated drug therapy which might be implicated? e.g.

Differentiation of SVT with aberrant conduction from ventricular tachycardia

	SVT with aberrancy	**Ventricular tachycardia**
First heart sound	Normal	Variable
ECG pattern	Usually RBBB	Bizarre wide QRS
Fusion beats	Absent	May be present
P waves	Synchronised with QRS	Not seen or dissociated
Onset of tachycardia	P wave preceding first wide QRS	No P wave preceding first bizarre QRS
Vagal manoeuvres	May slow ventricular response to reveal atrial activity	Ineffective
QRS duration	<140 msec	>140 msec
If in RBBB	rSR′ in V_1	Rsr′ in V_1
QRS axis	Normal	More negative than −30°
V leads complex polarity	Discordant (some positive, some negative)	Concordant (all positive, or all negative)

digoxin, sympathomimetics, tricyclic antidepressants, diuretics including hypokalaemia
• is there any underlying cardiac condition? e.g. mitral leaflet prolapse, recent myocardial infarction, sino-atrial disease, cardiomyopathy, aortic valve disease, etc.

In spite of all these points it may be impossible to identify the source of the tachycardia with certainty. An oesophageal electrode (easily swallowed as a 'pill on a wire') may help in identifying atrial activity from the left atrium. If this fails, more invasive electrophysiological recordings may be needed. It is very important to realise that the patients condition is no guide to the source of the tachycardia.

Clearing up these points will require echocardiography and probably exercise testing. Innocent ectopics tend to disappear with increasing heart rate. More pathological ones may increase in frequency with possible short salvos of ventricular tachycardia on effort (Fig. 10.2).

If full clinical examination is normal, echocardiography is normal, and an exercise test is negative (p. 394), then the patient should be reassured. Treatment will only be necessary if in spite of reassurance and avoidance of possible precipitating factors symptoms are still troublesome. Usually a small dose of a beta-blocking agent or disopyramide is effective, but should rarely be necessary.

Excessive zeal in trying to quench ectopic beats may result in drug side-effects being worse than the condition itself.

Ventricular premature beats following myocardial infarction

The treatment of ventricular premature beats following myocardial infarction is still controversial. Lown (1967) proposed certain types of premature beats were more likely to lead to VF and should be suppressed. These warning arrhythmias were:

• frequent VPBs
• multifocal VPBs

- R-on-T phenomenon
- salvos of VPBs (two or more)

Since then it has been established that as many as 50% of cases of VF post infarction occur with no warning arrhythmias at all. It has also been established that there is no case for routine use of anti-arrhythmic drugs in all patients entering a coronary care unit. There is no justification for a single drug policy for all patients.

Ventricular premature beats are possibly just a marker of the extent of myocardial damage and do not necessarily cause sudden death themselves. In an uncomplicated myocardial infarct, suppression of simple unifocal ectopic beats is usually not justified.

Suppression of ventricular premature beats following myocardial infarction:

- check K^+, other drugs (e.g. digoxin), acid–base state and blood bases (hypoxia, hypercapnia), and correct them if possible. K^+ should be 4.5–5.5 mmol/L
- consider prophylactic anti-arrhythmic drug if: poor haemodynamic state, frequent multifocal VPBs, R-on-T, or salvos of VPBs Lignocaine is given as an infusion, switching to an oral agent after 48 hours (flecainide or disopyramide)
- consider temporary pacing if ectopics are related to atropine-resistant bradycardia

6.14 Ventricular tachycardia (VT) (Fig. 10.2)

Available drugs

Commonly used drugs in the management of VT are shown in the table on p. 298. Many of the Class 1 agents (lignocaine, mexiletine, tocainide) have similar side-effects predominantly affecting the CNS (tremor, dizziness, confusion, cerebellar ataxia, fits) and the gastrointestinal tract (nausea, anorexia, vomiting). The large number of drugs testify to the failure of a single drug to work in all cases of VT, and often several drugs need to be used in prophylaxis.

Treatment of ventricular tachycardia depends on the patient's condition. In the very sick patient immediate DC cardioversion is necessary. If VT is well tolerated lignocaine 100–200 mg i.v. is given, followed by an infusion (4 mg/min for 30 min, 2 mg/min for 2 hours, then 1 mg/min is normally satisfactory). If lignocaine fails to control the tachycardia a second drug is tried (preferably from a different class in the Vaughan–Williams classification), e.g. disopyramide, flecainide, a beta-blocking agent or ajmaline if available.

Management and long-term prophylaxis

1 Check blood for K^+, acid–base balance and blood gases in all patients and correct if necessary (including artificial ventilation).

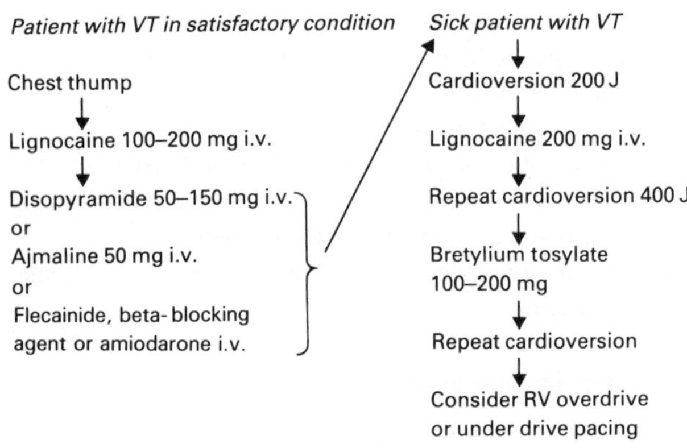

2 In the sick patient with low output state cardiac massage may help correct the arrhythmla.

3 Once successfully cardioverted prophylactic therapy is started orally. The effect of the chosen drug is monitored with 24-hour Holter taping. It is important to keep the serum K^+ between 4.5 and 5.5 mmol/L. If VT was secondary to myocardial infarction or acute myocarditis it is probably wise to continue drug therapy for three months in the first instance, and then

Drugs commonly used in ventricular arrhythmias

Drug	Oral dose	I.v. dose	Half life approx.	Therapeutic plasma level	Side-effects
Lignocaine (Xylocard)	—	100–200 mg i.v. bolus 4 mg/min for 30 min 2 mg/min for 2 hr: then 1 mg/min	30 min	1.5–6.0 µg/ml	Drowsiness + confusion, Paraesthesiae and numbness, dysarthria, fits
Quinidine (Kinidin, Kiditard, Quinicardine)	200 mg test dose 200–400 mg tds or qds Long acting preps bd	Rarely used 6–10 mg/kg over ½ hr (Quinidine gluconate)	7 hr	2–5 µg/ml	Visual disturbances, tinnitus, vertigo, thrombocytopenia, agranulocytosis, diarrhoea, paroxysmal VT or VF, half dose digoxin, warfarin, etc.
Procainamide (Pronestyl)	375 mg 4 hrly	100 mg over 5 min repeat up to max 1 g over 1 hr 2–5 mg/min infusion	3 hr	5–10 µg/ml	Hypotension, AV block, Insomnia, fever, rash, arthralgia, arteritis (Lupus syndrome), agranulocytosis
Disopyramide (Rhythmodan, Norpace)	100–200 mg (max) 6 hrly	50 mg i.v. over 5 min repeat to max 150 mg, and to 300 mg in 1 hour	6 hr	2–6 µg/ml	Dry mouth, blurred vision, urinary retention, constipation, hypotension, VT

Drugs commonly used in ventricular arrhythmias

Drug	Oral dose	I.v. dose	Half-life approx.	Therapeutic plasma level	Side-effects
Phenytoin (Epanutin)	100 mg tds to 200 mg bd	50 mg over 5 min, repeating to 500 mg	22 hr	10–18 μg/ml	Cerebellar signs, gum hypertrophy, megaloblastic anaemia (folate), lupus syndrome, bradycardia, hypotension
Mexiletine (Mexitil)	Loading dose 400 mg then 200 mg tds	100–250 mg over 10 mins 4 mg/min for 1 hr, 2 mg/min for 1 hr, then 0.5 mg/min	16 hrs	1–2 μg/ml	Anorexia, Nausea, vomiting, tremor, cerebellar signs, bradycardia, hypotension
Aprindine (Fiboran, Fibocil)	Loading dose 200 mg then 100–200 mg od	25 mg ovar 5 min repeated to 150 mg	12–66 hr 28 hr	1–3 μg/ml	Tremor, giddiness, diplopia, hallucinations, ataxia, agranulocytosis, jaundice (rare)
Tocainide (Tonocard)	400 mg tds to 800 mg tds	0.5–0.75 mg/kg/min over 15 min	14 hr	5–10 μg/ml	Nausea, vomiting, CNS disturbance, giddiness, cerebellar signs. Blood dyscrasias

Flecainide (Tambocor)	100–200 mg bd	1.5–2 mg/kg over 10 min	12–27 hr mean 20 hr	200–800 ng/ml	Avoid in paced patients. Giddiness. Blurred vision
Propranolol (Inderal)	40 mg tds (range 10–240 mg tds)	0.1–0.2 mg/kg over 5 min	3 hr	30–50 ng/ml oral 50–100 μg/ml i.v.	Hypotension, AV block, depression, LV failure, cold peripheries, bronchospasm
Amiodarone (Cordarone X)	200 mg tds for 1 week reducing to 200 mg od or less	5 mg/kg/ over 2–4 hr 10–20 mg/kg/day infusion	28 days	0.1 μg/ml	Photosensitivity, corneal micro deposits, thyroid dysfunction, sleep disturbance, etc., alveolitis, half dose digoxin, warfarin
Bretylium Tosylate (Bretylate, Bretylol)	Poorly absorbed	5 mg/kg over 10 min then 1–2 mg/min bolus dose if in VF	8 hr	0.5–1 μg/ml	Hypotension, dizziness, avoid in dig, toxicity
Ajmaline (Cardiorhythmine)	Not suitable as very short half life	5 mg over 2 min Repeated after 10 min	1–2 min	1–3 μ/ml	Caution if also on digoxin as may induce AV block

then repeat 24-hour monitoring both on the drug and after its withdrawal. In some cases more than one drug will be necessary and indefinite oral therapy may be required. Cardiac catheterisation is indicated to delineate an LV aneurysm if this is a suspected cause of recurrent VT.

Regimes of choice are one or more of these drugs:

Disopyramide 100 mg tds or qds
Mexiletine 200 mg tds
Amiodarone 200 mg tds for 1 week then reducing
Aprindine 100–200 mg daily if available (not in UK)
Beta-blocking agent
Flecainide 100–200 mg bd

Drugs of second choice may be added or tried separately if necessary:

Procainamide 375 mg 4 hourly
Quinidine durules two twice daily
Phenytoin 100 mg tds to 200 mg bd

The best combinations of the first group are those from different Vaughan–Williams classes (e.g. flecainide and amiodarone). There is some evidence that amiodarone is more effective than long-term beta-blockade in prevention of recurrent VT in patients with HOCM.

6.15 Wolff–Parkinson–White syndrome (WPW)

In normal sinus rhythm the ECG of patients with WPW syndrome is characterised by:

- short PR interval. Usually 0.1–0.12 sec
- delta wave. A slurred upstroke of the R wave
- a widened QRS complex due to the addition of the delta wave to the initial part of the QRS complex

The delta wave is due to the premature activation of part of the ventricular myocardium by the accessory pathway (Kent bundle). The portion of the ventricular myocardium activated depends on the site of the accessory pathway. The two most commonly recognised types are shown in the table below, but there are many possible accessory pathway sites and the surface ECG is of limited use diagnostically.

Type	**Site of accessory pathway**	**ECG appearances**
Type A	Posterior left atrial wall to left ventricle or paraseptal	Positive delta wave in leads V_1–V_6. Negative delta wave in lead I
Type B	Lateral right atrial wall to right ventricle	Biphasic or negative delta wave in leads V_1–V_3. Positive delta wave in lead I

The ECG complex in WPW is thus a fusion complex of abnormally activated and normally activated myocardium. The EGG appearances may mimic other conditions:
- LBBB (type B)
- true posterior infarction, or RV hypertrophy, or RBBB (type A)

Associated lesions

WPW syndrome may occur as an isolated condition or in association with other cardiac lesions (e.g. Ebstein's anomaly, hypertrophic obstructive cardiomyopathy, mitral valve prolapse), and paroxysmal tachycardia is a common problem in these conditions. WPW may be concealed and not obvious from the 12-lead surface ECG.

WPW tachycardia

The development of tachycardia results from unidirectional block in the accessory pathway (Fig. 6.6). A circus movement is set up with antegrade conduction down the AV node, and retrograde conduction in the Kent bundle (due to prolonged antegrade refractoriness of the Kent bundle). During tachycardia the delta wave is lost as ventricular activation occurs only via the

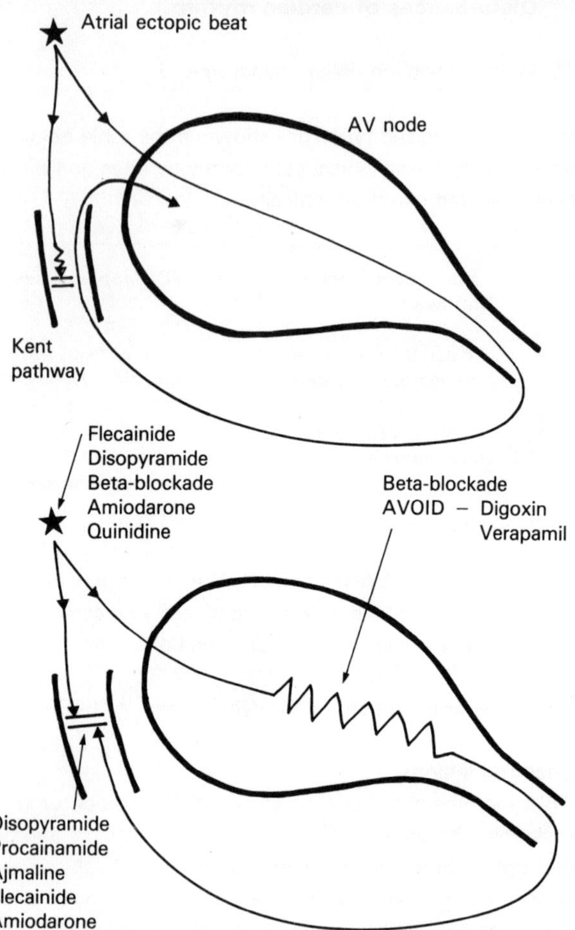

Fig. 6.6 Mechanisms and treatment of re-entry tachycardia in Wolff–Parkinson–White syndrome. The upper panel shows the re-entry circuit. A premature atrial beat (star) is blocked at the Kent bundle antegradely and conducted normally through the AV node. The Kent bundle is not refractory to retrograde conduction and the circus movement is set up. The lower panel shows the sites of drug action. The atrial premature beat can be abolished by disopyramide, beta-blockade, amiodarone, flecainide or quinidine. Antegrade conduction down the AV node is delayed by beta blockade. Retrograde conduction up the Kent pathway is blocked by disopyramide, amiodarone, flecainide, ajmaline and procainamide. Verapamil and digoxin are contra-indicated.

AV node, and the ECG and its axis may appear very different from the ECG in normal sinus rhythm. Very occasionally in small children the circuit is established the wrong way round (i.e. antegradely via the accessory pathway) and the QRS complexes are wide.

Drug treatment

Drugs can act in WPW at three sites in WPW tachycardia (see Fig. 6.6). Vagal manœuvres may help in some cases.

WPW tachycardia can be treated by i.v. disopyramide (50–150 mg) or i.v. propranolol (1–10 mg), or i.v. ajmaline (50–100 mg). Intravenous amiodarone is dangerous unless given very slowly (over 1–4 hours). Long term prophylaxis may require a combination of drugs (e.g. disopyramide + beta-blockade, amiodarone + beta-blockade). DC cardioversion should be used early if the tachycardia is poorly tolerated.

Digoxin and verapamil should be avoided in WPW tachycardia, as the drugs may accelerate antegrade conduction down the Kent bundle.

Electrophysiological studies

Patients who are unresponsive to simple medical treatment or who develop AF should be studied with electrophysiological methods. This should determine:

- the site of the accessory pathway
- the effective refractory period of the accessory pathway
- the response of the pathway to drug treatment

In a few rare cases completely refractory to medical treatment surgical ablation of the bypass, may have to be considered. Epicardial mapping of the sequence of ventricular activation is necessary prior to surgery. Atriotomy can be performed for laterally sited bypass tracts. Septal tracts can also be treated surgically but are more difficult. Electrical trans-catheter ablation is now possible for some of these tracts.

6.16 Problems with individual anti-arrhythmic drugs

Amiodarone

This iodine-containing compound has a very long half life and is strongly bound to plasma proteins. It is highly fat soluble and probably binds with phospholipids on the cell membrane and modifies adenyl cyclase activity.

Given orally it takes 5–10 days to saturate the tissues. It is of great value in both atrial and ventricular arrhythmias, as well as WPW syndrome where it acts by increasing the bypass anterograde effective refractory period (ERP).

Electrophysiological effects

It increases action potential duration (APD) in both sinus and AV nodes, but more so in the His-Purkinje system and ventricular muscle. It increases A–H interval without changing the H–V time. It slightly reduces the sinus node discharge rate and sinus node recovery time. It reduces conduction in WPW accessory pathway, and reduces anterograde ERP more than the retrograde ERP. It reduces excitability of all cardiac tissues, and the automaticity of SA and AV nodes is reduced. There is probably no chronic effect on contractility, although acute i.v. administration produces vasodilatation with afterload reduction which effects acute contractility measurements.

Drug interactions

The dose of digoxin and warfarin should be halved in patients starting amiodarone (displacement of digoxin from myocardial receptors increases plasma digoxin, but reduces the direct cardiac effect). Amiodarone can be used with verapamil or beta-blockers, but care is needed (effects on AV node).

Side-effects

These are common but rarely require stopping the drug. Patients should be warned about possible photosensitivity. They should shield themselves from the sun and use barrier creams if necessary.

Thyroid function is checked before starting the drug especially in patients with AF. It is best avoided in patients with known thyroid dysfunction.

Common side-effects	**Rarer side-effects**
Photosensitivity (more than 50% patients)	Peripheral neuropathy
Skin rash	Pulmonary fibrosis (fibrosing alveolitis)
Headache	Thyroid dysfunction (hypothyroidism more than hyperthyroidism)
Tremor	Slate grey skin and melanosis
Sleep disturbance, insomnia and nightmares	Hepatic dysfunction (raised enzymes)
Gut effects: nausea, constipation	Visual symptoms
Corneal microdeposits	Epididymitis
Increased prothrombin time	

Thyroid dysfunction (hypothyroidism) is due to inhibition of T_3 production and enhancement of reversed T_3 production (inactive). Corneal microdeposits are very common, but only visible on the slit lamp. They are reversible if the drug is stopped and regular eye checks are no longer needed. Only about 6% patients on the drug develop visual disturbance.

The drug is safe in moderate renal dysfunction.

Cardioversion on amiodarone

If the patient has sino-atrial disease care is needed (effect on reducing sinus node automaticity), but it is usually safe.

Dosage

- oral therapy. 200 mg tds for 1 week, reducing to 200 mg daily or less
- i.v. administration can be dangerous if given quickly (alpha-

blocking effect). It is avoided if possible in the elderly and patients with large hearts. In AF or VT it may restore sinus rhythm without the need for DC cardioversion in about 50% patients. Infusion dose is 5 mg/kg in 100 mls 5% dextrose (not N saline) over 1–4 hours. Maximum dose is 1200 mg in 24 hours. The abnormal rhythm may not be abolished immediately, sometimes reverting several hours after the infusion has stopped.

Disopyramide

A drug with both class 1a and class 3 actions, disopyramide also has an anticholinergic effect. The anticholinergic effect on the heart depends on the vagal tone present (in the normal heart disopyramide may occasionally increase heart rate slightly by this 'vagolytic' action).

About 90% is bioavailable taken orally, and with normal serum levels (2–6 μg/ml) about 30–50% is free in serum. Half is excreted unchanged in urine.

Electrophysiological effects

It prolongs atrial effective refractory period, it has a variable effect on AV node refractory periods, and prolongs ventricular refractory period. Conduction times in AV node and His-Purkinje system are little affected (unless there is pronounced vagal tone). It slows accessory pathway conduction.

It is a useful drug in atrial ectopics, prevention of AF, or paroxysmal SVT because it causes a rise in atrial ERP; WPW tachycardia because it causes a rise in accessory pathway conduction time; and ventricular ectopics or tachycardia because it causes a rise in ventricular ERP.

Dosage

Oral. Loading dose is 300 mg in adult (200 mg if <50 kg) followed by 150 mg 6 hourly (100 mg if <50 kg). Increase dose interval if renal dysfunction (e.g. once daily for creatinine clearance 15 ml/min or less).

I.v. 50 mg is given slowly over 5 min, and the dose may be carefully repeated up to 150 mg if necessary and contraindications have not appeared (see below).

Relative contraindications to disopyramide (where the drug has to be used with great care)

- congestive cardiac failure with a large heart, poor LV function or cardiogenic shock
- sino-atrial disease (prolongs atrial ERP)
- 2° or 3° AV block
- prostatic hypertrophy
- glaucoma
- hypokalaemia: rarely it may precipitate VT (torsades de pointes) as with quinidine.

Disopyramide toxicity on ECG: watch for lengthening QT interval, widening of QRS complex, bradycardia or conduction defects. Also watch for hypotension. More likely with too rapid i.v. administration, especially if the patient is also on beta-blockade, or other antihypertensive medication.

Side-effects

Common (anticholinergic)	**Less common**
Dry mouth, eyes, nose	Urinary retention
Blurred vision	Acute psychosis
Hesitancy in men with prostatic hypertrophy	Cholestatic jaundice
Constipation	Hypoglycaemia
Nausea	Agranulocytosis

In addition the following may also occur:

- a dry mouth is an expected side-effect and is neither a guide to plasma level nor drug toxicity
- occasionally the drug may potentiate warfarin
- it does not interact with lignocaine and can be used where lignocaine fails. It has only a weak negative inotropic effect.

Procainamide

A class 1 a antiarrhythmic with electrophysiological properties similar to quinidine. Up to 90% is absorbed orally and 15% only is protein bound. The drug is acetylated in the liver (first pass metabolism), and acetylator status is important in determining plasma levels and toxic side-effects. About 50% of the drug is excreted in the urine. The acetyl metabolite is also antiarrhythmic, and has a longer half life.

Dosage

• in the adult the drug is given 4 hourly. In some difficult cases this means waking the patient at night to maintain plasma levels (5–10 μg/ml)

• average adult dose is 375 mg 4 hourly (250–500 mg 4 hourly)

• slow release preparation: procainamide durules can be taken 8 hourly (dose 1–1.5 g 8 hourly)

• acetylator status

Fast acetylators. May not reach necessary plasma levels of procainamide, but acetyl metabolite is antiarrhythmic and less toxic

Slow acetylators. May have high plasma levels, and risk toxicity

• i.v. dose is 100 mg slowly i.v. over 5 min up to maximum 1 g in 1 hour

Electrophysiological effects of procainamide

Little effect on AV node conduction (A–H time), dose-dependent increase in His-Purkinje conduction (H–V time). Increase refractory period of Kent pathway making it useful in WPW tachycardia.

Side-effects

Make it a more useful drug in acute management of ventricular arrhythmias than in chronic suppression.

Intravenously it is a little safer than quinidine and can be tried if lignocaine fails. Side-effects following intravenous administration are:

- hypotension due to vasodilatation (reversed by phenylephrine)
- complete AV block. The drug should not be given in complete AV block as it may slow or extinguish the idioventricular rhythm
- in atrial flutter or fibrillation a vagolytic effect on the AV node may increase ventricular response (as with disopyramide). Procainamide is not usually used for atrial dysrhythmias although it may extinguish atrial ectopics

Long-term side-effects

- the lupus syndrome: rash, arthralgia, fever, arteritis, pleurisy and pericarditis, but not renal involvement. The effects resolve on stopping the drug. Antinuclear antibodies occur in half the patients receiving the drug
- agranulocytosis

Unless absolutely essential procainamide should be restricted to 3–6 months oral therapy.

Quinidine

The original anti-arrhythmic drug with class 1 a activity. The drug is completely absorbed orally and intravenous administration can be dangerous and is rarely used.

Unlike procainamide, 80% is protein bound, causing resulting drug interactions. The drug is hydroxylated in the liver, and in CCF liver congestion results in high plasma quinidine levels. Alkaline urine may result in toxic metabolic accumulation.

Quinidine may be tried in paroxysmal AF or other atrial arrhythmias, and may help keep a patient in SR after cardioversion. Atrial arrhythmias are the main indication for its use; it is rarely used for ventricular arrhythmias now, as less toxic drugs are available. It is contraindicated in sino-atrial disease, digoxin toxicity and complete AV block.

6.16 Problems with anti-arrhythmic drugs

Dosage

A test dose of quinidine sulphate of 200 mg is given to check for drug idiosyncracy (anaphylaxis).

Quinidine durules are then started initially two twice daily (= 500 mg quinidine bisulphate bd) to three times daily maximum. When starting treatment quinidine displacement of other drugs from plasma proteins necessitates reducing the doses of other drugs, so the dose of concomittant warfarin or digoxin should be halved.

Electrophysiological effects

As in procainamide: no change in A–H time (or even slight shortening due to vagolytic effect), plus lengthening of H–V time.

Surface ECG shows:

- widening QRS
- prolonged QT interval
- T wave changes

} these are useful guide to toxicity

QRS widening >120 msec is an indication to stop the drug.
With increasing toxicity the following may occur:

- atrial standstill
- ventricular tachycardia (torsade de pointes) (Fig. 10.2)
- VF

Side-effects

These are commonly gastrointestinal. Any others are indications to stop the drug.

- gastrointestinal: diarrhoea is expected, with nausea and vomiting
- cinchonism: tinnitus, vertigo, deafness, visual disturbances, blindness
- haematological: thrombocytopenia, purpura, agranulocytosis
- neuromuscular blocking effect: this may potentiate muscle relaxants. Its vagolytic action inhibits anticholinesterase activity in myasthenia

• quinidine syncope. This may be due to AV block, VT or VF. A prolonged QT interval plus an early ectopic (R on T) may be the cause

Lignocaine

A class 1 b antiarrhythmic which shortens the action potential duration. It differs from procainamide and quinidine in several respects:

	Class 1a: Procainamide Quinidine	**Class 1b: Lignocaine**
APD	Lengthened	Shortened
Peripheral vessels	Vasodilator	Vasoconstrictor
Oral preparation	Yes	No
Useful in atrial arrhythmias	Yes	No
Conduction of His-Purkinje system	Prolongs H–V time	Little effect
CNS toxicity	Uncommon	Common
Myocardial depression	In toxic doses	Minimal
Use in sino-atrial disease	No	Safe

It is the standard drug in use for ventricular arrhythmias in the CCU. It is rapidly metabolised in the liver allowing flexible control, and has to be given intravenously. Liver dysfunction or congestion (as in heart failure) require dose reduction. It is not protein bound.

Lignocaine metabolites are excreted in the urine and contribute to CNS toxicity. It is safer than i.v. procainamide in low output states, or in patients with degrees of AV block.

Dosage

There are numerous suggested schedules. One of the easiest is: 200 mg i.v. bolus over 5 min, followed by infusion of 4 mg/min for 30 min, then 2 mg/min for 2 hours, then 1 mg/min.

In low output states the initial 4 mg/min infusion period is omitted and the infusion is started at 2 mg/min. Plasma levels should be 1.5–6 μg/ml. Significant plasma levels can be obtained after intramuscular lignocaine (300 mg in the adult) after about 15 min. Lignocaine infiltration used for minor surgery, pacemaker insertion, etc. can also produce significant plasma levels.

Side-effects
These are primarily neurological especially in the elderly: numbness, drowsiness, confusion, nausea, vomiting, dizziness, dysarthria and eventually convulsions. Convulsions are managed with i.v. diazepam.

Lignocaine is safer in cardiac failure or cardiogenic shock than procainamide, provided lower infusion rates are used.

What to do if lignocaine fails

• check adequate infusion rate and drip still functional
• check plasma K^+: lignocaine is less effective in hypokalaemia
• check for additional drug therapy, possibly causing arrhythmias: digitalis, other inotropes, etc.
• gradually increase lignocaine infusion rate until early toxic signs appear
• if still ineffective switch to alternative drug, e.g. disopyramide, flecainide, amiodarone or bretylium tosylate

Mexiletine
A class 1b agent similar to lignocaine, but available for oral administration. Hepatic metabolism is slower than with lignocaine, and renal excretion is reduced if the urine is alkaline.

Electrophysiological effects are variable; the H–V time has been reported to increase or decrease. Generally it has little effect on AV conduction.

Dosage
Orally: 200–400 mg 8 hourly in the adult. Dosage i.v. is complicated as with lignocaine, since there is a small margin

between therapeutic effect and side-effects. Suggested i.v. regime: 100–250 mg i.v. over 10 min, 4 mg/min for 1 hour, 2 mg/min for 1 hour, then 0.5 mg/min.

Close attention is needed with i.v. mexiletine as the long half life compared with lignocaine means that fine tuning of the regime is much more difficult. Neurological side-effects are common with i.v. therapy. Chronic oral therapy is much easier, and side-effects are less likely.

Side-effects

As with lignocaine: dizziness, numbness, paraesthesiae, tremor, dysarthria, tinnitus, myoclonus, convulsions, nausea and vomiting, hiccoughs, bradycardia and hypotension. The bradycardia usually responds to atropine.

On oral therapy common complaints are nausea, anorexia and a continuous unpleasant taste in the mouth.

Tocainide

Also similar to lignocaine in structure and anti-arrhythmic effect but is available orally and has a longer half life (11–14 hours). 50% is protein bound. About 40% is excreted unchanged in the urine. Electrophysiological effects are similar to those of lignocaine.

As with lignocaine it is safe in low output states, but dosage should be reduced in patients with heart failure, renal disease or post myocardial infarction as the half life is prolonged (e.g. 17–19 hours) and twice daily dosage is sufficient in these patients.

Dosage

Oral: 400–800 mg 8 hourly, 400–600 mg 12 hourly in hepatic, renal disease or CCF

I.v. 0.5–0.75 mg/kg/min over 15–30 min, followed by oral therapy.

Side-effects are similar to lignocaine and mexiletine and

unfortunately as common. The main adverse effects are nausea, vomiting, dizziness and lightheadedness, tremors and paraesthesiae.

Recently neutropenia, agranulocytosis thrombocytopenia and aplastic anaemia have been reported. The drug should only be used for life-threatening arrhythmias and weekly blood counts are necessary while patients are on the drug.

Flecainide

A newer class 1c anti-arrhythmic agent of great value in long term therapy of ventricular tachycardia, multifocal ventricular extrasystoles, and reciprocating tachycardias involving accessory pathways (either intranodal or extranodal). It has some value in the management of paroxysmal atrial fibrillation or flutter. Like tocainide it has a long half life (approx 20 hours) and twice daily dosage is adequate. In common with other class 1c drugs, it does not prolong the action potential duration, but prolongs the refractory period in His–Purkinje and accessory by-pass tracts.

Dosage

Oral: 100–200 mg 12 hourly. Maximum daily dose 400 mg. The long-term dose should be reduced if possible, especially in the elderly.

i.v: 0.5–2.0 mg/kg slowly i.v. up to a maximum of 150 mg. Careful ECG monitoring needed if the patient is in VT. Inpatients with poor LV function it is safer to give the drug as a mini-infusion over 30 min.

Side-effects are not common and the drug is generally well tolerated. It is preferable to tocainide. Giddiness, light headedness and blurred vision are the commonest complaints. Like all anti-arrhythmic drugs there is a small number of patients (probably <10%) in whom a pro-arrhythmic effect occurs. It has a mild negative inotropic effect.

Flecainide should be avoided in:
- patients in cardiac failure
- patients with permanent pacing who do not have a programmable unit. The pacing threshold may rise and the pacemaker may need programming to a higher output voltage or pulse-width. A similar increase in pacing voltage may be needed with temporary wires
- 2nd or 3rd degree AV block
- sino-atrial disease

Propafenone
This is another class 1c agent still under evaluation and not yet available in the UK. As with flecainide, it is very valuable in the management of both supra-ventricular and ventricular arrhythmias, as well as those re-entrant arrythmias involving accessory pathway conduction. It blocks retrograde conduction in the accessory pathway.

Bioavailability is 50% and protein binding 90%. Half life is approx 4 hours. The drug is given 8 hourly. Dose: 150–300 mg tds.

Side-effect and contra-indications are similar to flecainide.

Adenosine
This purine nucleotide has a very short half-life (10–15 sec) and appears to be a safe and very effective agent in terminating refractory SVT. Adenosine has a more rapid action than verapamil in SVT but its effect are more transient and the arrhythmia may recur. It is a vasodilator and may have a mild negative inotropic effect. Care is needed in patients with poor LV function. The drug is given is given i.v. as 0.05 mg/kg increments up to 0.25 mg/kg maximum. It has also been effectively used in sick children.

Bretylium tosylate
A drug which tends to be used as a last resort in patients with VT or VF resistant to other anti-arrhythmic therapy. It is only

available i.v. or i.m. Its mode of action is not well understood, but it has both class II and III effects. 80% is excreted unchanged in the urine. Half life is about 8 hours.

Dosage
I.m., 5 mg/kg 8 hourly or 200 mg 2 hourly until the drug works (up to a maximum 2 g). Intravenously: Single bolus of 5 mg/kg for VF.

Side-effects
Hypotension, nausea, nasal stuffiness (sympathetic blockade); parotid pain with prolonged use; patients receiving bretylium should be lying flat, and hypotension (the commonest side-effect) can be reversed by volume loading and a pressor agent if necessary (e.g. phenylephrine).

7 Pericardial disease

7.1 Acute pericarditis

Inflammation of the parietal and visceral layers of the pericardium may be a primary condition or secondary to systemic disease.

Causes

• acute rheumatic fever
• other bacterial infections
• viruses, e.g. Coxackie group, EB virus
• fungal infections: patients on immunosuppressive agents
• uraemia
• trauma, e.g. RTA with steering wheel injury
• collagen vascular disease, particularly SLE, rheumatoid arthritis
• post-myocardial infarction (p. 185) acute
• post-cardiotomy syndrome, Dressler's syndrome (p. 19l)
• malignant disease
• radiotherapy
• hypothyroidism
• many cases are idiopathic

Pericardial pain and other symptoms

Pain is variable in intensity and site. It is usually retrosternal radiating to the neck, left shoulder, back, and around the left scapula. It may be epigastric only. It is often quite sharp in quality unlike the heavy sensation of angina. Its most important characteristics are:

• relation to position. It is relieved by sitting forward and made worse by lying flat, twisting the thorax, or lying on the left side
• relation to respiration. It is frequently worsened by deep inspiration, coughing, etc.

The pain does not necessarily improve as a pericardial effusion develops. Dyspnoea is a common symptom. The patient frequently taking small rapid breaths as any major respiratory movement causes pain.

An enlarging effusion increases dyspnoea. Other symptoms include and depend on associated condition, e.g. fever, dry cough, sweating, arthralgia, rash, pruritus, etc.

Physical signs

Venous pressure may be normal initially, rising as and if an effusion develops. Prominent x descent suggests tamponade (p. 324) may be developing.

Pericardial rub is best heard at the left sternal edge with the patient leaning forward. It is variable with respiration and often transient, coming and going over a few hours. It may be confused with and sound very similar to true cardiac murmurs (e.g. the to and fro murmur of aortic regurgitation). The heart sounds are soft, with a pericardial effusion.

Bronchial breathing at the left base with large effusions compressing the left lower lobe (Ewart's sign).

Signs of tamponade (p. 324).

Investigations

Obviously depend on the suspected aetiology but the list below is an example of the possible difficulties in making a diagnosis

FBC and ESR, U + E, creatinine
ASO titre, anti-DNAse B titre, etc., throat swabs
Blood cultures × 3
Viral titres: acutely and 2 weeks later. Urine + faecal samples
Paul Bunnell screen
Cold agglutinins (*Mycoplasma*)
LE cells, ANF, anti-DNA antibodies, immune complex titres, complement levels
T_4, T_3, TSH
Sputum culture and cytology
Mantoux test
Fungal precipitins
CxR, heart shape and size, lung pathology

ECG
Echocardiogram
Pericardial fluid for culture, Z-N staining, guinea-pig inoculation, cytology, and fungal culture.

ECG changes (p. 389) (Fig. 10.9)
Are often non-specific showing T wave inversion only. 'Saddle shaped' ST segment elevation may occur, and be confused with myocardial infarction, but in pericarditis the ST segment is concave upwards (convex upwards in infarction).

With the development of a pericardial effusion the voltage falls, and with very large effusions electrical alternans may occur.

Echocardiography (p. 423) (Fig. 10.23)
Is most valuable in confirming the presence of an effusion, its site and size. Left ventricular function is assessed regularly for possible deterioration, e.g. associated myocarditis.

Cardiac catheterisation
Is rarely necessary now. RA cineangiography prior to pericardial aspiration will confirm the diagnosis with an obviously thickened pericardium.

Management
Analgesia and bed rest are the main forms of therapy. Soluble aspirin or non-steroidal anti-inflammatory agents are very successful in relieving pain in most cases. A short course of steroids (e.g. 2 weeks) will also work, but care must be taken to follow the patient carefully following cessation of treatment, as the symptoms may recur. Idiopathic benign recurrent pericarditis is treated symptomatically.

Aspiration of the effusion is indicated for diagnosis and/or the relief of symptoms or tamponade. Patients with recurrent effusions not settling on medical treatment should have surgical drainage with a pericardial window and direct histology may be helpful. Specific therapy is necessary for the possible associated condition.

Recurrent loculated effusions may require extensive pericardectomy

7.2 Tamponade

An acute situation which requires quick diagnosis and pericardial aspiration. Patients, if conscious, complain of dyspnoea, a dull central chest pain, facial engorgement, abdominal and ankle swelling. A chronic form of Tamponade does occur.

Acute causes

- myocardial infarction with rupture of ventricular wall
- aortic dissection into pericardial cavity
- Following cardiac surgery
- chest trauma
- following trans-septal puncture at cardiac catheter
- uraemic patients undergoing haemodialysis (and heparinisation)
- malignant disease and/or radiotherapy
- patients on anticoagulants
- associated with acute pericarditis

Chronic pericardial effusion may in addition occur with collagen diseases, Dressler's syndrome, viral, bacterial, or tuberculous pericarditis. Chylous effusions can occur with lymphatic obstruction.

Diagnosis of tamponade should be considered in any patient with a low output state, high venous pressure, oliguria or anuria who is not responding to inotropes.

Physical signs

JVP: Raised with prominent 'x' descent (systolic). Forward flow from the cavae only occurs during ventricular systole. No 'y' descent (Fig.1.1). Inspiratory filling of the neck veins is not common.

BP: Low. May be undetectable on inspiration

Pulse: Low volume

Pulsux paradoxus. An abnormally excessive reduction in pulse volume on inspiration. The exact mechanism is still debated, but increased venous return on inspiration fills the right heart, and left heart filling is less possible with increased RV volume occupying more space in the 'rigid box'. Other factors also contribute (e.g. the normal inspiratory reduction of intra-thoracic pressure transmitted to the aorta, and a relative failure of intra-pericardial pressure to fall much on inspiration). Diaphragmatic traction on pericardium is now thought irrelevant.

Normally there is a slight reduction of systolic pressure on inspiration (e.g. about 5 mmHg). Reduction of systolic pressure of >10 mmHg is suggestive of pulsus paradoxus.

Other causes of pulsus paradoxus are

- constrictive pericarditis (less commonly)
- status asthmaticus (exaggerated pressure swings within the thorax transmitted to the aorta)

Heart sounds: Soft.There may be a pericardial rub in tamponade.

Oliguria or anuria rapidly develops with tamponade, and a brisk diuresis occurs when tamponade is relieved.

Other help in diagnosis

ECG: shows progressive reduction in voltage, and sometimes electrical alternans.

CxR: Shows a symmetrical globular enlargement of the heart.

Echocardiography confirms large pericardial fluid collection (Fig. 10.23, p. 423).

Right atrial cineangiogram: confirms diagnosis but is not necessary now with 2D echocardiography.

Management

Pericardial needle aspiration may be life-saving, but usually is only of temporary benefit. Insertion of a surgical drain or creation of a pericardial window is frequently necessary.

Needle aspiration is best performed via the xiphisternal route with the patient supine using ECG control if screening is not available. The 'V' lead of a standard ECG is attached to the aspiration needle with a crocodile clip. The needle is inserted ½ inch below the xiphisternum and, keeping it horizontal, the tip is rotated 45° to the left (towards the left shoulder tip). The cardiac pulsation can usually be felt at the end of the needle, but if the needle penetrates myocardium itself ST segment elevation occurs ('injury potential').

Pericardial fluid should be sent for cytology if no obvious diagnosis is apparent. Creation of a pericardial window allows a pericardial biopsy to be taken. Removal of even a small amount of fluid from the pericardial sac (e.g. only 50–100 ml) can produce a considerable improvement in haemodynamics as the intrapericardial pressure falls sharply.

Instillation of chemotherapeutic agents is possible in confirmed malignant disease with reaccumulation of fluid (e.g. 5-fluorouracil, nitrogen mustard or ^{32}P). Instilling tetracycline in patients with recurrent malignant pericardial effusions may help obliterate the pericardial space.

7.3 Chronic constrictive pericarditis

Constrictive pericarditis and restrictive cardiomyopathy usually present in a similar way with signs and symptoms of both right-and left-sided heart failure. However there is no history of hypertension, angina is rare, and the heart is not grossly enlarged (as in dilated or congestive cardiomyopathy). Clinically right-sided signs are prominent with marked elevation of venous pressure, hepatomegaly and often ankle oedema or ascites. The cause is often not identified. It is probably the result of haemorrhagic pericarditis resulting in fibrosis with organisation of the exudate.

7.3 Chronic constrictive pericarditis

Possible causes

- viral
- radiotherapy and/or malignancy
- tuberculosis
- collagen/autoimmune disease, rheumatoid arthritis
- other bacterial infections
- rarely uraemia, drugs (procainamide, hydralazine), trauma

Physical signs

JVP: The most important sign is appearance of prominent 'x' and 'y' descents (Fig. 1.1) in the venous pressure. This is an important differential diagnostic point from tamponade. These two prominent descents can be seen even if the patient is in AF. Forward flow occurs during ventricular systole and on tricuspid valve opening. Inspiratory filling of the neck veins may occur (Kussmaul's sign) but it is not a particularly reliable sign.

Pulsus paradoxus: is uncommon in constrictive pericarditis.

Ankle oedema and ascites are common, as is hepatosplenomegaly.

Heart sounds are soft. There may be an early third sound associated with rapid early ventricular filling (pericardial knock). AF is common.

Although the condition is chronic, the development of oedema and ascites may be acute and sudden.

Conditions clinically similar to chronic pericardial constriction

- chronic pericardial effusion (see table on p. 328)
- restrictive cardiomyopathy: amyloidosis, endomyocardial fibrosis, Loffler's eosinophilic endocarditis
- congestive cardiomyopathy (COCM)
- mitral stenosis with pulmonary hypertension and tricuspid regurgitation
- HOCM involving RV and LV

- thromboembolic pulmonary hypertension
- ischaemic CCF

The heart is large in COCM and ischaemic CCF but tends to be smaller or normal in constrictive pericarditis and restrictive cardiomyopathy.

Left ventricular systolic function is usually normal in restrictive cardiomyopathy and often normal in constrictive pericarditis. It grossly reduced in COCM, and ischaemic CCF.

Severe pulmonary hypertension is not a feature of constriction or restriction, but is frequently found in the other conditions listed above.

Cardiac catheterisation may be the only way to reach a definitive diagnosis.

Similarities and differences in tamponade and pericardial constriction

	Tamponade	Constrictive pericarditis
JVP/RA pressure	Prominent 'x' descent	Prominent 'x' and 'y' descents
Kussmaul's sign	Usually absent	May be present
Pulsus paradoxus	Invariable	Not common
Atrial pressures	Equal	Equal
LVEDP/RVEDP	Equal	Equal
Diastolic dip and plateau waveform	Absent	Present

Investigations

Are usually unrewarding. There is little point in viral titres in such a chronic disease. The important point is a vigorous search for tuberculosis, e.g.

- Mantoux, early morning sputum and urine
- ANF, DNA antibodies, rheumatoid factor
- CxR, calcification of the pericardium strongly suggests a

tuberculous aetiology

• Echocardiography shows normal LV size with rapid early filling and diastasis (best seen on posterior wall movement). Cardiac catheterisation is necessary to differentiate the condition from restrictive cardiomyopathy. Atrial pressures are high and equal with prominent x and y descents. LVEDP = RVEDP (or virtually so) at any phase of respiration and both are high. Systolic function is usually normal in constriction, but may be impaired in severe cases (the constricted pericardium may involve the epicardium). There is a typical diastolic plateau waveform in both ventricles (rapid early filling then diastasis) (Fig. 7.1).

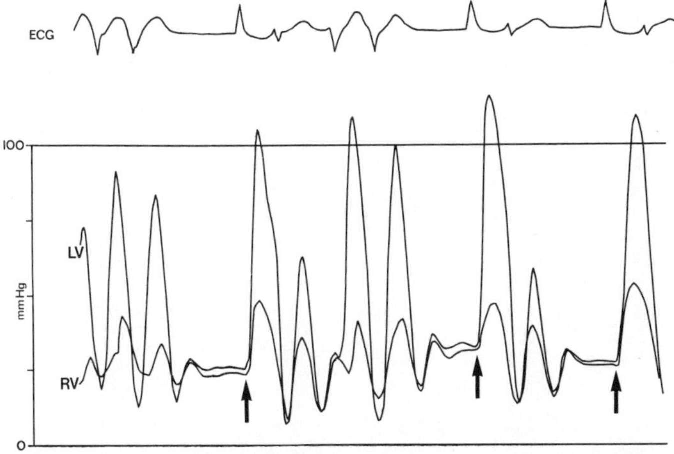

Fig. 7.1 Simultaneous recording of left and right ventricular pressures in chronic constrictive pericarditis. On longer R–R intervals there is a dip and plateau wave-form in diastole. The end-diatolic pressures of both ventricles is high and virtually equal (arrowed). This helps distinguish the condition from restrictive cardiomyopathy.

Management

Although diuretic therapy may be of temporary benefit, pericardectomy is usually necessary. As much of the anterior wall of both ventricles as possible is freed. It is a procedure not without difficulties as the pericardium may be strongly adherent to the epicardial muscle. Freeing the AV groove is important if at all possible. The pericardium should be sent for histology and culture. A year's course of anti-tuberculous therapy may be necessary.

8 Infective endocarditis

8 Infective endocarditis

This is no longer termed sub-acute bacterial endocarditis as non-bacterial organisms are becoming an increasing cause of the condition. Infective endocarditis is a changing disease, but the advent of newer antibiotics has made little effect on mortality figures. The changes in the type of disease are due to several factors:

- the decline in rheumatic fever
- increasing incidence in older patients
- increased survival of patients operated upon for congenital heart disease
- prosthetic valve endocarditis
- different organisms: increasing number of staphylococcal and fungal infections
- antibiotic resistance
- drug addicts with tricuspid valve endocarditis

Overall mortality is still said to run at about 30%. Prosthetic valve endocarditis is now a major therapeutic problem, with a higher mortality (approx 60%), and further surgery usually required as part of the management.

8.1 Predisposing cardiac lesions

These are shown in the table on p. 334. The haemodynamic situation which appears to predispose to infection is a high pressure jet into a lower pressure system through a narrow orifice resulting in endothelial wear and tear. Thus infective endocarditis is much more likely on a VSD than ASD. Bacterial colonisation occurs and platelet, fibrin, and cellular accumulation follows surrounding bacteria in a 'protective cocoon'.

There seems little doubt now that infective endocarditis can occur on a previously normal valve. In spite of this the logistics of antibiotic cover for dental procedures, etc. are such that it is at present advised only for those patients with known predisposing lesions listed above.

Other predisposing factors should also be remembered: patients at higher risk of infection from general medical conditions

8 Infective endocarditis

8.1 Predisposing cardiac lesions

Commonly in	Less commonly in	Virtually never in
Aortic valve disease (Bicuspid or rheumatic)	HOCM and subaortic stenosis	ASD Pulmonary valve stenosis
Mitral valve disease: Regurgitation > stenosis, Floppy valve	Previously normal valve	Divided PDA
Coarctation	Jet lesion AV fistula Mural thrombus e.g post infarct	
Patent ductus arteriosus		
VSD		
Prosthetic valves Tricuspid valve in drug addicts		

(e.g. diabetes, renal failure, haemodialysis, and alcoholism) i.v. drug abusers are also at high risk.

8.2 Portals of entry

This is often unknown, but careful history-taking may reveal one of the following in the previous few months:

• *Dental work* of any type: extraction, fillings, or even scaling. Patients with poor dental hygiene are at risk and this is often the elderly, the immunosuppressed, patients with polycythaemia (congenital heart disease) or gingivitis associated with gum hypertrophy (e.g. phenytoin or nifedipine). Badly fitting dentures or dental braces may also be dangerous. Retained dental roots are a particularly common source of infection and the teeth are still the most common portal of entry.

• *Urinary tract infection*. Cystoscopy. Catheterisation.

• *Respiratory infection*.

• *Enterococci* may gain access to the circulation via carcinoma of the colon, and present with infective endocarditis (e.g. *Streptococcus bovis*). Endoscopy is still contentious. It is unlikely following standard gastroduodenoscopy, or even sigmoidoscopy.

- *Skin disease*. Purulent lesions. Burns.
- *Intravenous cannulation*. This is particularly a problem with CVP lines and may be a cause of infective endocarditis soon after valve replacement. It is particularly likely in patients requiring CVP lines for more than 48 hours and in those with additional medical problems (e.g. jaundice, uraemia, additional steroid treatment). Strict aseptic procedures necessary for all CVP line insertions.
- *Gall bladder disease*
- *Surgery*
- *Abortion*. operative > spontaneous
- *Parturition*. Although a theoretical likely portal of entry this is probably less of a risk factor than once thought.
- I.v. drug abusers
- Fractures

The fact that the portal of entry is often unknown has led to virtually every invasive procedure being incriminated as a possible cause. As a result many probably 'innocent' procedures (e.g. gastroscopy) have been included. Sigmoidoscopy is possibly a cause of bacteraemia, and rectal biopsy should also be covered by antibiotics (see below). Basically all endoscopy procedures should be covered by antibiotics in patients with known predisposing lesions.

8.3 Organisms responsible

Bacterial

- *Streptococcus viridans* group. Still the commonest although less so than in the past. Probably accounts for 50% of cases now.

Streptococcus viridans group now comprises four types: *Streptococcus milleri, S.mutans, S. mitis* and *S. mitior*. *Streptococcus milleri* is present in mouth. gut and vagina.

It tends to form abscesses more frequently than other types.

- Enterococci group. Approx 10% cases.
- *Staphylococcus aureus*
- *Staphylococcus epidermidis* } approx 25% cases
- Diptheroid bacilli
- Microaerophilic streptococci } especially post cardiac surgery
- Much rarer bacterial organisms can cause infective endocarditis, e.g. *Haemophilus aphrophilus* (not *H. influenzae*), *Streptobacillus moniliformis*, anaerobic Gram-negative bacilli (Fusobacterium, bacteroides), Cardiobacterium, *Listeria monocytogenes, Brucella abortus* and many others.
- *Coxiella burneti* (Q fever)
- *Chlamydia psittaci, Chlamydia trachomatis*

Fungal

- *Candida, Aspergillus, Histoplasma*

Other organisms

- ? viral infection (as yet unproven)

8.4 Diagnosis and physical signs

An awareness of the possibility of infective endocarditis is vital as the condition may occur in the absence of a fever or a murmur initially, especially if the patient is elderly or has received recent antibiotic therapy.

Infective endocarditis is also the great mimic, as the wide variety of physical signs may be mistaken for conditions as diverse as a collagen vascular disease, rheumatic fever, a non-specific viral infection, a primary neurological condition, mild haemolytic anaemia, left atrial myxoma, or brucellosis.

Presentation

Typically the condition presents with

- *Signs of infection*: Fever, night sweats, rigors. Weight loss and general malaise. Anaemia is expected. With chronic untreated infection there is additional clubbing and splenomegaly

• *Signs and symptoms of immune complex deposition*: Microscopic haematuria is common and there may be frank glomerulonephritis. A generalised vasculitis can affect any vessel (e.g. brain, skin, kidneys, etc). A toxic encephalopathy may occur. Retinal haemorrhages are common (flame or boat-shaped) Roth spots (boat-shaped haemorrhages with a pale centre) on the retina occur in more fulminating or in untreated cases. Splinter haemorrhages on finger or toe nails. Arthralgia. Osler's nodes–painful pulp infarcts on fingers or toes, or on palms or soles. Janeway lesions–less common than Osler's nodes: Painless flat erythema on palms or soles.

• *Signs of the cardiac lesion*: A new murmur is very significant, as is a change in the nature of an existing murmur. Auscultation daily is necessary in patients with infective endocarditis. Mild aortic or mitral regurgitation may not be audible.

• *Emboli*: These may be followed by abscess formation in the relevant organ. Common sites are; cerebral, retinal, coronary, splenic, mesenteric, renal or femoropopliteal arteries. In patients with right-sided endocarditis pulmonary infarcts are often followed by lung abscesses. A mycotic aneurysm may follow a cerebral embolus and present with subarachnoid haemorrhage. Possibly Osler's nodes have an embolic element also. Large emboli are common in fungal endocarditis. Embolic events may occur during or after antibiotic treatment, even in an apparently 'cured' case. Secondary abscess formation prevents bacteriological cure.

• *Complications of valve destruction or abscess formation*: This may result in increasingly severe valve regurgitation. Abscess formation can result in the dehiscence of the prosthetic valve sewing ring. A septal abscess (e.g. aortic valve endocarditis) produces a long PR interval leading to complete AV block. Aortic root abscesses may produce a sinus of Valsalva aneurysm, or involve the coronary ostia. Large fleshy vegetations may cause valve obstruction (e.g. aortic fungal endocarditis).

• *Left ventricular failure*: This is one of the commonest causes of death in infective endocarditis. Primary involvement of the myocardium occurs with reduction in contractility, and non-specific ST–T wave changes on the ECG. There may be an associated pericardial effusion or even pyopericardium. Left ventricular failure is exacerbated by additional valve dysfunction.

Investigations

• Six blood cultures from different venous sites and at peak fever. Culture-negative cases are usually caused by common bacteria, but those are inaccessible due to the age of the lesion or prior antibiotic treatment.

There is little point in performing arterial or marrow cultures if venous blood cultures are negative. Approximately 20% of cases are culture negative. Blood should also be cultured through a CVP line if there is one *in situ*. The CVP line is then removed and the tip cultured.

• Routine full blood count and ESR. Normally the condition is associated with an anaemia, neutrophil leucocytosis and high ESR. None of these are absolute. A rising haemoglobin and falling ESR are useful signs of therapeutic success. Routine biochemistry, liver function tests, creatinine.

• Microscopy of fresh urine for red cells. Microscopic haematuria is common early in the disease and should regress during treatment. MSU if indicated.

• Swabs of any skin lesion, drip site. Nasal swab.

• Dental x-rays. OPG + special views as indicated.

• ECG and CxR at regular intervals (at least weekly).

• A lengthening PR interval on the ECG suggests an aortic root and septal abscess.

• Weekly echocardiography. Vegetations are not visualised until >3 mm in size (see echocardiography section).

• Immune complex titres.

If initial blood cultures are negative then the following investigations should be considered in addition:

- Q fever antibodies (CFT)
- *Aspergillus* precipitins, fungal cultures
- Culture for L-forms
- *Brucella* agglutinins
- *Candida* antibodies are less helpful: they are elevated in most cases of endocarditis (anamnestic response). A rising titre is more important

8.5 Treatment management

There is nothing to be gained by waiting to see if cultures are positive. If the condition is suspected, and investigations have been performed treatment should start immediately.

If dental extractions are required these are ideally performed at the start of the course of antibiotics. This is not always practical and additional antibiotic cover is usually required in the middle of an established course. Culturing teeth is rarely useful as a large spectrum of oral flora results.

If a systemic embolus occurs it should be cultured and examined for hyphae.

Route

Intravenous therapy is essential initially. The choice rests between central and peripheral lines. Both have their advantages and must be inserted with strict aseptic techniques.

The central line (subclavian or internal jugular) should be changed weekly. The best central line is a tunnelled subclavian inserted via the infra-clavicular route. The tunnel helps prevent spread of infection from the skin entry site. The catheter should be soft, pliable, and not reach as far as the right atrium. The catheter in RA or SVC may cause infected mural thrombus. A stiff central line in the right atrium may perforate the wall. The central line skin entry site should be covered by a steri-drape (e.g. 'Op-site'). Covering with other dressings is not advised and povidone iodine on the entry site does not prevent infection.

Peripheral lines are less dangerous but more inconvenient

and painful. The peripheral line should be changed every 72 hours if possible even if the vein has not thrombosed. This helps preserve the life of peripheral veins. The arm is immobilised, dilute antibiotic solution is used, and a heparin flush (500 units in 5 ml 5% dextrose) given after each infusion helps preserve the vein.

The giving set should be changed daily with either system.

Length of course

There is no definite length of course and this depends on response, patient tolerance, and access availability. The following are suggested minimal lengths of courses:

- *Streptococcus viridans* group on native valve, 6 weeks
- *Staphylococcus epidermidis*, 2 months
- Prosthetic valve endocarditis, 2 months
- *Staphylococcus aureus*, 3 months
- Q fever endocarditis, 3 months followed by indefinite oral therapy
- Fungal endocarditis, 3 months initially

These figures are for intravenous therapy. If valve replacement is necessary the course follows surgery.

Choice of antibiotic regime

Guidance from the bacteriologist is essential and depends on the sensitivity of the organism. Antibiotic levels are necessary to check both the dose and the risk of toxicity (especially with the aminoglycosides and antifungal agents).

Plasma antibiotic levels are measured at trough (pre-dose) and peak (15 min post i.v. dose).

Minimum inhibitory concentration (MIC) is estimated and provides a guide to dosage and drug choice. Therapy should aim to reach trough levels of at least 10 × MIC. In *Streptococcus viridans* infection if MIC is > 0.01 mg/litre then the addition of an aminoglycoside to penicillin should be considered.

Do not stop an antibiotic if the temperature fails to settle in a few days. This may take 2 weeks, even with drug-sensitive organisms. Persistent fever may be an indication to add a second antibiotic.

A bactericidal antibiotic is used except in rare circumstances: tetracycline therapy in Q fever endocarditis, and high dose erythromycin if there is penicillin and cephalosporin allergy. Probenecid is no longer used to raise plasma penicillin levels.

The clinical response is a most useful guide to therapy. The regimes set out below are the doses suggested in a 70 kg adult with normal renal function. Doses must be reduced in smaller patients, elderly patients, and those with renal failure. It will be seen that high doses of penicillin are recommended (12 g/day ≡ 20 mega units/day).

Streptococcus viridans group
Benzyl penicillin 3 g i.v. 6 hourly. Add gentamicin if organism is less sensitive, and MIC is > 0.01 mg/L.

Streptococcus faecalis and culture-negative endocarditis
Benzyl penicillin 3 g i.v. 6 hourly
Gentamicin 80 mg i.v. 8 hourly initially.

Staphylococcus epidermidis
Benzyl penicillin 3 g i.v. 6 hourly or flucloxacillin 2 g i.v. 6 hourly (depending on sensitivities), plus fusidic acid 500 mg i.v. 8 hourly. Gentamicin may be added if necessary. *Staphylococcus* is not a 'benign' endocarditis and should not be treated with a single drug.

Staphylococcus aureus
Flucloxacillin 2–4 g i.v. 6 hourly
Fusidic acid 500 mg i.v. 8 hourly
Gentamicin 80 mg i.v. 8 hourly initially.

Gram-negative organisms
Ampicillin 2–4 g i.v. 6 hourly
Gentamicin 80 mg i.v. 8 hourly initially
Metronidazole 500 mg i.v. 8 hourly is added for uncontrolled anaerobic organisms (e.g. Fusobacterium, or Bacteroides endocarditis).

Q fever (*Coxiella burneti*)
Tetracycline 500 mg i.v. 12 hourly followed by indefinite oral therapy.

Candida albicans or other yeast organisms
5-fluorocytosine (Flucytosine) 3 g i.v. 6 hourly. (50 mg/kg 6 hourly). If resistant cases of *Candida* are encountered or this fails add amphotericin B 250 µg/kg/day initially, increasing if renal function is satisfactory. Miconazole 600 mg i.v. 8 hourly is an alternative if renal function is poor.

Aspergillus or other non-yeast fungi
Amphotericin B 250 µg/kg/day i.v. or miconazole 600 mg i.v. 8 hourly if poor renal function. In most cases of fungal endocarditis it is probably better to use two drugs.

Antimicrobial side-effects and other problems
Penicillin
Allergy (fever, urticaria, arthralgia, rash); angioneurotic oedema; interstitial nephritis; sodium loading; encephalopathy; hypokalaemlc alkalosis; neutropenia.

The last four are dose-dependent side-effects, usually quickly reversible on stopping the drug. They are rare, and are possible if > 24 g/day penicillin is used. With a history of penicillin allergy there is roughly a 10% chance of cross-sensitivity to cephalosporins.

Fusidic acid
Nausea and vomiting, jaundice and hepatotoxicity, microbial resistance.

Nausea and vomiting are very common, even with i.v. therapy, and may make the drug impossible to use. Liver damage is reversible if the drug is stopped early. Microbial resistance develops quickly if the drug is used alone.

Aminoglycosides
Ototoxicity, nephrotoxicity.
About 10% of patients on these drugs develop VIIIth nerve damage. If long-term treatment is required weekly audiometry is essential with calorics to detect early damage. Either the vestibular or auditory component may be damaged first or in isolation. High frequency deafness may occur early without the patient noticing any side-effects. Beware the patient using the drip pole as a support, concealing ataxia. The suggested dose schedule is shown below. Doses are reduced in renal impairment.

Nephrotoxicity is exacerbated by concomittant use of frusemide, ethacrynic acid, cephaloridine and possibly some other cephalosporins. Frequent tests of renal function are necessary (serum creatinine three times per week). The urine is tested daily for protein, and urine microscopy performed to look for casts at regular intervals.

Guide to gentamicin dosage
• Adults with normal renal function: 160 mg i.v. initially followed by 80 mg i.v. 8 hourly. Maximum dose is 5 mg/kg/day.
• Children with normal renal function: 3 mg/kg i.v. initially followed by 2 mg/kg i.v. 8 hourly.
• With renal impairment the dose is reduced. Until drug levels are known the dose is regulated corresponding to blood urea levels:

7–17 mmol/l: 80 mg 12 hourly
17–33 mmol/l: 80 mg daily

> 33 mmol/l: 80 mg alternate days

• Drug levels. Blood for these is taken from the opposite arm if a peripheral line is used. They are performed initially on the 3rd day of treatment.

Trough level: taken just prior to gentamicin dose. The trough level is the most important measurement of all and must always be < 2 μg/ml. Levels of 2–5 μg/ml mean drug accumulation and the dose interval should be increased.

Peak level: Taken 15 min after i.v. dose. The level should be < 10 μg/ml. Preferably 6–10 μg/ml. The dose is reduced if the level exceeds this.

It is safest to restrict gentamicin therapy to just the first 2 weeks of treatment if possible.

Other drugs of great value in bacterial cases

1 *Amikacin*: In gentamicin-resistant cases. 15 mg/kg/day in 2 doses 12 hourly.

2 *Tobramycin*: In mild renal impairment, as it is less nephrotoxic than gentamicin. Up to 5 mg/kg/day in 3 doses 8 hourly (similar to gentamicin).

3 *Vancomycin*: In any degree of uraemia. May be used as a single antibiotic. Maximum adult dose 2 g/day. Start with 500 mg i.v. 6 hourly. May be reduced to as little as 1 g/week in uraemia associated with endocarditis. Infusion may cause histamine release and the red man syndrome.

4 *Rifampicin*: Not just an anti-tuberculous drug, but toxicity in 20% cases: Shock, renal failure, thrombocytopenia, hepatotoxicity, influenzal and respiratory symptoms. Oral therapy 450–600 mg daily before breakfast.

5 *Netilmicin*: This drug is less ototoxic than gentamicin or tobramycin and may supersede both. Dose for average size adult with normal renal function: 150 mg i.v. 12 hourly (total 4–6 mg/kg/day).

Second line drugs

1 *Lincomycin and clindamycin*: Very effective staphylococcal (and some anaerobic) infections. Pseudomembranous colitis limits their use. If it develops vancomycin is effective given orally.
2 *Cephalosporin group*: May be useful in penicillin hypersensitivity. Nephrotoxicity a reputed problem with many and concomitant aminoglycoside use best avoided.
3 *Erythromycin*: Bacteriostatic in low doses. May be useful in penicillin hypersensitivity.
4 *Chloramphenicol*: Best avoided in long courses unless desperate. Causes leucopenia, thrombocytopenia, irreversible aplastic anaemia, peripheral and optic neuritis, gut side-effects, erythema multiforme.

Monitoring therapy effects

1 Daily patient examination. The most important of all to detect new signs.
2 Daily weight.
3 6 hourly temperature chart.
4 Daily urine testing. Microscopy for RBCs and casts.
5 FBC, U + E, and LFTs twice weekly as minimum. A steady or rising haemoglobin and falling ESR are good signs. The ESR is often the last variable to return to normal after a long antibiotic course in infective endocarditis. It may only return to normal a month or so after the course has finished.
6 Antibiotic drug levels.
7 Weekly echocardiogram. Although vegetations are frequently not seen on the echo, a gradual change in valve configuration may be detected.

8.6 Other interventions and infective endocarditis

Anticoagulants and endocarditis

This is controversial with the risk of haemorrhage at the site of embolus impaction (e.g. mycotic embolus and subarachnoid

Nephrotoxicity guide with antibiotic use in endocarditis

	Renal excretion	Site of damage	? Use in renal disease
Penicillin G	90% proximal tubular secretion	*Rare* Hypokalaemic alkalosis Hypersensitivity Interstitial nephritis	Yes with dose reduction 1–2 g 6 hourly
Gentamicin	All glomerular filtration	Tubular necrosis 2–10% Binds to renal tissue	Yes with great care taking drug levels. Cephalosporins probably best avoided
Tobramycin	All glomerular filtration	Tubular necrosis in 1–2% Less than gentamicin	Safer than gentamicin in renal damage
Vancomycin	80% renal excretion	None	Yes with dose reduction levels, from 1 g/day to 1 g/week
Amikacin	95% renal excretion	Probably similar to gentamicin	As with gentamicin levels
Cephalothin	70–80% renal excretion	Tubular necrosis	Aminoglycosides probably best avoided. Care in renal disease
Cephaloridine	85% renal excretion	Tubular necrosis	Avoid
Tetracyclines	Principally renal excretion	'Antianabolic effect' increases uraemia Old tetracyclines: Fanconi syndrome	Avoid (except doxycycline)
Fusidic acid	Principally biliary excretion	None in kidney	Yes, no dose adjustment necessary
Amphotericin B	Slow renal excretion	Reduces renal blood flow (arteriolar constriction) Nephrocalcinosis, Tubular damage. RTA. Potassium wasting	Reduce dose (e.g. 0.25 mg/kg alternate days)

haemorrhage). Anticoagulation does not prevent the development of vegetations.

It is best reserved for: patients with prosthetic (non-tissue) valves, pelvic vein thrombosis or gross DVT, pulmonary embolism. Patients with mixed mitral valve disease and endocarditis already on anticoagulants should be continued on anticoagulants with a control BCR of 2:1 approximately.

Cardiac catheterisation

This is usually not necessary and was once thought to be absolutely contra-indicated with the risk of dislodging friable vegetations. However it may be useful in cases of aortic valve endocarditis with suspected abscess formation to get more information of the anatomy of the root by an aortogram with the catheter well above the valve. Also the significance of mitral regurgitation in the course of infective endocarditis may require cardiac catheterisation with left ventricular angiography. Intravenous digital subtraction angiography of the aortic root can provide information about possible aortic root abscesses.

Indications for surgical intervention

- aortic or mitral regurgitation not responding quickly to medical therapy
- development of an aneurysm of the sinus of Valsalva
- lengthening P-R interval and development of a septal abscess
- failure of antibiotic therapy to control the infection
- relapse of infection after a full medical course of antibiotics
- valve obstruction with large fleshy vegetations
- fungal endocarditis usually responds best to valve replacement and antifungal therapy

If possible a few days' antibiotics are given prior to surgery, but in very severe cases this may be only a few doses.

After valve replacement for infective endocarditis a full course of medical therapy should be given, of a length detailed earlier.

8.7 Prevention of infective endocarditis

Much of the evidence on which recommendations are made is based on animal work. The American Heart Association's recommendations of 1977 have been modified to allow a simpler regime which is more likely to be followed. This prophylaxis is necessary for:

- any dental work
- any surgical procedure
- cystoscopy and urinary tract instrumentation
- prostatic biopsy (transrectal)
- insertion of permanent pacemakers

Prophylaxis is not necessary prior to cardiac catheterisation. There is no hard evidence that it is necessary prior to gastroscopy or sigmoidoscopy but is advisable. It is usually used prior to rectal or colonic biopsy and also prior to delivery.

It is safer to advise patients to have antibiotic prophylaxis prior to every dental appointment. If several visits to the dentist are required it is easier if these are spaced out over several months. The same antibiotic should not be used twice within a month to cover dental visits. The regime is shown in the table.

8.8 Non-infective endocarditis

Non-infective thrombotic endocarditis (marantic endocarditis)

Non-infective vegetations may occur on heart valves. This is sometimes called marantic endocarditis. They may, if large, be identified on echocardiography (> 5mm in size) and may embolise. These vegetations occur in:

- mucinous adenocarcinomas of pancreas and upper gastrointestinal tract
- other malignant disease, e.g. bladder, lung and lymphomas
- associated with a thrombotic tendency, and peripheral microthrombi in small vessels in adult respiratory distress syndrome

Dental or surgical prophylaxis for infective endocarditis

Type of case procedure	Not sensitive to penicillin	Penicillin hypersensitivity
Dental treatment for rheumatic or congenital heart disease under local anaesthetic	*Amoxycillin* 3 g sachet orally on an empty stomach 1 hour before the procedure. A second 3 g dose is given 8 hours after the procedure. For children age 5–10 use 1.5 g	*Erythromycin stearate* 1.5 g orally 1 hour pre-dentistry followed by 500 mg 6 hourly for two doses
Dental treatment for rheumatic or congenital heart disease requiring general anaesthesia	*Triple penicillin* (Triplopen) 1 vial i.m. about 20–30 min before the procedure. No other dose necessary	*Erythromycin lactobionate* 1 g i.v. just before the procedure followed by erythromycin stearate 500 mg 6 hourly for 2 doses or *Vancomycin* 1 g slowly i.v. 30 min before the procedure. No other dose necessary
Patients with prosthetic heart valves needing dental treatment or any patient at risk needing gut or urinary tract surgery	*Triple penicillin* 1 vial i.m. plus *gentamicin* 80 mg i.m. 20 min before the procedure, followed by gentamicin 80 mg i.m. 8 hourly for 2 doses	*Vancomycin* 1 g slowly i.v. plus *gentamicin* 80 mg i.m. 20–30 min before the procedure

In cases with malignant disease there may be an associated migratory thrombophlebitis, disseminated intravascular coagulation and microangiopathic haemolytic anaemia. Often the condition is only discovered at autopsy.

Libman–Sacks endocarditis

This has been called an active 'verrucous' endocarditis with verrucae or vegetations commonly affecting the aortic or mitral valves, chordae, papillary muscles and ventricular endocardium. It occurs as part of the spectrum of organ involvement of systemic lupus erythematosus (SLE) and rarely scleroderma. As with non-infective thrombotic endocarditis valve regurgitation is uncommon and the condition may only be appreciated at autopsy. Valve cusps contain a large amount of mucopolysaccharide and it has been suggested this is due to steroid therapy.

Although aortic and mitral valves are more commonly affected the tricuspid valve may also be involved. Very occasionally valve replacement is indicated.

9 Other important cardiac conditions

9.1 Pulmonary hypertension (PHT)

Pulmonary hypertension exists when the PA pressure exceeds 30/20 mmHg. This is due either to an increase in flow through the pulmonary vascular bed, or to a reduction in calibre of pulmonary arterioles.

Common causes

- left atrial hypertension: aortic and mitral valve disease, ischaemic heart disease, congestive cardiomyopathy, hypertrophic cardiomyopathy
- chronic pulmonary disease: chronic bronchitis and emphysema, pulmonary fibrosis
- chronic thrombo-embolism
- high flow—reactive PHT, e.g ASD, VSD, PDA

Rare causes

- primary pulmonary hypertension
- left atrial conditions: myxoma, cor-triatriatum
- pulmonary veno-occlusive disease, pulmonary vein stenoses
- peripheral pulmonary artery branch stenoses
- chronic hypoxia: pickwickian syndrome, high altitude, pharyngeal obstruction, neuromuscular disorders, e.g. polio, myasthenia
- restrictive cardiomyopathy and constrictive pericarditis

There is a considerable fall in pulmonary vascular resistance in the first 24 hours of life when the ductus closes and the PVR continues to fall for the first few months.

Chronic PHT is associated with intimal thickening ('onion' skinning) of pulmonary arterioles, and medial hypertrophy in larger arteries. Vessels may be totally occluded by the endothelial proliferation and secondary thrombosis occurs.

Variability of PHT

Various factors may alter pulmonary artery pressure and these are relevant to treatment. The most important is the role of oxygen in regulating pulmonary vascular tone.

Increasing PHT	Decreasing PHT
Hypoxia, high altitude	Oxygen
Acidosis	Acetyl choline
Hypercapnia	Hydralazine
High haematocrit	α-blocking agents
Prostaglandin $F_2\alpha$ and A_2	Prostaglandin E and I_2
? Histamine	Pirbuterol
α-agonists	Calcium antagonists
	Nitrates

High haematocrit is important in patients with cyanotic congenital heart disease and Eisenmenger syndrome.

9.2 Pulmonary embolism

Symptoms

- dyspnoea. Acute onset dyspnoea is typical. In retrospect mild dyspnoea may precede the acute attack by a day or two. In a few cases dyspnoea presents as acute bronchospasm
- pain. Sudden onset pleuritic chest pain probably occurs with smaller emboli. Involvement of the diaphragmatic pleura causes shoulder tip pain. Pain may be primarily abdominal
- cough. Persistent dry cough is common
- haemoptysis. Streaky or frank. Haemoptysis may persist with resolution of the infarcted segment
- sweating, fear and apprehension
- syncope occurs with massive pulmonary embolism. Overall mortality is approximately 8–10%

Signs

A restless, centrally cyanosed, sweaty, distressed and dyspnoeic patient.
JVP raised with prominent 'a' wave if in SR.

Tachycardia, low volume pulse, transient rhythm disturbance.
RV: $S_{3/4}$ gallop
Accentuated delayed P_2
Fever
Chest signs: rales, later a pleural rub.
Leg signs: only about one-third of patients have evidence of DVT with phlebitis, oedema, etc.
Cardiac arrest and sudden death.

Many of these signs are non-specific and a high index of suspicion should be maintained for patients at risk, e.g.

- history of previous DVTs
- patients on prolonged bed rest
- post-myocardial infarction (p. 186)
- patients on diuretics—haemoconcentration
- patients with CCF—low flows
- post-operative patients: especially pelvic, prostatic hip and leg surgery
- polycythaemic patients
- pelvic inflammatory or malignant disease

Smaller pulmonary emboli may be missed clinically, presenting as a flick in the temperature chart, mild dyspnoea and transient AF, SVT or just ventricular ectopic beats.

ECG changes (not specific for pulmonary embolism)

Typical acute right ventricular strain shows as: S_1 Q_3 T_3 pattern in standard leads, incomplete or complete RBBB, T wave inversion in anterior chest leads (see Fig. 10.8).

Other possibilities to note are: right axis shift. Rhythm changes: ectopic—atrial or ventricular, AF or SVT. ST–T changes with ST depression over inferior leads.

All these changes may be transient.

CxR changes

There may be very little to see on the CxR of patients with small pulmonary emboli.

Features to look for include in the acute stage: elevated hemi-diaphragm, pulmonary oligaemia in one or more segments, large pulmonary artery conus, or enlargement of a single hilar artery with rapid pruning or tapering.

Later on (24 hours – 1 week) if pulmonary infarction occurs the CxR may show: pulmonary infiltrates, plate atelectasis, small pleural effusions or pleural thickening.

Superadded infection in an infarcted segment may cause cavitation.

Making the diagnosis

This may be difficult. Small emboli may be easily missed. Diagnosis is based on:

- patient at risk
- history and physical signs
- ECG
- CxR
- *blood gases:* The PaO_2 should be <80 mmHg due to ventilation/perfusion (V/Q) mismatch. Large pulmonary emboli result in severe hypoxia, hypocapnia and metabolic acidosis—a 'mixed' picture
- *ventilation/perfusion scan:* This is a useful test for recurrent small emboli which may be missed by pulmonary angiography. The ventilation scan must be normal. The diagnosis is difficult in the presence of chronic obstructive airways disease, severe emphysema or bronchopneumonia. Segmental perfusion defects in the presence of normal ventilation scan are strongly suggestive of pulmonary emboli.

Tomography of the perfusion study in various planes is useful. The CxR should be available to the interpreter of the scan. Follow up scans may show rapid resolution of the perfusion defects due to lysis of the thrombus.

- *pulmonary angiography:* This is generally performed in the sicker patient in whom the diagnosis is still uncertain or who will probably require streptokinase therapy as the catheter can be left in the PA for 48–72 hours following angiography if necessary.

Angiograms should show vessel 'cut offs' or obvious filling defects in the artery. There should be segmental filling defects in addition. Chronic thromboembolic pulmonary hypertensive patients will have large proximal arteries with tortuous distal vessels with peripheral pruning.

Investigations of less value

- *cardiac enzymes.* Pulmonary infarction causes elevation of LDH and sometimes SGOT (aspartate aminotransferase) and bilirubin
- *leg venograms,* ^{125}I fibrinogen scanning, Doppler ultrasonography. Tests to document peripheral leg vein thrombus merely prove an association. They cannot make a diagnosis of pulmonary emboli.

Differential diagnosis

The commonest condition to be confused with acute pulmonary embolism is inferior myocardial infarction. Both cause chest pain, elevated neck veins and similar ECG changes. Transmural inferior infarction causes ST segment elevation, and pulmonary embolism more commonly causes ST segment depression in inferior leads. Patients with inferior infarcts are generally not dyspnoeic.

Other causes of pulmonary hypertension should be considered.

9.3 Management of pulmonary embolism

The acute attack is managed with anticoagulation, and thrombolytic therapy in more severe cases. Pulmonary embolectomy is rarely necessary. Attention is then focused on preventive measures.

General measures

Oxygen and analgesia are usually required. The severe apprehension associated with large pulmonary emboli will require opiate analgesia.

Volume loading. In more severe cases plasma or colloid substitutes should be given even with a raised venous pressure. This may help increase right ventricular stroke volume in severely compromised patients. Start with 500 ml plasma and repeat if necessary.

Anticoagulation

This is all that is required with mild-to-moderate embolisation as natural lysis occurs in the lung spontaneously. Heparin is not directly thrombolytic.

Heparin 10 000 units i.v. stat followed by heparin 5000 units i.v. 2–4 hourly. A continuous infusion of heparin probably reduces bleeding complications (dose = 1000 units/hour). After one week if no further emboli have occurred then oral anticoagulants are started and the heparin stopped two days later. Heparin dose is monitored by thrombin time estimations. Oral anticoagulants are continued for 3 months only in the first instance unless there are recurrent emboli.

Recurrent emboli are rare in patients treated with anticoagulation alone.

Thrombolytic therapy

This is reserved for more serious cases who appear unlikely to survive 24–48 hours or who have two or more lobar arteries occluded on angiography.

Thrombolytic therapy has been shown to resolve emboli faster than heparin, to lower the pulmonary artery pressure more than heparin and appearances on repeat pulmonary angiography and lung scanning show greater improvement with thrombolytic therapy than with heparin.

The improvement is greatest with massive pulmonary emboli. No trial has shown a greater reduction in mortality of thrombolytic therapy over heparin.

Urokinase is more expensive than streptokinase, but may be necessary if streptokinase reactions occur (fever, rashes and allergic reactions are more common with streptokinase).

Prior to streptokinase therapy blood is taken for the following tests: full blood count, haematocrit; platelet count; PT, PTT; thrombin time; fibrinogen titre and FDPs. Tests are repeated during therapy (every 4 hours if possible).

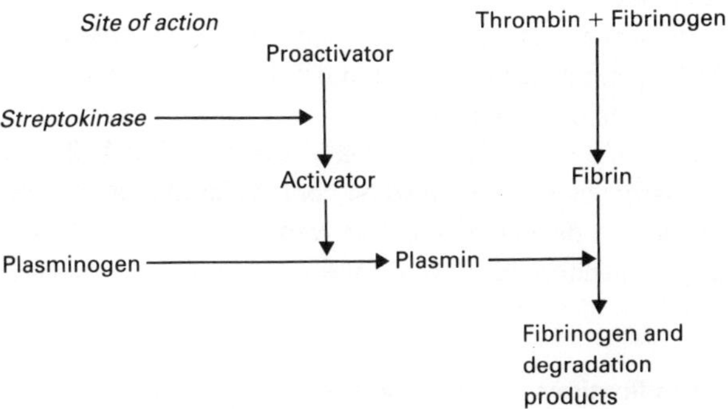

Streptokinase dose (Kabikinase, Streptase)
Hydrocortisone 100 mg i.v. stat. Streptokinase 250 000 units in 100 ml N saline infused into PA over 30 min. Then: streptokinase 100 000 units hourly up to 72 hours maximum. Heparin is then gradually restarted over the next 12 hours.

The streptokinase dose is controlled by the fibrinogen titre. A titre falling below 1:4 in saline may require a decrease in streptokinase dose (e.g. by 50 000 units/hour). The thrombin time should be prolonged by 2–4 times normal value.

The main control however is the clinical state. Prolonged thrombin times do not predict bleeding complications.

Complications of streptokinase

• Allergic reactions are common. Rise in temperature is expected; rashes, and pruritus are common. Nausea, vomiting, flushing and headaches may occur. Acute hypotension may occur with the first dose. Hydrocortisone and volume replacement are necessary.

• Bleeding complications. Local bleeding at catheter entry sites is expected, and a fall in haemoglobin is common on treatment. Heparin increases the bleeding risk. Pressure on a local bleeding site is all that is generally necessary. A pledget soaked in EACA may help.

Streptokinase is stopped with major bleeding complications and fibrinogen replacement started (fresh frozen plasma, cryoprecipitate or fresh blood).

The effects on stopping are usually reversed after 1–2 hours when emergency surgery could be contemplated if absolutely necessary. In a desperate situation with continued bleeding fibrinolytic inhibitors (EACA) or kallikrein inactivator (Trasylol) can be tried.

Contra-indications to streptokinase

See **5.9**.

Urokinase (Abbokinase, Ukidan)

If this is available and streptokinase has produced unacceptable side-effects or there has been a known recent streptococcal illness, urokinase can be substituted (it is not antigenic).
Urokinase 4400 i.u./kg/hour infusion over 12 hours.
Approximately 15 ml solution/hour, up to 200 ml.

Fibrin specific thrombolytic agents (see **5.9**)

rt-Pa and APSAC are two fibrin specific thrombolytic agents with fewer bleeding complications than streptokinase. Used primarily for coronary thrombolysis, they should be considered in patients with large pulmonary emboli who have had streptokinase in the last 6 months.

Pulmonary embolectomy

This is rarely necessary. It carries a high mortality (23–57%) in various series especially if the operation is performed very early. (Two-thirds of patients who die from PE do so in the first 2 hours anyway.) Surgical mortality is lower if no cardiac arrest has occurred.

It should be considered in patients with cardiogenic shock who: have had 1 hour maximum medical therapy; in whom streptokinase is contra-indicated; are unlikely to survive the next hour.

Cardiac massage should be prolonged in an arrest due to massive pulmonary embolism as it may help to fragment the thrombus. Pulmonary embolectomy can only remove large proximal thrombus, while streptokinase may in addition deal with smaller peripheral thrombi.

Prevention of pulmonary emboli

Low dose subcutaneous heparin has been shown in several trials to prevent pulmonary emboli following surgery (e.g. 5000 units s.c. 2 hours pre-operatively, then 5000 units s.c. 8 hourly for 7 days). A combination of dextran 70 given at the end of surgery plus the use of pneumatic leggings has also been shown to reduce post-operative pulmonary emboli. Early mobilisation is vital.

Most cases of recurrences of pulmonary emboli will be prevented by oral anticoagulants.

Various operations on the IVC below the renal veins have attempted to prevent PE (plication, ligation, filters, umbrellas, etc.). This is only of temporary benefit as large collateral channels rapidly develop. It may be life-saving in rare instances.

9.4 Anticoagulants in pregnancy

Heparin does not cross the placenta, however coumarin derivatives cross the placenta and are teratogenic. In addition there is a risk of fetal haemorrhage induced by birth trauma.

However subcutaneous or intravenous heparin throughout pregnancy is impractical. Long term i.v. heparin can cause osteoporosis. A compromise regime is generally accepted.

First trimester: Heparin s.c. The mother can be taught to administer this herself (10 000 units bd)
12th—37th week: oral anticoagulants. Aim to keep BCR (prothrombin time ratio) 2–2.5
37th week to 6 hours before delivery: heparin. 10 000 units 12 hourly s.c.)
6 hours post-delivery: restart heparin
48 hours post-delivery: switch to oral anticoagulants.

The baby will be bottle-fed as coumarin derivatives appear in the breast milk. Alternatively vitamin K supplements will be necessary.

This regime should prevent haemorrhagic complications to the fetus, and the teratogenic effects of warfarin in the first trimester. This is a complex regime. It may be felt reasonable to accept the teratogenic effect of warfarin and use it throughout pregnancy. The risk of spontaneous abortion on warfarin is high, and the chance of having a live deformed baby are probably 10–30%.

9.5 Primary pulmonary hypertension

Is fortunately rare as there is no specific treatment for a completely idiopathic disease. It is more common in women.

Factors implicated include: chronic small pulmonary emboli; collagen vascular disease (association with Raynaud's phenomenon); allergic vasculitis (drugs, polyarteritis nodosa); drugs—aminorex fumarate (anorexic agent); bush tea—*Crotalaria fulva* alkaloid ingestion by West Indians; hormonal influences (female sex predominance, association with the pill, etc.); association with cirrhosis.

Symptoms are similar to patients with pulmonary emboli. Signs to note are: prominent 'a' wave in JVP; RV heave (left parasternal); RV. S_4; S_3 in later stages; palpable pulmonary artery pulsation in second left interspace; pulmonary ejection click, soft systolic ejection murmur and accentuated P_2; signs of RV failure. Secondary tricuspid regurgitation.

Management

The condition is usually fatal within 3 years of making the diagnosis. Patients should be anticoagulated.

Acetylcholine infusion into the pulmonary artery lowers the pressure. On the basis of this vasodilators have been tried, but all lower systemic vascular as well as pulmonary vascular resistance. Hydralazine, diazoxide and phenotolamine have all been reported as successful in a few cases. Recent reports however suggest hydralazine may be harmful and care is needed in its use. Nifedipine and diltiazem have been used with limited success. Intravenous prostacyclin (PGI_2) is expensive, but can be used intermittently or as a low dose continuous infusion. It successfully lowers pulmonary vascular resistance. In severe cases it buys time prior to heart–lung transplantation which offers the only hope for long-term survival.

Spontaneous improvement is very rare but does occur.

9.6 Systemic hypertension

Definition

Blood pressure rises with age, with cold environment or anxiety, with effort, and varies with the time of day (lowest at 4.00 am rising rapidly by 9.00 am). With mild hypertension the blood pressure (BP) is taken twice or more before calling a patient 'hypertensive'. With more severe hypertension this is not necessary. Systolic and diastolic pressure are of equal importance.

9.6 Systemic hypertension

Age	Normal	Borderline	Definite
17–40	<140/90	150/95	>160/100
41–50	<150/90	160/95	>160/100
60+	<160/90	165/95	>170/100

Pitfalls in measurement

A long cuff is needed to encircle the arm. Too small a cuff or too fat an arm records spuriously high readings. Patient should be calm having had five minutes rest, and no preceding coffee or cigarette. Korotkow phase 4 (muffling) is probably better than phase 5 (disappearance). In UK phase 4 is recorded. In USA phase 5 is recorded. Check BP in both arms on first occasion.

Beware digit preference: random zero equipment avoids this problem.

Significance of hypertension

Hypertension is associated with an increased risk of CVA, cardiac failure, myocardial infarction, occlusive peripheral arterial disease and renal failure. Each increment of 10 mmHg systolic pressure reduces life expectancy. Successful BP control reduces mortality from CVA and renal failure (but not definitely myocardial infarct deaths).

Mild hypertension should be treated even if there is no organ damage.

Typical symptoms

Headache: frontal or occipital are typically worse in the morning. May have migraine. Dyspnoea on effort progressing to orthopnoea or PND. Angina (increase muscle mass + coronary disease) and/or claudication. Nocturia even if off diuretics. Possibly haematuria and/or dysuria in history. History of transient ischaemic attacks. Mild visual disturbance. Epistaxes.

Signs to note

BP in both arms. Synchrony of radial and femoral pulses. Check all peripheral pulses. Arterial bruits: carotid, aortic, renal. LV hypertrophy. ? S_3 present. Fundal examination: AV nipping, haemorrhages, exudates, papilloedema.

Causes

- essential: 95% of cases
- renal disease, glomerulonephritis, pyelonephritis, polycystic disease, hydronephrosis
- renal artery stenosis (atheromatous plaques or fibromuscular hyperplasia)
- coarctation of the aorta
- phaeochromocytoma
- primary hyperaldosteronism (Conn's syndrome)
- Cushing's syndrome
- iatrogenic drug therapy: glucocorticoids, carbenoxolone, MAO inhibitors, sympathomimetics, oestrogens
- acromegaly
- hypercalcaemia
- CNS disturbances: raised intracranial pressure, familial dysautonomia
- post-operative: especially cardiopulmonary bypass
- pre-eclampsia

Investigations

Almost all patients will have essential hypertension (? family history) and the necessary investigations are: FBC, U & E, creatinine (preferably U & E off diuretics). Urine testing: protein, blood, sugar (if positive, urine culture) CxR, ECG.

A routine IVP is not necessary. It should be considered in patients with a history of renal disease and in those who are most likely to have renovascular hypertension:

- onset of hypertension under the age of 30 years

• accelerated hypertension or rapidly deteriorating renal function
• hypertension after renal trauma, or an episode of renal pain
• presence of a renal bruit

The estimation of 24-hour urine VMA is expensive and the test should be done in all cases of hypertension + glycosuria, patients with a history of paroxysmal hypertension, sweating, palpitations, episodes of hypotension, or the young patient. Three 24-hour urine VMAs are required with the patient on a vanilla-free diet and preferably off all drugs (normal range up to 35 μmol/24 hours). Urine saves must be done before the IVP.

Renovascular hypertension

Features suggesting this on an IVP are a disparity of renal size by >2 cm, delayed appearance of dye on the affected side with increased density of dye later on that side. With a positive IVP the following investigations may be necessary to confirm that the abnormal kidney is the cause of the hypertension:
• radioactive renography
• renal arteriography: preferably digital subtraction from venous injection if available rather than selective arterial injection
• plasma renin activity (peripheral blood) lying and after one hour standing
• renal vein renin ratio: simultaneous sampling with the patient off beta-blockade. A ratio of >1.5:1 (abnormal: normal) is significant. Differential ureteric sampling is only rarely required now

Phaeochromocytoma

24-hour urine VMA needs repeating on several occasions as hormone release may be pulsatile. Metadrenalines in urine may be measured. The diagnosis is confirmed by:
• CT scan and/or ultrasound of adrenals. 5% of the tumours are multiple and approx 5% malignant
• plasma adrenaline and noradrenaline after a period of rest

• IVP with tomography of the adrenals. It is important to collect the 24-hour urines before the IVP
• pentolinium test (if doubtful case. Excludes false positives)
• MIBG scan. Iodine–123 meta-iodobenzylguanidine is a guanethidine analogue, and is taken up by pre-synaptic adrenergic neurones. Dense uptake occurs in phaeochromocytoma tissue. It is useful for detecting extra-adrenal phaeochromocytomas.

More dangerous investigations such as arteriography, or adrenal venous and IVC sampling are only performed under adequate α-and β-blockade with intra-arterial pressure monitoring. Pre-investigation therapy: a minimum of phenoxybenzamine 10 mg tds and propranolol 80 mg tds is needed. Further control of hypertension is managed during investigation by i.v. phentolamine, hydralazine or trimetaphan (see pp. 196–7). Rarely associated lesions include neurofibromatosis, medullary carcinoma of the thyroid and hyperparathyroidism. Calcitonin assay, calcium studies and a more extensive endocrine screen may be necessary.

Treatment

General measures
Weight reduction. Discourage adding salt to food. Advise women on the pill to change to a different type of contraception.

Drug treatment scheme

	Mild Hypertension	**Moderate hypertension**	**Severe hypertension**
	(<160/110)	(<170/120–130)	(<170/130)
Initial therapy	Thiazide diuretic	Thiazide diuretic Beta–blocking agent	Bed rest, thiazide, Beta–blocker, vasodilator
Additional therapy if necessary	Beta–blocking agent	Vasodilator, e.g. nifedipine retard	Switch to captopril + frusemide

Diuretics
Thiazides increase salt and water excretion but can cause hyperuricaemia, hypercalcaemia, hypokalaemia, hypertriglyceridaemia and lower HDL cholesterol. They may cause impotence. Frusemide is not a good drug for hypertension unless used wth captopril, or unless there is a degree of renal failure. Spirolactone is most useful for primary hyperaldosteronism. Vasodilators and beta-blocking agents are discussed in Chapter 5.

Surgery
Is necessary for coarctation, phaeochromocytoma, uncontrolled primary hyperaldosteronism and some cases of renal artery stenosis. Cases of renal artery stenosis may be controlled medically, and renal artery angioplasty via the femoral artery obviates the need for surgery now in some centres.

Surgery involves either renal endarterectomy, saphenous vein bypass or nephrectomy. Removal of a small kidney does not necessarily result in an improvement in BP.

9.7 Dissecting aneurysm of the thoracic aorta

This commonly occurs in men aged 40–70 years and is frequently fatal if untreated. More than 50% die within 5 days and 90% within 6 months. It is more common in hypertensive negroes than caucasians, but rare in the oriental races.

Predisposing conditions include:

- Marfan's syndrome
- coarctation of the aorta
- hypertension

A history of trauma is not common. It rarely occurs at surgical aortotomy sites.

Pathophysiology
A combination of high intraluminal pressure and medial damage seem to be the prime factors (e.g. cystic medial necrosis in

Marfan's syndrome). Syphilis causes saccular aortic aneurysms not dissections, and atheroma is usually associated with saccular aneurysms. The cause of the medial damage is unknown (a genetic mucopolysaccharide deficiency in Marfan's, possibly ischaemic necrosis due to occlusion of vasa vasorum in other cases).

Presentation

• *pain.* The commonest form of presentation. A sudden onset literally tearing sensation felt in chest. Usually restrosternal radiating through to the back, neck and left chest. The pain may be similar to ischaemic cardiac pain. It is very severe. Leaking dissections will produce pleuritic pain in addition. Dissection round a coronary ostium may produce an additional myocardial infarct

• *symptoms from arterial involvement:*

CNS. Monoplegia, paraplegia (spinal artery occlusion), hemiplegia, stupor to loss of consciousness, visual disturbances, speech disturbance

gastrointestinal: abdominal pain (mesenteric artery dissection), haemorrhage (bowel infarction or aorto-intestinal fistula), dysphagia (oesophageal compression)

renal: renal pain, haematuria (renal artery dissection) or anuria

limb: pain and pallor in any limb

• *pleuritic pain:* aneurysm leaking may also cause haemoptysis

• *giddiness or syncope:* either cerebral effect or secondary to effective volume loss, e.g. retroperitoneal haematoma

• *dyspnoea* (LVF, massive haemothorax, pleural effusions, pulmonary haemorrhage)

Aortic dissection may thus mimic clinically a wide variety of conditions from a CVA, acute appendicitis, acute pancreatitis, perforated peptic ulcer, saddle embolism as well as myocardial infarction, or pulmonary embolism. A patient may present with one ischaemic and one paralysed limb simultaneously.

Physical signs and examination

The patient may be in great pain, shocked, cyanosed and sweating profusely. The BP may be high normal or low.

The most important things to check are:

the blood pressure in both arms; all peripheral pulses, their presence and equality (a change in the nature of the pulses may be a valuable clue); there may be arterial bruits, arterial tenderness or palpable aneurysms:

the presence of aortic regurgitation;

signs of tamponade (p. 324), pericardial rub itself is not common. SVC obstruction rarely confuses the issue, as it is commoner with saccular aneurysms;

signs of LVF, presence of pleural effusions; staining of chest or abdomen (haemorrhage from leaking aneurysm is an ominous sign);

abdominal signs, rigidity, palpable mass—? pulsatile, abdominal tenderness is common;

CNS signs, fundal examination, hypertensive changes; Horner's syndrome; Urinary retention; Limb movement and sensation; General state of consciousness; ? Marfan habitus.

Chest x-ray

Widening of the upper mediastinum is strongly suggestive of a dissection, but not diagnostic. An unfolded aorta with a tortuous descending aorta may resemble a dissection.

Fluid in the left costophrenic angle associated with a wide mediastinum is a particularly ominous sign.

Classification

The original De Bakey classification is shown in Fig. 9.1.

Type I. The ascending and descending aorta are involved usually into the abdomen. The 'walking stick' distribution.

Type II. Involvement of ascending aorta only. The least common. May occur in Marfan's syndrome.

Type III. Involvement of descending aorta only distal to the left subclavian downwards. The most favourable type prognostically.

This classification was proposed in 1965 and is still widely used. More recently Shumway has proposed a more simple classification into two types only:

Type A	(proximal). Ascending aorta involved	Shumway classification
Type B	(distal). Ascending aorta not involved	

The Shumway classification has largely taken over from the De Bakey.

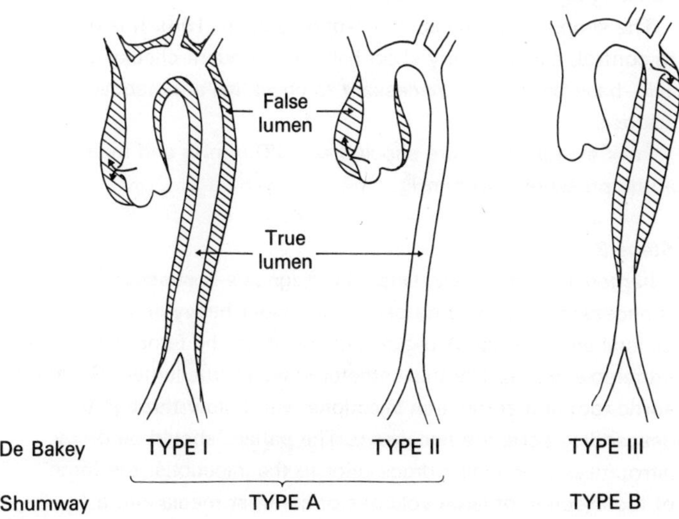

Fig. 9.1 Thoracic aorta dissection — classification.

Management

Stage 1

Pain relief, i.v. diamorphine as required. ECG monitoring, chest x-ray. Establish two CVP lines and radial artery pressure if possible. Cross match 10 units blood as volume replacement may be necessary if aneurysm leakage has occurred. Plasma should be given initially, followed by whole blood. Dextran 70 may have to be used. Echocardiography is used to visualise aortic root and to check for pericardial fluid.

Stage 2

Correction of hypertension if present. Wheat in 1965 realised the importance of lowering both mean systolic pressure and the dP/dt. This he accomplished by trimetaphan i.v. 1–2 mg/ml, guanethidine 50 mg bd and reserpine 1–2 mg i.m. A variety of other drugs have been used since e.g. methyl-dopa, beta-blocking agents, and diuretics.

The simplest regime is i.v. nitroprusside (p. 194). It is easier to control, having a very short half life. Frequent checks on acid–base balance are necessary to check for a metabolic acidosis.

Peak systolic pressure should be <120 mmHg and mean aortic pressure <90 mmHg.

Stage 3

Emergency aortography. Once the diagnosis is suspected this is necessary. It should be performed under heavy sedation or general anaesthesia. A pigtail catheter from the femoral route is preferable and usually this catheter stays in true lumen. Separate aortic root and aortic arch injections with follow through to descending aorta are necessary. The patient should be on i.v. nitroprusside or similar drugs prior to the injections: the force of the injection of large volumes of contrast media into a dissected root has occasionally proved fatal.

Digital subtraction angiography

When generally available this will probably prove to be the safest, quickest and most reliable method of diagnosis. Only venous cannulation is needed and the danger of an aortic injection is avoided.

Renal films should be taken at the end of the procedure.

CT scan

This investigation is proving increasingly useful in aortic dissection but is not always available on an emergency basis. A double lumen can be visualised and the dissection flap. It may not however be quite as good as aortography in visualising the origin/point of entry of the dissection, but is very helpful in making the diagnosis and determining the extent of the dissection. It is obviously safer than aortography.

Transoesophageal echocardiography

This is proving very useful in the diagnosis of dissection and is particularly good at visualising the dissection flap in the descending aorta.

Stage 4

Medical or surgical management. Types I and II (De Bakey) or Type A (Shumway). It is now agreed surgery is the treatment of choice in any case involving the ascending aorta.

Type I. Cardiopulmonary bypass with coronary perfusion. The ascending aorta is transected, the two cuffs of true and false walls are sutured together at both sides of the transection and then end-to-end anastomosis is performed.

Type II. Aortic root replacement using a Dacron graft with coronary cuff anastomosis to graft. Aortic valve replacement is often necessary using a tube valve conduit. The original aortic wall is buttressed around the graft.

Type III. Medical management initially unless complications develop. If the dissection re-enters at or above the diaphragm, replacement of the descending aorta with a Dacron graft is possible (using a temporary proximal to distal aortic bypass). The difficulty with this operation is the distal anastomosis, and the possibility of paraplegia due to damage to anterior spinal arteries.

Involvement of the abdominal aorta in a type III dissection is much more of a problem, and medical treatment is advocated initially. However local surgery at the aortic bifurcation may be necessary to save ischaemic legs.

9.8 Cardiac myxoma

This may occur in any cardiac chamber but most commonly in the left atrium. It is typically a gelatinous friable tumour attached to the atrial septum by a short pedicle. It is three times more common in the left atrium than the right. Untreated, it is usually fatal, although disease progression may be very slow over a period of years. The tumour often prolapses through the mitral or tricuspid valve and can cause sudden obstruction to blood flow. Fragments of the tumour easily break off and cause systemic emboli. Multiple tumours occur vary rarely. There is also a very rare familial form associated with Lentiginosis (multiple freckles) or HOCM.

Symptoms

The atrial myxoma commonly presents in one of four ways in order of frequency:

- *dyspnoea*. This may be of gradual onset or sudden severe pulmonary oedema
- *systemic emboli*. Any organ may be involved, e.g. brain (fits, hemiplegia etc.), myocardial infarction, acute ischaemia of a limb, etc.

• *constitutional upset.* Weight loss, fever, myalgia, (low albumen and raised globulin with a high ESR are often associated)
• *sudden death.* The atrial myxoma is found at post mortem occluding the mitral valve orifice

Physical signs

The left atrial myxoma most closely mimics mitral stenosis but there are one or two pointers suggesting a myxoma:
• the patient is in sinus rhythm. Atrial dysrrhythmias are rare
• signs of mitral stenosis may be transient and only occur if the tumour approaches the mitral valve orifice. Sometimes postural changes will influence the murmur
• there is no opening snap
• there may be an early diastolic plop as the tumour prolapses through the valve

Right atrial myxomas are more difficult to pick up clinically. There may be signs suggesting right ventricular dysfunction (raised JVP, oedema, etc.) or pulmonary infarction from emboli. A tricuspid diastolic flow murmur is often difficult to hear.

Investigations

Chest x-ray shows a small heart with enlargement of the left atrial appendage and possible pulmonary oedema. There is no mitral valve calcification. In long-standing cases calcification may occur in the tumour itself.

Echocardiography is diagnostic. 2D echocardiography (Fig. 10.18b) will be diagnostic in almost all cases of prolapsing myxoma. Transoesophageal echocardiography will give more accurate information of the size and site of the myxoma.

Cardiac catheterisation is now virtually never required. In cases of left sided myxomas where there is diagnostic doubt after echocardiography, pulmonary angiography with follow through to the left heart may help. Direct left heart catheterisation should be avoided as this may dislodge friable material from the myxoma. With right sided myxomas if there is doubt following echocardiography; digital subtraction angiography from a peripheral venous injection is helpful.

Histology. This may be obtained from analysis of peripheral embolic material. Although the tumour embolises frequently it does not grow in its peripheral site.

Differential diagnosis

The following conditions should be considered in a patient with a mitral murmur, mild pyrexia, weight loss, abnormal plasma proteins and high ESR:

- rheumatic mitral stenosis
- infective endocarditis
- systemic lupus erythematosus
- reticulosis
- cor triatriatum
- left atrial thrombus

Treatment

Following echocardiographic diagnosis, surgical removal of the myxoma should be performed as soon as possible using cardiopulmonary by-pass. Occasionally atrial septectomy and an interatrial patch is required. Recurrence of the myxoma is extremely rare but patients should be followed up for the first 5 years.

10 Cardiac investigations

10.1 Electrocardiography

The electrical axis

The normal mean QRS axis in the frontal plane is –30° to + 90°. The normal T wave axis in the frontal plane should be within 45° of the mean frontal QRS axis, i.e. the QRS–T angle should be <45°. The hexaxial reference system is shown below.

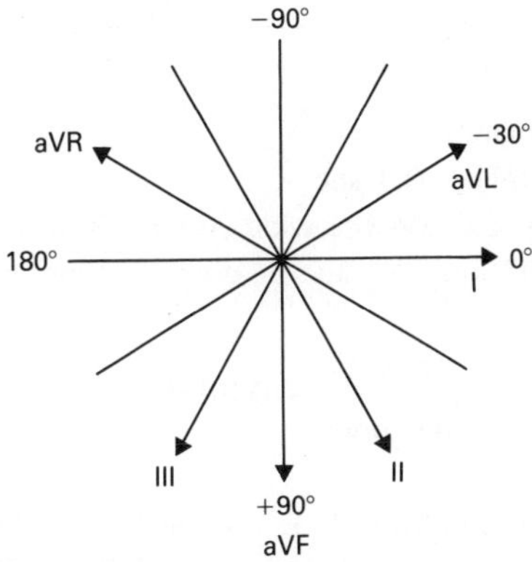

The following gives a quick calculation of the mean frontal QRS axis: find the isoelectric lead; the QRS axis is at right angles to this. Find the lead at right angles to the isoelectric lead from the hexaxial reference system. If the QRS is positive this lead is the electrical axis, if it is negative the axis is 180° away.

Left axis deviation = –30° to –90°.
Right axis deviation = +90° to +180°.
The quadrant –90° to 180° = extreme right or extreme left axis deviation.

10.1 Electrocardiography

Right axis deviation	Left axis deviation
Infancy	Left anterior hemiblock
RV hypertrophy	LV hypertrophy
Acute RV strain: pulmonary embolism	LBBB
Cor pulmonale	Primum ASD
Secundum ASD	Tricuspid atresia
RBBB	Cardiomyopathies
Fallot, severe PS	
TAPVD	

Intervals

Normal PR interval: 0.2 sec

Normal QRS duration: 0.1 sec

Normal Q wave is <0.04 sec wide and <25% of the total QRS complex. The QT interval must be corrected for heart rate (QTc)

$$\text{Normal QTc} = \frac{\text{QT}}{\sqrt{\text{R–R interval}}} = 0.38\text{–}0.42 \text{ sec}$$

Heart rate calculation from R–R interval. At standard paper speed of 25 mm/sec each big square = 0.2 sec. Count the number of 'big squares' between each R wave.

R–R interval (sec)	Number of large squares	Heart rate/min
0.2	1	300
0.4	2	150
0.6	3	100
0.8	4	75
1.0	5	60
1.2	6	50
1.4	7	43
1.6	8	37

For intra-cardiac electrophysiological measurements see **6.8**.

Hypertrophy

Atrial hypertrophy and the P wave

The normal P wave axis is +30° to +80° in the frontal plane. It is normally <2.5 mm in height. Right atrial depolarisation occurs first and causes the initial P wave deflection. Left atrial depolarisation causes the terminal deflection.

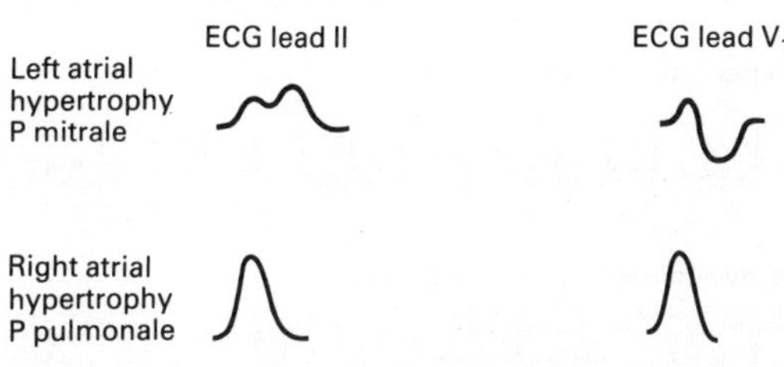

Ventricular hypertrophy

There is no single marker of ventricular hypertrophy on the ECG. Several factors are taken into consideration (electrical axis, voltage, delay in the intrinsicoid deflection, and ST-T wave changes) and then the ECG is correlated with the patient's condition. Relying on a single marker of ventricular hypertrophy, e.g. ventricular voltage, may not be reliable. A thin chest wall in young men results in a large voltage. A fat chest may mask it.

Factors influencing chest lead voltage

- LV cavity size
- LV muscle mass
- presence of pericardial fluid
- lung volume in front of heart
- chest wall thickness

10.1 Electrocardiography

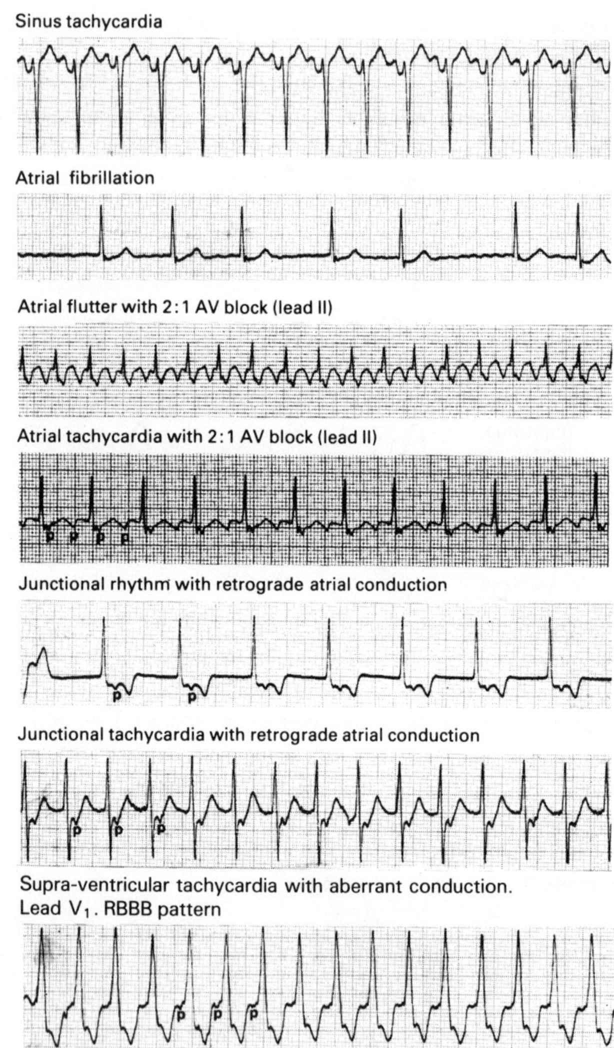

Fig. 10.1 Common atrial rhythms.

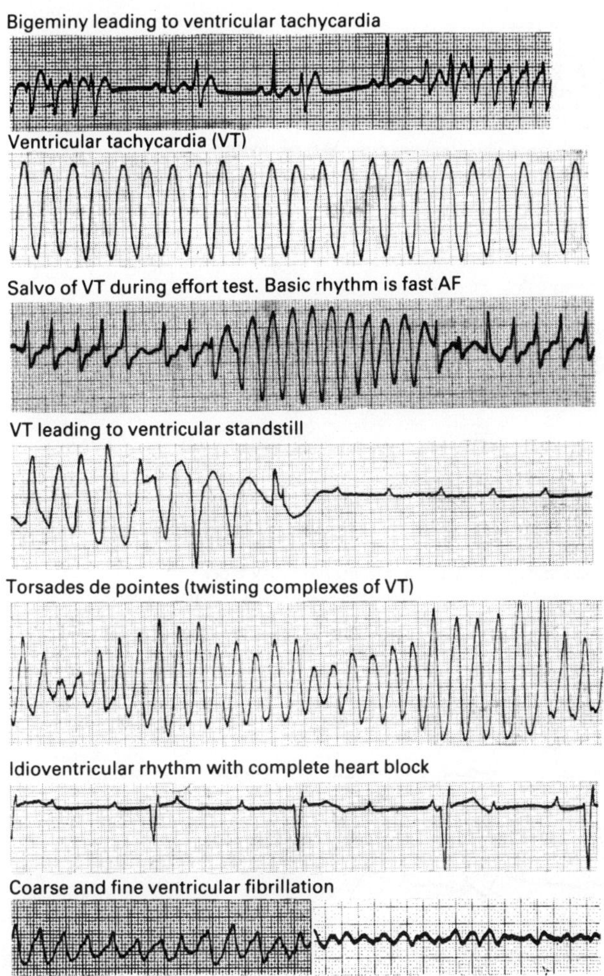

Fig. 10.2 Common ventricular rhythms.

10.1 Electrocardiography

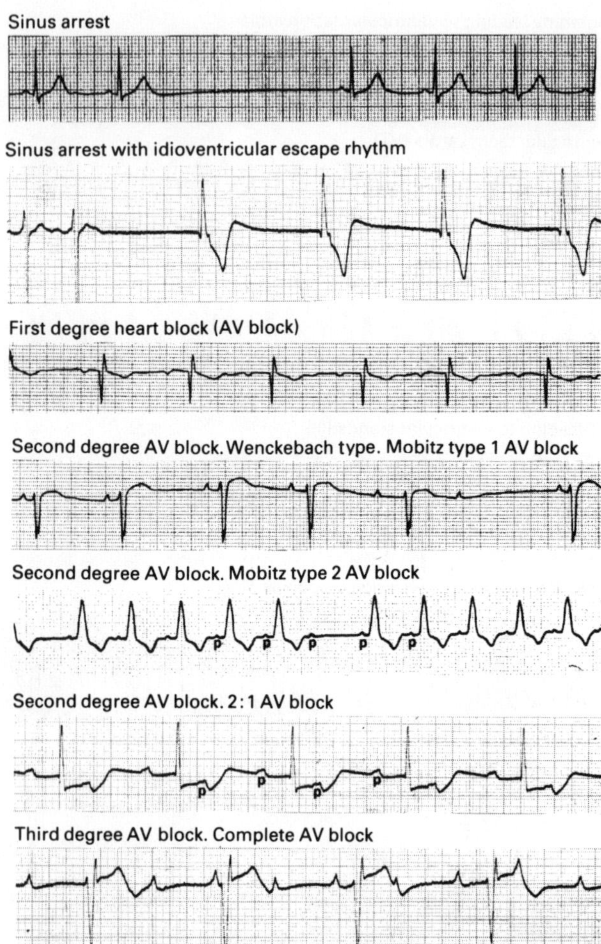

Fig. 10.3 Examples of conduction disturbances.

10.1 Electrocardiography

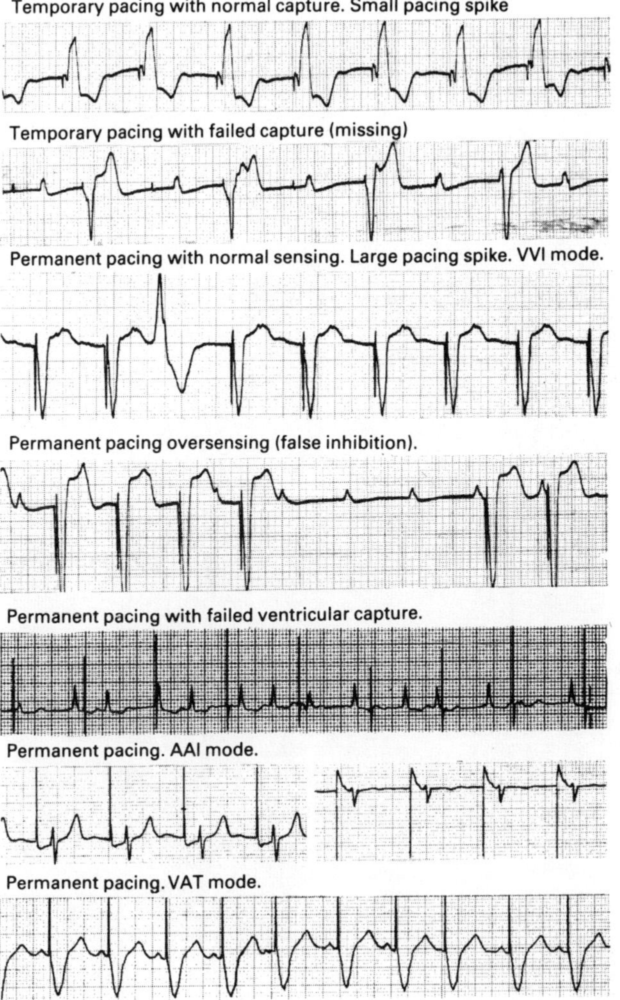

Temporary pacing with normal capture. Small pacing spike
Temporary pacing with failed capture (missing)
Permanent pacing with normal sensing. Large pacing spike. VVI mode.
Permanent pacing oversensing (false inhibition).
Permanent pacing with failed ventricular capture.
Permanent pacing. AAI mode.
Permanent pacing. VAT mode.

Fig. 10.4 Examples of common pacing ECGs.

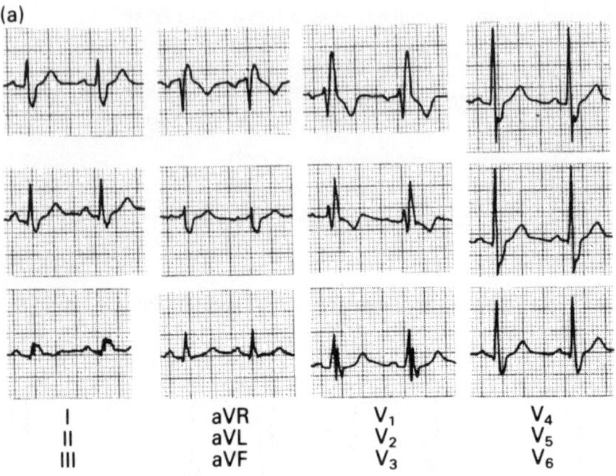

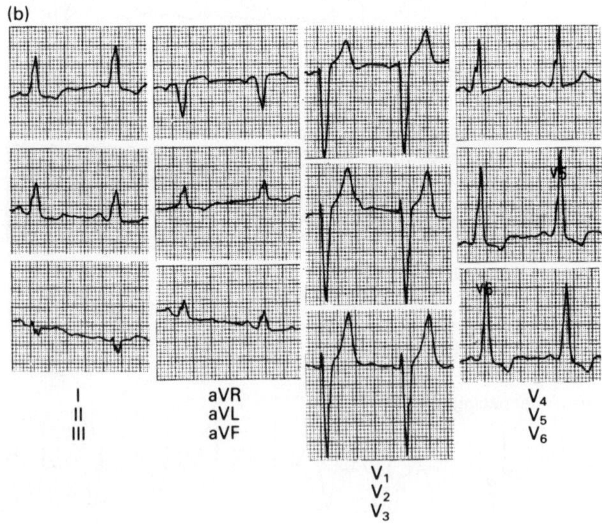

Fig. 10.5(a) Right bundle branch block. (b) Left bundle branch block.

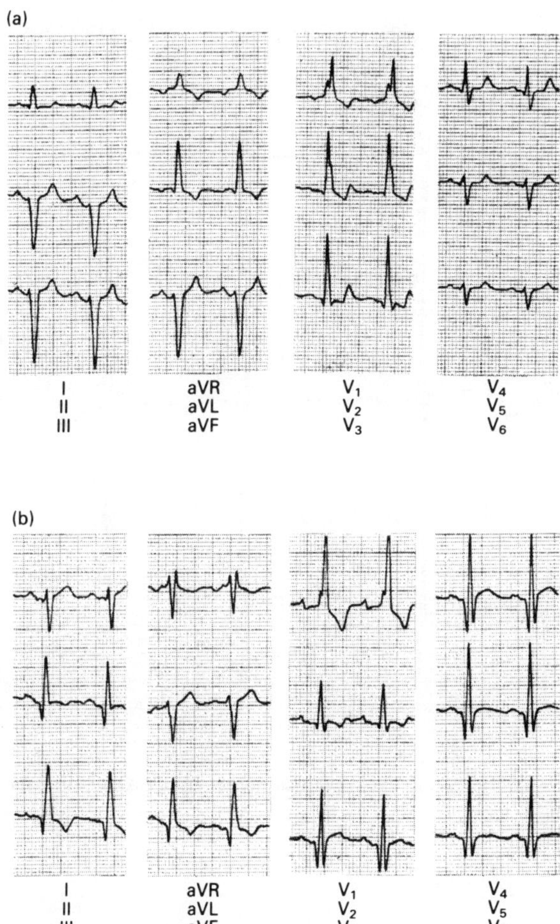

Fig. 10.6 Bifascicular blocks. (a) Right bundle branch block and left anterior hemiblock. (b) Right bundle branch block and left posterior hemiblock.

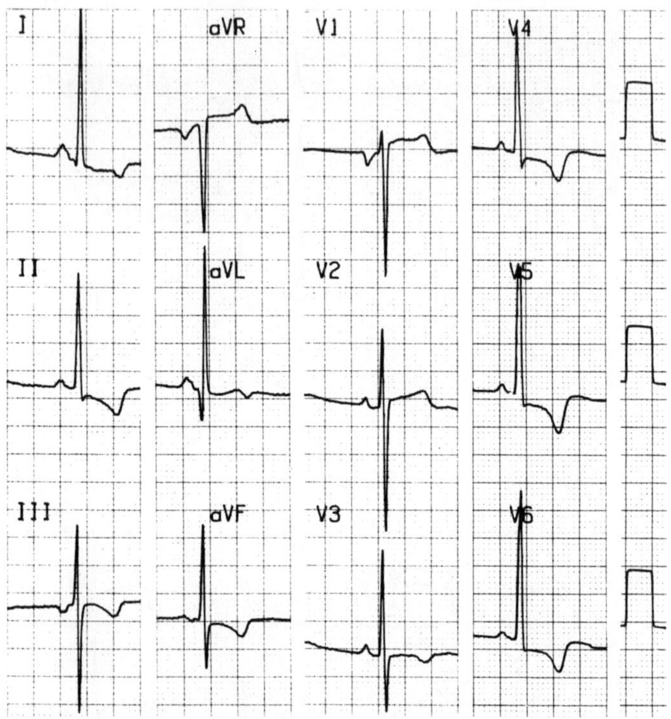

Fig. 10.7 ECG in severe left ventricular hypertrophy taken from patient with HOCM.

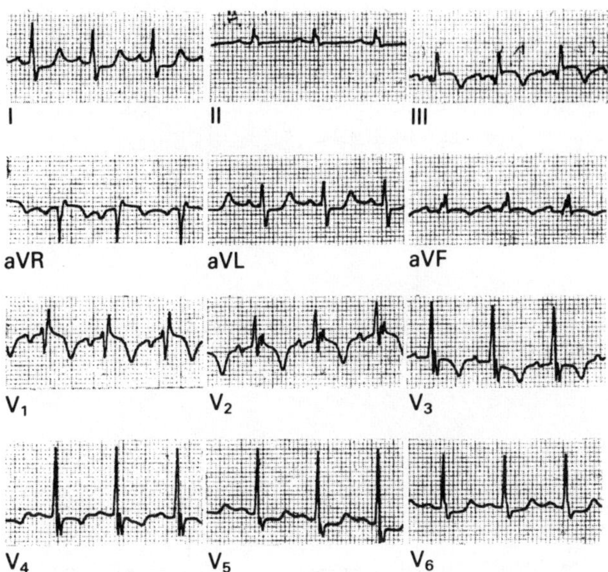

Fig. 10.8 ECG in acute pulmonary embolism. S_1, Q_3, T_3 pattern with incomplete RBBB and T wave inversion V_1, – V_4 (RVstrain).

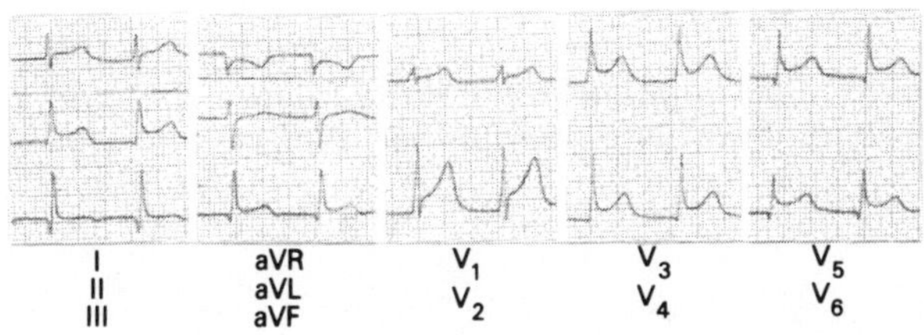

Fig. 10.9 Acute pericarditis. This shows typical 'saddle-shaped' ST segment elevation.

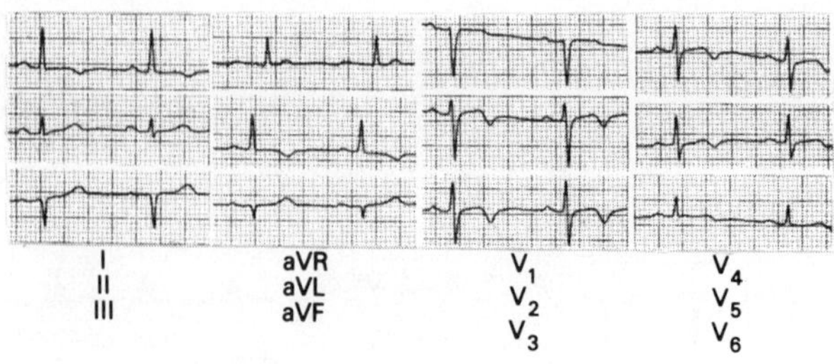

Fig. 10.10 Acute anterior subendocardial ischaemia. Anterior T wave changes only due to severe LAD stenosis. Enzyme elevation needed with this type of ECG to document infarction.

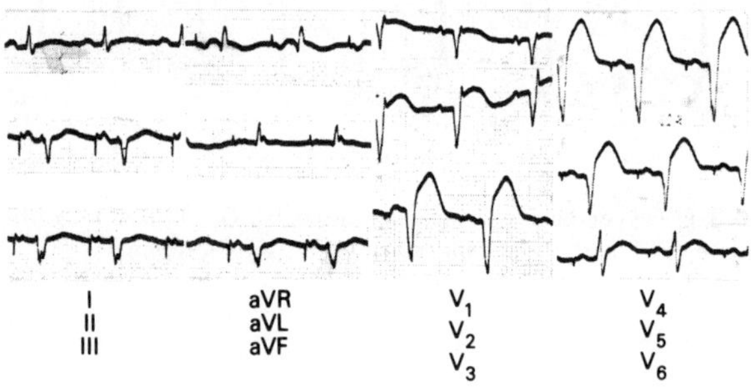

Fig. 10.11 Acute transmural anterior myocardial infarction. Typical anterior Q waves with ST segment elevation. Atrial pacing.

10.1 Electrocardiography

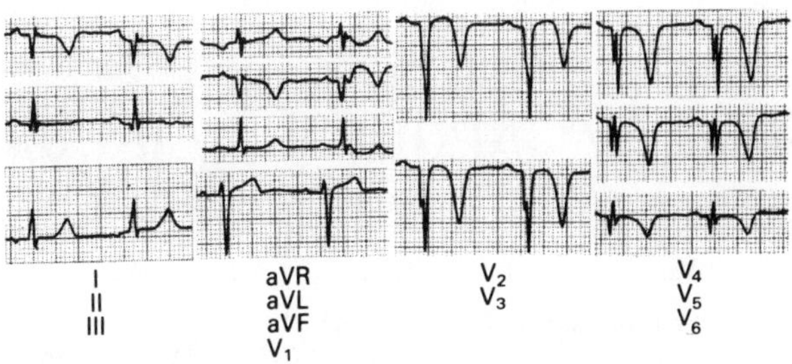

Fig. 10.12 Recent transmural anterior myocardial infarction.

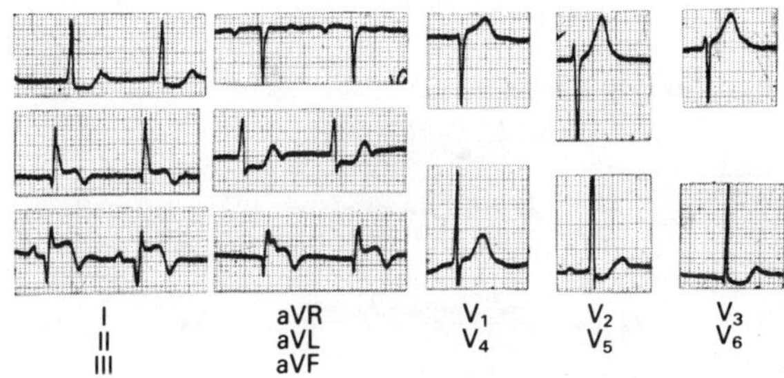

Fig. 10.13 Acute transmural inferior myocardial infarction. This shows typical Q waves and raised ST segments in inferior leads. There is variable sinus and nodal rhythm. Reciprocal or mirror image ST depression in I and aVL .

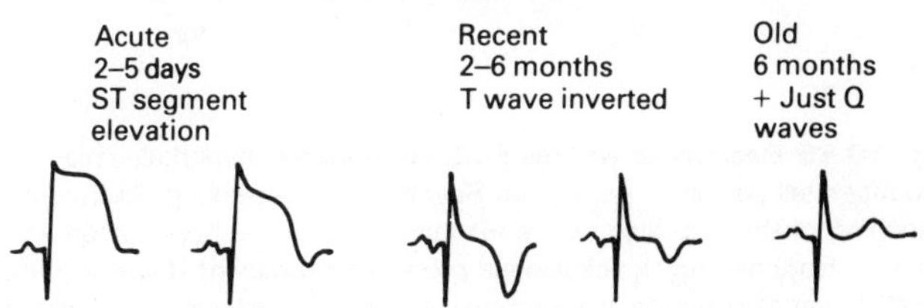

Fig. 10.14 Evolution of ST segments following myocardial infarction. Persistent ST segment elevation after 3 months suggests an LV aneurysm.

10.1 Electrocardiography

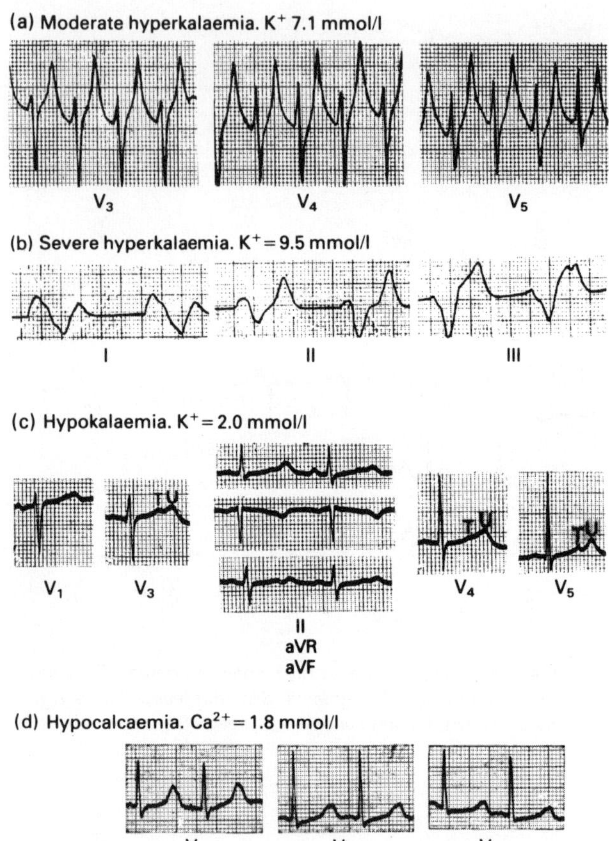

Fig. 10.15 Electrolytes and the ECG. (a) Moderate hyperkalaemia produces tall peaked T waves. (b) Severe hyperkalaemia produces gross widening of the QRS also with a resulting 'sine wave' appearance. P waves disappear. (c) Hypokalaemia produces prominent U waves with small T waves resulting in an apparently long QT interval. The T wave is often lost in the U wave. (d) Hypocalcaemia produces a long QT interval with small T waves, while hypercalcaemia produces a short QT interval with normal T waves.

10.1 Electrocardiography

Right ventricular hypertrophy	Left ventricular hypertrophy
Right axis deviation > 90°	Left axis deviation > −30°
$RV_1 + SV_6 > 11$ mm	SV_1 or $V_2 + RV_5$ of V_5 or $V_6 > 40$ mm
RV_1 or $SV_6 > 7$ mm	SV_1 or V_2 or RV_5 or V_6 > 25 mm
R/S $V_1 > 1$	$R_I + S_{III} > 25$ mm
R/S $V_6 > 1$	R in I or aVL > 14 mm
T wave inversion $V_1 - V_{3\ \text{or}\ 4}$ ST depression	T wave inversion in I, aVL ST depression $V_4 - V_6$
Delay in intrinsicoid deflection in $V_1 > 0.05$ sec	Delay in intrinsicoid deflection in $V_6 > 0.04$ sec
P pulmonale	P mitrale

Examples of acute RV strain are seen in Fig. 10.8, and LV hypertrophy in Fig. 10.7

Right ventricular hypertrophy in children

The neonate has right ventricular predominance on the ECG with dominant R waves in V_1 and aVR and deep S waves in V_6. The pattern gradually swings leftward through childhood and has reached adult configuration by the age of 15 years. By the end of the first week T waves are negative in V_1 and V_2 and positive in V_5 and V_6. By 1 month the positive R wave in aVR has disappeared. The dominance of the RV in the first 3 months makes the diagnosis of pathological RV hypertrophy difficult and serial ECGs may be needed.

RV hypertrophy 1 month to age 15

Presence of a Q wave in V_1
Delay in intrinsicoid deflection in $V_1 > 0.04$ sec in the absence of RBBB
R/S or R/Q in aVR > 1
QRS axis > 120°
P pulmonale with P wave > 3 mm in II
R/S in V_1 7 (at 3 months)
R/S in V_6 0.5 (at 3 months)

10.1 Electrocardiography

Combined ventricular hypertrophy

The effects of both RV and LV hypertrophy on the ECG may cancel each other out and the QRS complexes appear normal. Suspect it if:

LV hypertrophy + right axis.
RV hypertrophy + left axis.
LV hypertrophy + dominant R in V_1 and aVR and deep S in V_5.
RV hypertrophy + large Q and R waves in V_5 and V_6.

10.2 Exercise testing

The reliability, limitations and uses of exercise testing have been carefully established in recent years. Although the sensitivity and specificity of treadmill exercise testing has been widely studied it has also been realised that the results of an exercise test must be interpreted with reference to Bayes' theorem. The prevalence of coronary artery disease in the population under study is very important. The predictive accuracy of a positive test increases with increasing prevalence of the disease in the population. For a definition of terms see table on p. 396.

Assume exercise test with 80% sensitivity and 75% specificity

Patient	Pre-test likelihood of coronary disease	predictive accuracy of positive test
Asymptomatic man	5%	14–36%
Man with angina pectoris	90%	97%

Use in asymptomatic patients

It can be seen that exercise testing is of little value in screening asymptomatic subjects. The ST segment response to exercise in this group has a poor predictive accuracy. In this group with a low pre-test likelihood of coronary disease a positive test is often a false positive test.

Use in symptomatic patients
In the high risk group (e.g. men with angina) a positive test confirms a clinical diagnosis. A negative test may well be a false negative test and has a low correlation with the absence of coronary disease.

Thus exercise testing in patients with cardiac symptoms has major limitations from the diagnosis point of view (coronary disease vs. normal coronaries). Nevertheless it has great value in the assessment of cardiac function and the evaluation of symptoms.

Uses of exercise testing

- confirmation of a diagnosis of coronary disease in a group with a high pre-test likelihood of the disease
- evaluation of cardiac function and exercise capacity
- prognosis following myocardial infarction
- serial testing in evaluation of medical or surgical treatment
- detection of exercise-induced arrhythmias
- useful in rehabilitation and patient motivation

Patient safety
The patient should have avoided cigarettes or a recent meal prior to the test. A physician should be present at all exercise tests. The procedure is extremely safe provided strict criteria for stopping the exercise test are followed. Reported mortality rates are <1 in 10 000 tests.

A defibrillator should be instantly available. A complete trolley of cardiac resuscitation equipment should be on-hand, including intubating equipment and full range of cardiac drugs. Although cardiac resuscitation is very rarely necessary during or after exercise testing, occasional patients may develop refractory ventricular tachycardia requiring cardioversion.

Definition of terms

Term	Explanation	How calculated
Sensitivity	Percentage of all patients with coronary artery disease who have an abnormal exercise test	$\frac{TP}{TP + FN} \times 100$
Specificity	Percentage of negative exercise tests in normal patients without coronary artery disease	$\frac{TN}{TN + FP} \times 100$
Predictive accuracy	Percentage of positive exercise tests that are true positives	$\frac{TP}{TP + FP} \times 100$
False positive response	Percentage of total positive exercise tests that are false positives (occurring in normal patients)	$\frac{FP}{TP + FP} \times 100$ (or 100%–predictive accuracy)
False negative response	Percentage of total negative exercise tests which are false negatives (occurring in patients with coronary artery disease)	$\frac{FN}{TN + FN} \times 100$ (or 100%–sensitivity)
Risk ratio	Predictive accuracy related to false negative response (predictive error)	$\frac{TP}{TP + FP} / \frac{FN}{TN + FN}$
TN	Total negatives	
TP	Total positives	
FN	Total false negatives	
FP	Total false positives	

10.2 Exercise testing

Contra-indications to exercise testing

Exercise testing should be avoided in patients with

- severe aortic stenosis
- acute myocarditis or pericarditis
- any pyrexial or 'flu'-like illness
- severe left main stem stenosis or its equivalent
- left ventricular failure or congestive cardiac failure
- adults with complete heart block
- unstable or crescendo angina
- frequent fast atrial or ventricular arrhythmias
- renal failure
- orthopaedic or neurological impairment
- dissecting aneurysm
- uncontrolled hypertension
- thyrotoxicosis
- the test is obviously avoided in any frail, elderly or sick patient
- recent acute myocardial infarction. In patients who are fully mobile and capable of climbing one flight of stairs exercise testing may be performed under careful supervision at about 7–10 days post-infarction, i.e. the day before hospital discharge

What exercise test?

It is now known that graduated treadmill exercise testing is superior to bicycle ergometry or step testing. Greater limits of exercise are achieved and maximal oxygen uptake is higher with treadmill testing than with other methods. Some patients are unable to pedal a bicycle efficiently, and many stop with 'tired legs' before reaching desired target heart rates.

There are numerous treadmill protocols with variations in increasing speed and gradient. Many centres start the exercise test with a preliminary 'warm up' period of 3 min (1.0 mph at 5% elevation).

There is no particular advantage of one protocol over another. Many centres use the Bruce protocol as its higher stages

Table of standard treadmill protocols

Name		Bruce		Sheffield		Naughton		Ellestad		Balke 3.0		IMC 3.4		Rehabilitation	
Speed/Elevation		mph	%	mph	%	mph	%	mph	%	mph	%	mph	%	mph	%
Stage	1	1.7	10.0	1.7	0.0	1.0	0.0	1.7	10.0	3.0	6.0	3.4	0.0	2.0	0.0
	2	2.5	12.0	1.7	5.0	2.0	0.0	3.0	10.0	3.0	8.0	3.4	4.0	2.5	0.0
	3	3.4	14.0	1.7	10.0	2.0	0.0	4.0	10.0	3.0	10.0	3.4	8.0	2.5	3.0
	4	4.2	16.0	2.5	12.0	2.0	3.5	5.0	10.0	3.0	12.0	3.4	12.0	2.5	6.0
	5	5.0	18.0	3.4	14.0	2.0	7.0	5.0	15.0	3.0	14.0	3.4	16.0	2.5	9.0
	6	5.5	20.0	4.2	16.0	2.0	10.5	6.0	15.0	3.0	16.0	3.4	20.0	2.5	12.0
	7	6.0	22.0	5.0	18.0	2.0	14.0			3.0	18.0				

Stage 3 of the Sheffield protocol onwards is the same as Stage 1 onwards of the Bruce protocol

(6 and 7) are much more demanding than some other protocols. (More gradual protocols are available for less fit patients, e.g. those used in cardiac rehabilitation.) Most tests now are performed continuously. The blood pressure is recorded at every stage.

ECG leads and lead systems

Many exercise tests are spoiled through inadequate skin preparation. The shaved skin should be cleaned with alcohol or acetone-soaked gauze. The cleaned skin is gently abraded with dry gauze, sand-paper, sterile needle or dental burr. Silver/silver chloride pre-gelled electrodes are then applied (e.g. Cambmac medicotest, or Sentry medical products). The electrodes and leads are secured by micropore tape. Electrically screened leads should be used.

The sensitivity for recording significant ST depression increases as more leads are used. Cardiac centres have now moved from a standard V_5 lead to 10 or 12-lead ECG recording:

ECG lead	**% of all positive cases of ST segment depression post-exercise recorded using these leads**
V_5 alone	89%
V_5 V_6	91%
V_4 V_5 V_6	93%
V_3 V_4 V_5 V_6	95%
11 V_3 V_4 V_5 V_6	96%
11 AVF V_3 V_4 V_5 V_6	100%

Oxygen consumption

The relation between heart rate and oxygen consumption is linear for most patients during exercise. The slope of the relation is less for the fitter and more athletic patients (i.e. greater oxygen consumption for less increment in heart rate). Maximum oxygen consumption is a good measure of maximum cardiac performance and is usually measured in ml O_2/kg/min or METS equivalent. Resting O_2 consumption is approx 3.5 ml O_2/kg/min which = 1 METS.

In a male athlete VO_2 max is approx 70–80 mls O_2/kg/min, and 60 mls O_2/kg/min for a female athlete.

Table of oxygen consumption at stages of exercise in various protocols in ml O_2/kg/min

Stage	Bruce	Sheffield	Balke 3.0
1	17.5	8	18.0
2	24.5	12	21.0
3	34	17.5	24.0
4	46	24.5	28.0
5	56	34	32.0

Thus at stage 5 of the Bruce protocol (≡ Stage 7 of Sheffield protocol) oxygen requirement is 56 ml O_2/kg/min or 16 METS.

End points and when to terminate the exercise test

1 The test should be stopped when target heart rate has been achieved. This may be maximum heart rate for age or sub-maximal (commonly 85% of maximum predicted heart rate).

Age adjusted target heart rates

Age	Sub-maximal HR (85% max)	Maximal HR
30	165	194
35	160	188
40	155	182
45	150	176
50	145	171
55	140	165
60	135	159
65	130	153

A useful mental guide for heart rate (maximum) is for women, 220 – age; for men, 210 – age.

2 The test should be stopped prior to maximum or sub-maximal heart rate if any following symptoms or signs occur:

- progressive angina pectoris
- undue dyspnoea
- vasoconstriction with a clammy sweaty skin
- fatigue
- musculoskeletal pain
- feeling of faintness
- atrial fibrillation or atrial tachycardia
- premature ventricular contractions with increasing frequency
- ventricular tachycardia
- progressive ST segment depression } with or without chest pain
- progressive ST segment elevation } with or without chest pain
- failure of HR or BP to rise with effort. This is very important and applies even in patients on beta-blocking agents
- excessive rise in peak systolic pressure (>230 mmHg)
- electrical alternans
- development of LBBB
- development of AV block

Sometimes the greatest ECG abnormalities occur during the recovery period when the patient is lying down. Young unfit patients may develop a profound vagal bradycardia post exercise requiring atropine. A period of 10–15 min is usually long enough for recovery. All haemodynamic criteria (HR and BP) and ECG should have returned to the pre-exercise state before the patient is moved.

Exercise testing and drugs

Digoxin frequently causes a false positive exercise test and ST segment changes at rest are common. If possible the drug should be stopped at least 1 week prior to exercise. Digoxin is not thought to cause false negative responses.

Beta-blocking agents. These do not need to be withdrawn prior to exercise, and sudden withdrawal may be dangerous. The maximum heart rate response and maximum work load achieved will be reduced from normal. However there is evidence that beta-blockade may help in converting false positive results to negative, and allow true positive results to remain positive. A single dose of a beta-blocking agent (e.g. 80 mg oxprenolol) is taken 1½–2 hours prior to the exercise test. Beta-blockade appears to increase the specificity and predictive value of exercise testing.

Exercise testing following myocardial infarction

In the absence of the contra-indications listed, exercise testing may be safely performed following myocardial infarction and before hospital discharge (at about 10 days post-infarction), although exercise testing is usually delayed until about 1 month post-infarction. Early studies suggest that a limited treadmill test may be useful in predicting sudden early death or recurrent angina within 1 year of infarction. Poor prognostic signs are shown on p. 406.

What represents a positive test?

1 *ST segment depression* (see Fig. 10.16)

There must be 1.0 mm or more ST segment depression 80 msec after the J point, using the PQ segment as the baseline in 6 consecutive cycles. If the J point is not clearly visible the nadir of the S wave may be used instead. It does not matter if the ST segment is downsloping, horizontal or upsloping at the 80 msec point. Sometimes all 3 may occur in the same patient in different leads, and the ST segment changes should preferably be seen in more than 1 lead anyway. Some centres prefer to use 1.5 mm ST depression 80 msec after the J point if the ST segment is upsloping. If 1.5 or 2.0 mm ST depression is taken as the necessary hallmark of a positive test the sensitivity of the test will fall, but the predictive accuracy increase. T wave inversion alone is valueless.

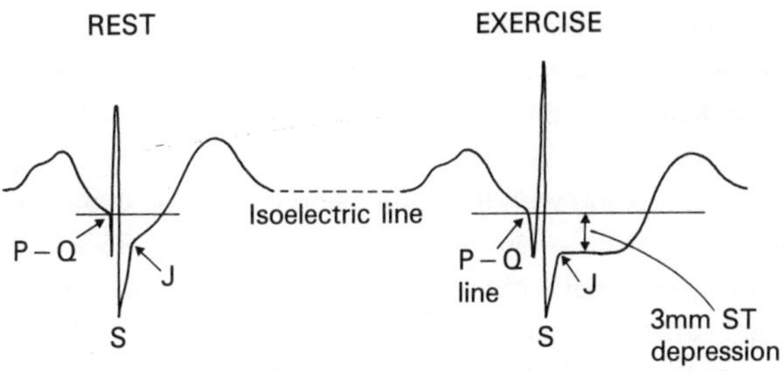

Fig. 10.16 ECG at rest (on left) and on exercise (on right). The PQ junction line is below the isoelectric line and is taken as the baseline for ST segment analysis. The complex on the right shows 3 mm ST segment depression 80 msec after the J point. If the J point is not clearly seen the nadir of the S wave may be used.

The PQ junction is taken as the baseline as this junction is normally depressed on exercise below the classical isoelectric line. The Ta wave (P wave repolarisation) on exercise may extend through the QRS and influence the ST segment even in normals. Hence the need for the 80 msec delay after the J point for test interpretation.

Although the degree of ST segment depression is the diagnostic hallmark of a positive exercise test it is also important to note

- how many and in which leads it occurs
- the heart rate at which it first appears
- its persistence in the recovery period

Some equipment now integrates the area of ST segment depression (in microvolt seconds). It is also possible to run exercise tests using signal averaging of the QRS complex. This produces clear recordings with no electrical or myographic interference. However the equipment is expensive, and meticulous attention to satisfactory electrode placement is all that is really necessary. Typically positive exercise tests are shown in Fig. 10.17.

ST segment elevation
May occur during exercise in leads with Q waves, and has the same significance as ST depression in other leads.

2 *Chest pain*
Taken in association with ST depression chest pain increases the sensitivity of the exercise test to approximately 85% in a cohort of symptomatic patients. The nature of the pain is important. Unilateral chest pain is unlikely to be angina. Patients who experience 'walk through' or 'second wind' angina do not normally do so on an exercise test as the work load is progressive and not steady.

Other criteria discussed below are not as useful as the ST segment in predicting coronary disease. However they are important correlates of a positive test and said to increase the sensitivity of the exercise test still further when combined with ST segment analysis.

3 *Increase in R wave voltage* (Fig. 10.17 bottom panel)
In the normal patient R wave voltage decreases during exercise. Immediately post exercise R wave voltage is at its smallest and then gradually returns to normal during the recovery period. The reduction in R wave voltage is thought to be due to the reduction of left ventricular end-diastolic volume with increasing exercise in the normal patient. The relation of QRS voltage to LV blood volume is the Brody effect. LV volume also decreases on standing from the supine position.

In patients with coronary disease R wave voltage usually remains unchanged or increases, especially in those with poor LV function. R wave changes may be useful in patients with LBBB where ST changes lack sensitivity or specificity.

Unfortunately the R wave is not only related to LVEDV but to other factors also (e.g. respiration). R wave voltage is best averaged for several cycles and leads rather than taking a mean of a single lead (e.g. V_5).

4 *Inverted U waves*
Leads in which U waves are well seen may show U wave

10.2 Exercise testing

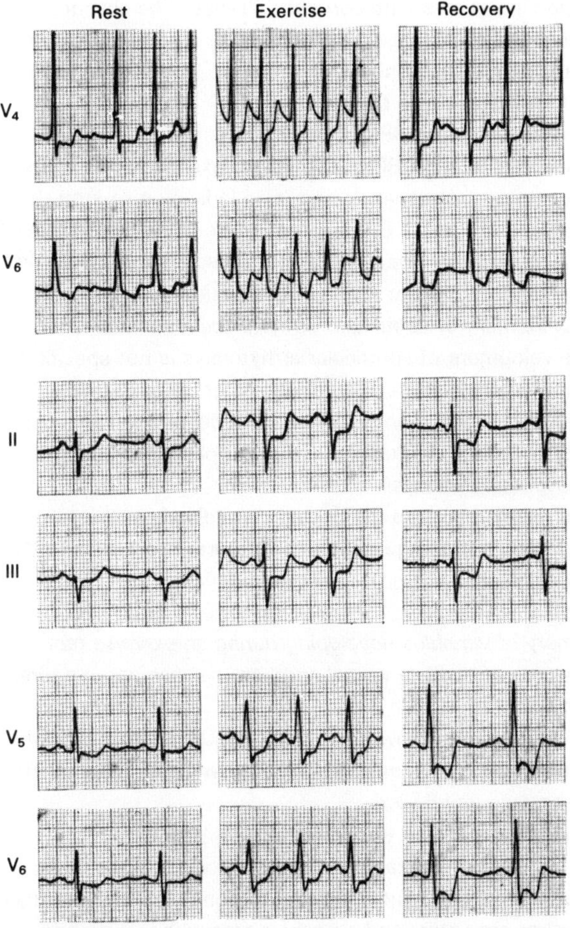

Fig. 10.17 Changes in ST segments. This shows three examples of positive ST segment depression. The top panel shows upsloping and downsloping ST segment depression in different leads. The second panel shows a positive test persisting after β-blockade. The bottom panel shows ST segment depression getting progressively worse into the recovery stage.

inversion in patients with coronary disease. The changes may be transient and at peak exercise only. They are characterised by a concave depression in the T–P segment. The U wave is usually overlooked in exercise testing.

5 *Abnormal systolic BP response*

Failure of the systolic BP to rise during exercise is an important indicator of an abnormal LV and is an indication to stop the test. A decrease in systolic BP during exercise is even more specific of severe coronary artery disease — assuming there are no valve lesions, and the patient is not on vasodilators.

6 *Development of ventricular arrhythmias* (Fig. 10.2)

The development of ventricular arrhythmias is not specific for coronary artery disease. Ventricular ectopics (>10/min), multifocal ectopics, ventricular tachycardia, etc., associated with ST segment depression and chest pain are more specific.

7 *Auscultating changes*

Auscultation should be performed immediately in the recovery period. New mitral regurgitation or a fourth heart sound (S_4) are highly significant.

Summary of variables developing during an exercise test suggestive of multiple vessel coronary disease and a poorer prognosis

• ST depression: at low heart rate (<130/min off β-blockade), greater than 2 mm in several leads, downsloping, persisting >5 min into recovery period.

• BP response: failure to rise or falling >10 mmHg

• ventricular arrhythmias developing at low exercise load

• poor exercise tolerance: inability to complete Bruce protocol Stage II or equivalent and a positive test with inappropriate tachycardia

Patients with these results are generally referred for coronary angiography.

False positive results

An enormous number of conditions may be associated with false positive exercise tests. They are particularly common in patients with a low pre-test likelihood of coronary artery disease (e.g. asymptomatic young women). Known associations of false positive results in patients with normal coronaries are:

- hyperventilation
- prolapsing mitral valve
- hypertrophic cardiomyopathy
- congestive cardiomyopathy
- hypertension with LV hypertrophy
- aortic stenosis
- young women with chest pain
- WPW syndrome
- drugs, e.g. digoxin, antidepressants
- anaemia
- coronary artery spasm
- hypokalaemia
- hypersensitivity to catecholamines
- observer variability

Hyperventilation as a cause of a false positive test can be excluded by asking the standing patient to hyperventilate for 30 sec prior to the exercise test. Patients with sympathetic over-activity, emotional liability and resting tachycardia are very likely to have a false positive test. This functional condition has been called the hyperkinetic heart syndrome. Beta-blockade may abolish resting T wave abnormalities on the ECG in these patients and will increase the specificity of the test by preventing the false positive result.

10.3 Echocardiography

Echocardiography is now a standard non-invasive cardiac investigation following the early pioneering work of Edler and Hertz in 1953.

Pulsed ultrasound of high frequency is generated by a piezoelectric crystal which acts as both transmitter and receiver. Transmitted pulses of sound are produced by the transducer and reflected sound is converted back to an electrical signal and recorded.

The higher the frequency of the ultrasound used the greater the resolution of the image (with the shorter wavelength), but tissue attenuation (absorption of ultrasound) is greater.

Properties of ultrasound commonly used in cardiology

Frequency: 2.25 MHz in adults
5 MHz in children (where tissue attenuation is less)

Focal length: 7.5 cm
10 cm for more obese patients, or patients with emphysema

Repetition rate: 1000/sec. Each transmitting and receiving period lasts for 1 msec only. Of this period only 1 microsec is taken up in transmission, and the rest in 'listening'.

Velocity of sound in human tissue: 1540 m/sec. Distances can be recorded in cm rather than time.

Velocity of sound in silastic (ball valve): 980 m/sec.

Types of scan (Fig. 10.18)

A-mode (Amplitude modulation). The returned ultrasound signals are displayed on the oscilloscope as a series of vertical lines. The amplitude/height of each line represents the strength of the returning signals. The base is represented as cm distance from the transducer.

B-mode (Brightness modulation). The peaks of the A-mode scan are represented as a series of linear dots whose brightness represents the echo intensity.

M-mode (Motion mode). The B-mode scan is displayed on light sensitive paper moving at constant speed to produce the conventional permanent record—a single dimension/time image.

Two dimensional ('Real time'). A two dimensional image of a segment of the heart is produced on the screen: a cine image or moving tomographic cut which can be stored on videotape. Frozen images can be hard copied. The 2D image is produced either by rotating the scanning head rapidly through 80–90° (single crystal) or a phased array (multicrystal) scanning head. In the phased array system the ultrasound crystals are excited in sequence or phase to produce a fan-shaped wave front.

The original multicrystal head in linear format (as used in abdominal ultrasound) is unsuitable for cardiac imaging as the ribs interfere with the ultrasound beams.

2D echocardiography cannot be covered in this book. Several conditions are much better visualised by a 2D study than by M-mode. These include most congenital heart disease, LV aneurysm, intraventricular thrombus, LA myxoma, septal defects and small shunts which can be detected by 5% dextrose microbubble injection technique. An example of an LA myxoma seen on a 2D scan is shown in Fig. 10.18(b).

Several views are needed in a single 2D study. The commonest four are long axis and short axis views, the four chamber view and the sub-costal view. Suprasternal views are useful in children for visualising the great vessels.

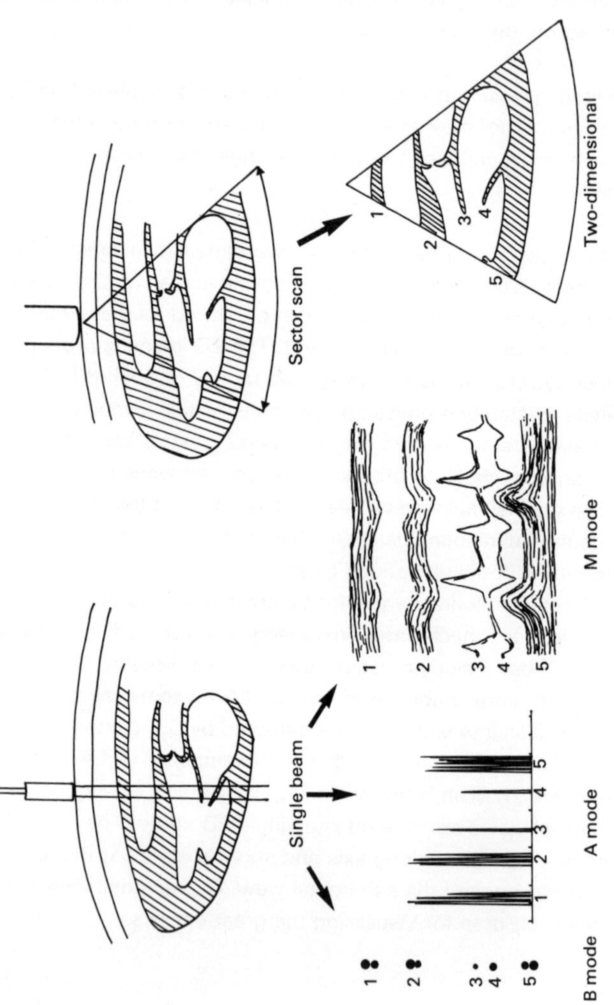
Single beam
Sector scan
1
2
3
4
5
B mode
A mode
M mode
Two-dimensional

(a)

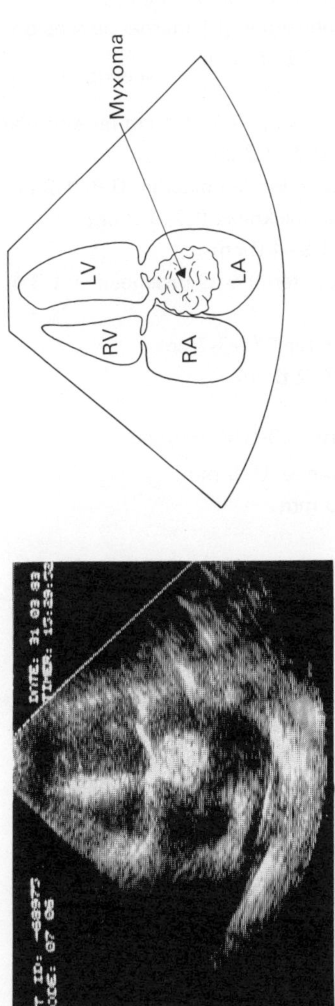

Fig. 10.18(a) Diagrammatic representation of types of echocardiogram. The numbers refer to the same structure in each type of scan: 1 = anterior right ventricular wall; 2 = interventricular septum; 3 = anterior mitral leaflet; 4 = posterior mitral leaflet; 5 = posterior left ventricular wall. **(b)** An example of a 2D scan in the four chamber view, showing a left atrial myxoma.

Normal echocardiographic values in an adult

Ventricular and atrial dimensions: (ID internal dimension)

- LVIDd (end diastole): 3.5–5.6 cm } see Fig. 10.19
- LVIDs (end systole): 1.9–4.0 cm } see Fig. 10.19
- Posterior LV wall thickness: 0.7–1.1 cm (at end diastole)
- RVID (end diastole): 0.7–2.6 cm
- Posterior LV wall excursion (amplitude): 0.8–1.2 cm
- Interventricular septal thickness 0.7–1.2 cm
- LAID (end systole): 1.9–4.0 cm
- Ratio of septum to posterior wall thickness = 1.3:1

Aorta and aortic valve:

Aortic root internal diameter 2.0–3.7 cm

Aortic valve opening 1.6–2.6 cm

Mitral valve:

- E–F slope (closure rate) 70–150 cm/sec
- E point to septal distance: 0–5 mm
- D–E distance: 20–30 mm

Ventricular function

- Ejection fraction 0.62–0.85
- Velocity of circumferential fibre shortening of LV (Vcf) = 1.1 – 1.8 circ/sec

Formulae used in echocardiographic calculations of left ventricular function

LVEDV = $(\text{LVIDd})^3 = (\text{Dd})^3$ ml (for normal ventricles)

LVESV = $(\text{LVIDs})^3 = (\text{Ds})^3$ ml

Stroke volume = $\text{Dd}^3 - \text{Ds}^3$ ml

$$\text{Ejection fraction } \frac{\text{Dd}^3 - \text{Ds}^3}{\text{Dd}^3} \times 100\%$$

$$\text{Vcf} = \frac{\text{Dd} - \text{Ds}}{\text{Ds} \times \text{LVET}} \text{ circ/sec}$$

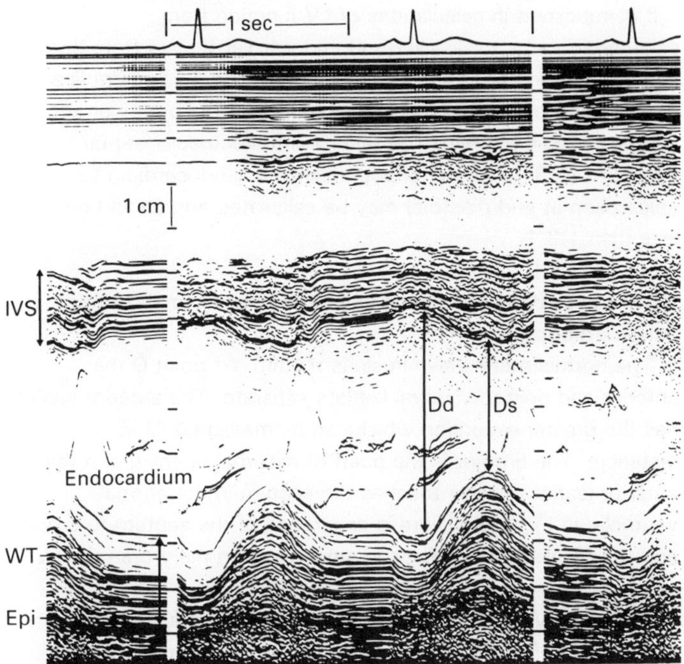

Fig. 10.19 Echocardiograph in an adult to show measurement of ventricular dimensions.

LVET is measured from carotid pulse (see systolic time intervals)

Example from Fig. 10.19

Dd = 5.0 cm $\quad Dd^3 = 125$

Ds = 2.9 cm $\quad Ds^3 = 24.4$

Dd is taken at the maximum diastolic diameter at the point of augmentation due to the 'a' wave—at the timing of the R wave of the ECG (see Fig. 10.19).

$$\text{Ejection fraction} = \frac{125 - 24.4}{125} \times 100\% = 80\%$$

It is important in calculations of LV function from echocardiograms to obtain good endocardial echoes from both septum and posterior left ventricular wall. The epicardium is a denser band of echoes visible at the back of the posterior left ventricular wall (PLVW). The ratio of interventricular septal thickness (IVS) to posterior wall thickness (endocardium to epicardium at end-diastole) may be calculated and should be less than 1.3:1.

Common patterns of mitral valve movement on M-mode echocardiogram

1 The normal mitral valve in sinus rhythm. At point D the anterior and posterior mitral leaflets separate. The anterior leaflet has the greater excursion which can be measured (D–E distance). The E point is the point of maximal opening and the anterior leaflet virtually touches the septum in the normal ventricle. In LV failure there is separation of the septum to E point and the greater the E point to septal distance the worse the LV function.

The mitral valve immediately starts to close again to the F point. The E–F slope is a measure of the rate of mitral valve closure. Normal E–F slope is 70–150 cm/sec. It is reduced in mitral stenosis. The mitral valve re-opens at end-diastole with the A wave. The leaflets meet at point C at the onset of systole. The movement of the posterior leaflet mirrors the anterior leaflet, but its excursion is less. It is more difficult to record on the M-mode echo.

2 The normal mitral valve with a slower heart rate in sinus rhythm. The movements are as in 1, but an extra excursion is seen in mid-diastole after the F point. This is normal and just represents mid-diastolic flow into LV.

3 The normal mitral valve in AF. Here the A wave disappears and the excursion of the E point varies depending on the R–R interval. Little fibrillation waves may be seen between the main mitral excursions.

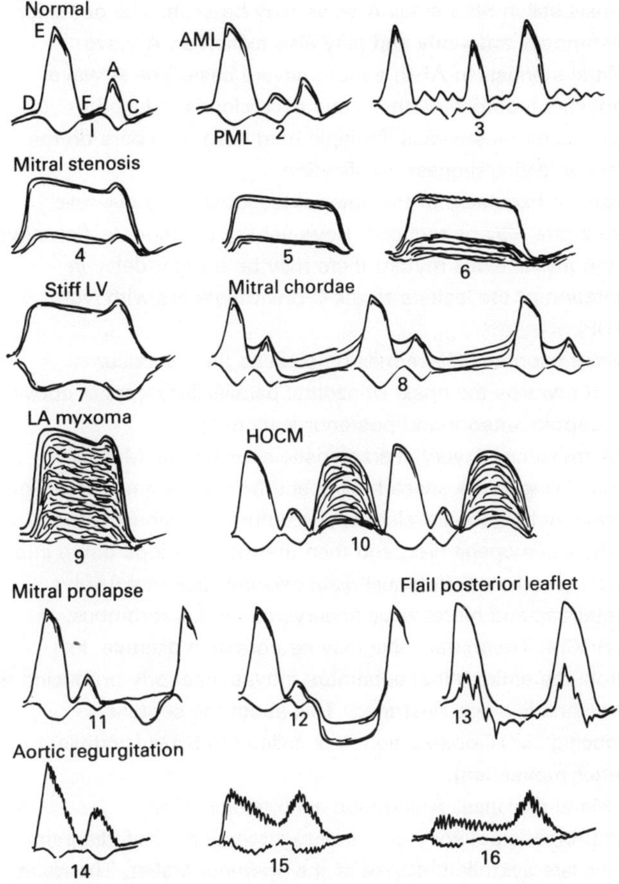

Fig. 10.20 Common patterns of mitral valve movement on M-mode echocardiogram.

4 Mitral stenosis in sinus rhythm. The mitral anterior leaflet excursion is reduced. The slope of mitral valve closure (E–F slope) is greatly reduced and in severe cases may be horizontal, giving a castellated appearance to the mitral valve. In mobile mitral stenosis still in SR a small A wave may be seen. The posterior leaflet moves anteriorly and may also exhibit an A wave.

5 Mitral stenosis in AF in a more severe case. The A wave disappears (compare with 4), and excursion is reduced.

6 Calcific mitral stenosis. Multiple hard horizontal bars on the posterior leaflet suggest calcification.

7 Stiff LV Excursion of the anterior leaflet and the diastolic closure rate may be reduced. However the Posterior leaflet moves posteriorly. In sinus rhythm there may be a slight delay in coaptation of the leaflets to the C point (patients with high LVEDP).

8 Mitral chordae. These may be seen as the tranducer is angled towards the apex. Horizontal parallel lines appear above the coapted anterior and posterior leaflets.

9 LA myxoma. A very characteristic appearance. Multiple echoes filling in the space behind and below the anterior leaflet. There may be an initial clear space before the echoes appear, i.e. the valve opens first, and then the tumour plops down into the mitral orifice. Differential diagnosis includes mitral valve vegetations and mitral valve aneurysm, and LA thrombus.

10 HOCM. The mitral valve may be normal in diastole. In systole the entire mitral apparatus moves anteriorly producing the characteristic bulge illustrated. This abuts the septum producing LVOT obstruction. It is called the SAM (systolic anterior movement).

11 Mitral prolapse. A common echo finding in an asymptomatic patient (see mitral regurgitation). This diagram shows late systolic prolapse of the posterior leaflet. The point of separation of the anterior and posterior leaflets in mid-systole will coincide with the mid-systolic click if present. The late systolic murmur follows.

12 Pansystolic prolapse. This is a more severe variety and is associated usually with symptomatic mitral regurgitation.

13 Flail posterior leaflet. Ruptured chordae can result in chaotic movement of the posterior leaflet. The important diagnostic point

is anterior movement and fluttering of the posterior leaflet in diastole.
14–16 Grades of aortic regurgitation: mild, moderate and severe. Mild aortic regurgitation causes diastolic fluttering of the anterior leaflet only, with normal mitral valve excursion. As regurgitation becomes more severe mitral valve excursion is reduced (premature mitral valve closure) and both anterior and posterior leaflets flutter. In very severe cases the mitral valve hardly opens until the A wave.

Common patterns of aortic valve movement on M-mode echocardiogram (Fig. 10.21)
1 Normal. The aortic cusps in diastole form a central closure line (CL). With left ventricular ejection the cusps separate to the edge of the aortic wall: the right coronary cusp anteriorly (RCC) and the posterior non-coronary cusp (PCC) posteriorly. The aortic valve in systole assumes a parallelogram shape. The left ventricular ejection time can be measured from the point of cusp opening to cusp closure if good echoes are obtained.
2 Normal. In this diagram the left coronary cusp is included and is rarely seen. Systolic fluttering of the aortic cusps is not necessarily abnormal and may occur with high or low output states, or causes of turbulence (e.g. sub valve stenosis).
3 Low output state. Separation of the aortic cusps is limited, but the cusps are normal. Anterior and Posterior movement is diminished—the aorta is barely swinging compared with 1 and 2).
4 and **5** Bicuspid aortic valve. Although the cusps separate normally the closure line is eccentric and may be either anterior (**4**) or posterior (**5**), Approximately 15% of bicuspid valves have a central closure line, and this sign cannot be relied on diagnostically. In addition a tricuspid aortic valve with a sub aortic VSD and prolapsing right coronary cusp may produce an eccentric closure line. Once a bicuspid valve is heavily calcified it cannot be distinguished from a tricuspid calcified valve by echocardiography.

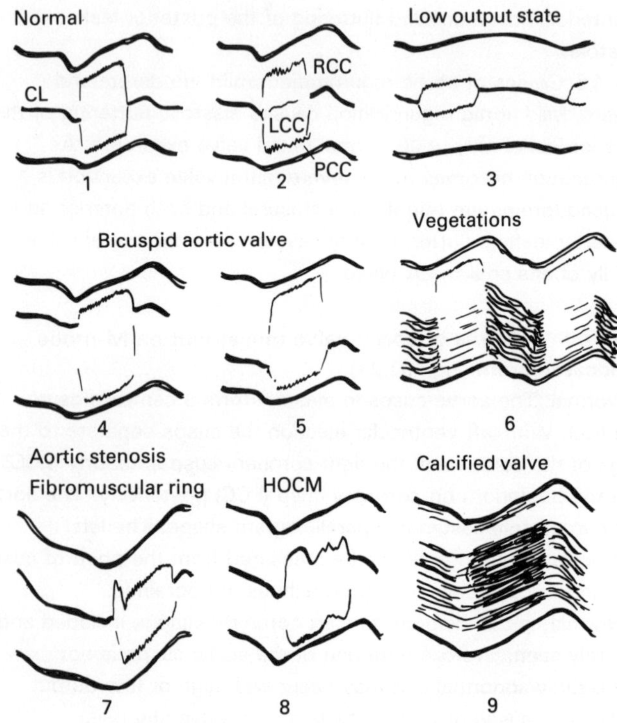

Fig. 10.21 Common patterns of aortic valve movement on M-mode echocardiogram.

6 Vegetations. These will only be visualised echocardiographically if they are larger than 3 mm. Small granular vegetations will be missed. Large aortic valve vegetations will be seen in both systole and diastole as dense horizontal lines. They may be confused with aortic valve calcification. Usually aortic valve vegetations are not continuous in systole and diastole, and are often seen only in diastole. Aortic valve calcification usually produces denser more continuous linear echoes. Unfortunately there is no absolute guide to their distinction.

7 Fibromuscular ring (discrete sub-aortic stenosis). There is immediate systolic closure of the aortic valve, best seen on the right coronary cusp. Often valve opening never returns to normal during the rest of systole. Compare this with hypertrophic obstructive cardiomyopathy (**8**) where premature aortic valve closure also occurs, but later in mid-systole.

8 HOCM. Premature aortic valve closure occurs in mid-systole when septum and mitral apparatus meet to produce LVOT obstruction. Mid-systolic aortic valve closure *per se* is not diagnostic of HOCM. It may occur in other conditions (e.g. mitral leaflet prolapse, aortic regurgitation, COCM, VSD, DORV).

9 Calcific aortic stenosis. Dense linear echoes usually continuous through systole and diastole are produced by one or more cusps. In more severe cases the entire aorta may be filled with these echoes and no discrete cusp movement is visible.

The pulmonary valve

This is the most difficult valve to visualise with the echo. Usually the posterior leaflet only is seen, and during pulmonary valve opening the echo often disappears to reappear as the valve closes.

Diagrammatic examples of pulmonary valve movement are shown in Fig. 10.22.

1 Normal. Atrial systole is transmitted to the pulmonary valve and causes a small posterior movement or 'a' wave. Systolic opening occurs next (B–C). The valve drifts slightly anteriorly to point D later in systole and then closes rapidly (D–E). In diastole the valve drifts slowly posteriorly (E–F slope) in the presence of a low PA pressure before the next 'a' wave.

2 Pulmonary hypertension. The 'a' wave disappears and so does the normal posterior drift of the EF slope. The E–F line is horizontal or may even be reserved. There is frequently coarse systolic fluttering of the pulmonary valve and mid-systolic closure.

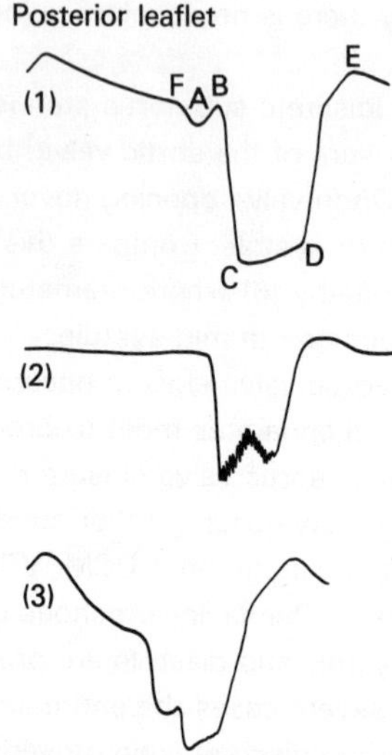

Fig. 10.22 Pulmonary valve appearances on M-mode echocardiogram. (1) Normal, (2) Pulmonary hypertension, (3) Pulmonary stenosis.

3 Pulmonary stenosis. The 'a' wave becomes increasingly prominent as the pulmonary stenosis becomes more severe. Unfortunately the size of the 'a' wave is not a completely reliable guide to the severity of the pulmonary stenosis.

Infundibular pulmonary stenosis produces diastolic and systolic fluttering of the pulmonary valve from turbulence. The 'a' wave disappears as the sub-pulmonary obstruction prevents its transmission to the valve.

The tricuspid valve

Is only visualised successfully on M-mode in conditions where the right heart is dilated. Usually the anterior leaflet only is seen. Its movement is very similar to mitral valve movement but slightly delayed. Tricuspid valve closure occurs normally up to 40 msec after mitral closure. With wide right bundle branch block closure may be delayed up to 65 msec. In Ebstein's anomaly, in which tricuspid and mitral echoes are often seen well at the same time, tricuspid closure is delayed still further.

Many features of mitral valve disease echocardiographically also apply to the tricuspid valve (e.g. visualisation of vegetations, posterior tricuspid leaflet prolapse).

In primum ASD with A–V canal defect there may be a free floating leaflet across the ventricular septal defect component. Either the mitral or tricuspid component of the valve may be seen to cross into the septum.

Septal movement

The septum normally acts as part of the left ventricle with posterior movement in systole (see example under LV function). Some conditions result in paradoxical septal motion in which the septal's posterior movement is delayed; it moves anteriorly in systole acting as part of the RV. The main causes are:

- RV volume overload: atrial septal defect, tricuspid regurgitation, pulmomary regurgitation, partial or total anomalous pulmonary veins, Ebstein's anomaly.
- Delayed or abnormal activation: LBBB, Wolff–Parkinson–White syndrome, ventricular ectopics.
- Septal abnormalities: ischaemic heart disease, congestive cardiomyopathy.
- Pericardial disease: pericardial effusion, constrictive pericarditis, congenital absence of pericardium.
- Open heart surgery: even in the absence of a conduction defect.

Paradoxical septal movement is divided into:

Type A: anterior systolic movement of the septum.

Type B: a horizontal septum with no net anterior or posterior movement in systole.

The echo sweep

Continuous recording of the echocardiogram is performed starting at the aortic valve and sweeping the transducer downwards and to the left towards the apex passing the mitral valve.

This technique is used to check:

• Aortic mitral continuity. The posterior wall of the aorta should be continuous with the anterior mitral leaflet on sweeping towards the apex. Absence of aortic mitral continuity is seen in double outlet right ventricle, some patients with Fallot's tetralogy and truncus arteriosus. It is not diagnostic of DORV as was originally thought.

• The left ventricular outflow tract. A difficult area to visualise. A prolapsing aortic cusp may be seen, or large vegetations in the LVOT flicking in and out of sight just above the anterior mitral leaflet. A discrete subvalve fibromuscular ring is easier visualised by 2D echocardiography.

• Aortic septal continuity. The anterior aortic wall is normally continuous with the interventricular septum. Over-riding of the aorta in Fallot's tetralogy can be shown with aortic septa discontinuity on M-mode echo.

• Which AV valve is continuous with which great vessel? In transposition of the great vessels (TGA) the posterior AV valve (mitral) is continuous with the posterior pulmonary artery. The anterior tricuspid valve is continuous with the aorta. Distinction of the great vessel depends on size (larger aorta in adults), venous injections of contrast in children (5% dextrose), and the recognition of a possible end-diastolic 'a' wave on the pulmonary valve. Unfortunately both AV valves may look identical so the distinction of the great vessel is important.

Pericardial effusion

The echocardiogram is very useful in detection of pericardial effusion. Pericardial fluid accumulates anterior to both ventricles and anterior and lateral to the right atrium. The pericardial reflection behind the left atrium limits the extension of effusion behind the left atrium and the pericardium tends to be adherent posteriorly. Pericardial fluid tends to be limited on the left side at the A–V groove.

Thus an echo taken at ventricular level may show fluid in front of the RV wall and behind the posterior LV wall (Fig. 10.23). Smaller effusions may only be visualised posteriorly. Usually an echo at the level of the aortic valve shows fluid anteriorly, but none behind the left atrium for the reasons given above.

The effect of the swinging heart inside the bag of fluid may produce paradoxical septal motion, pseudo-mitral prolapse, and electrical alternans on the ECG.

False positives may be obtained by incorrect gain settings. Posterior effusions should be seen in both systole and diastole. Increasing the reject setting to identify the pericardium is

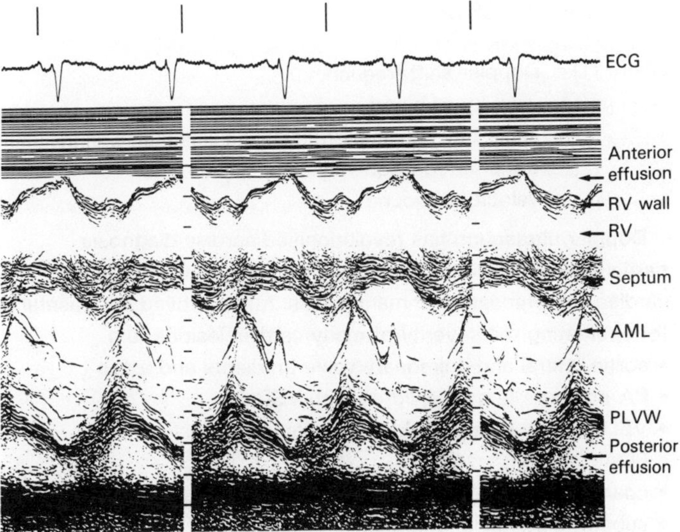

Fig. 10.23 Pericardial effusion seen both anterior to the RV wall and posterior to the LV wall.

important. In the presence of an effusion the posterior percardium is relatively static compared with the posterior LV wall.

Estimation of the size of an effusion is not reliable from an M-mode echo. The 2D echo grading should be small medium or large. Quantitation is inaccurate and unhelpful.

Doppler ultrasound

Doppler echocardiographic equipment compares the frequency of transmitted ultrasound with the received ultrasound frequency reflected off moving blood cells. Cells moving directly towards the transducer will result in a higher frequency ultrasound, and cells moving away from the transducer, a lower frequency.

This doppler shift frequency is used to estimate the velocity of blood.

i.e. $$fD = \frac{2f(V\cos\theta)}{c}$$

where fD = Doppler shift frequency,
V = velocity of blood,
θ = angle between transmitted and reflected sound,
f = transmitted frequency,
c = velocity of sound.

Doppler ultrasound has revolutionised cardiac diagnosis particularly in paediatric cardiology and has obviated the need for cardiac catheterisation in many cases. It has proved very useful for estimating the severity of many cardiac lesions, e.g.:

- aortic, mitral and pulmonary valve gradients and areas
- PA pressure (e.g. in children with VSDs)
- VSD closure (rising peak velocity of jet)
- PDA
- coarctation
- subaortic stenosis. Infundibular stenosis
- pulmonary artery branch stenosis
- severity of valve regurgitation

Modes of Doppler ultrasound used in cardiology

1 Pulsed wave (PW). Useful for identifying the exact site of stenosis, leak, etc. Not useful however for quantitative measurements. Pulsed Doppler cannot detect high frequency Doppler shifts as the pulse repetition frequency is limited. This results in 'aliasing' in which the signal may wrap around and appear on the other side of the base-line. This may introduce confusion as to the true direction of flow.

2 Continuous wave (CW). Needed to quantitate valve stenoses, etc. Aliasing does not occur. Blood flowing away from the transducer is represented as a spectral display below the base-line, and blood flowing towards it as a display above the base-line.

3 Colour Doppler. This colour codes for the direction of ultrasound shift:

e.g. red indicating blood moving towards the transducer, blue indicating blood moving away from the transducer.

This enables the echo technician to localise much more quickly the site and direction of abnormal blood flow (e.g. prosthetic valve regurgitation). It is not so useful in quantitating the severity of lesions.

The normal Doppler examination

Normal blood velocity: In adults (and children) in m/sec.

- tricuspid valve 0.3–0.7
- pulmonary valve 0.5–1.0
- mitral valve 0.6–1.3
- aortic valve 0.9–1.7

Children with innocent murmurs have higher velocities in ascending aorta. Low velocity in the ascending aorta is due to a low cardiac output or a wide aorta (e.g. Marfan syndrome). Higher velocities occur in higher flow situations (e.g. post exercise, anxiety) or in the right heart with left to right shunts.

10.3 Echocardiography

Normal valve regurgitation:
Doppler examination has establised that a very mild degree of regurgitation occurs through normal pulmonary and tricuspid valves. This regurgitation has a low peak velocity (e.g. <1 m/sec through the pulmonary valve). Tricuspid and pulmonary regurgitation are more common in cases with pulmonary hypertension, older children or RBBB.

Laminar vs turbulent flow: With laminar flow all the velocities of the blood cells are similar and a thin wave form with minimal spectral broadening is produced. With turbulent flow multiple different velocities are recorded and the Doppler signals is filled in with marked spectral broadening. See Figs. 10.26 and 10.27.

Estimation of PA pressure: First a good recording of tricuspid regurgitation is obtained using CW Doppler. Peak velocity of the tricuspid regurgitation is measured (say 2 m/sec). Then peak RV pressure $= 4V^2$ of peak tricuspid regurgitation velocity ($=16$). Add an extra 5 for estimated RA pressure, then peak RV pressure = 21 mmHg = peak PA pressure assuming no pulmonary stenosis.

Valve gradients
With good apical views using continuous wave, Doppler aortic and mitral valve gradients can be estimated. Suprasternal view of aortic valve needed in children (not possible in adults). Even using continuous wave Doppler, it is possible to underestimate aortic valve gradient if the cardiac output is low, the maximum jet is not recorded, or the angle between the ultrasound beam and the blood jet >20 degrees.
- Aortic valve: peak gradient. See Fig. 10.24.

Peak systolic gradient $= 4\ V\text{max}^2$ where Vmax is measured peak velocity in m/sec.
- Mitral valve: peak gradient $= 4\ V\text{max}^2$. Use CW from the apex.

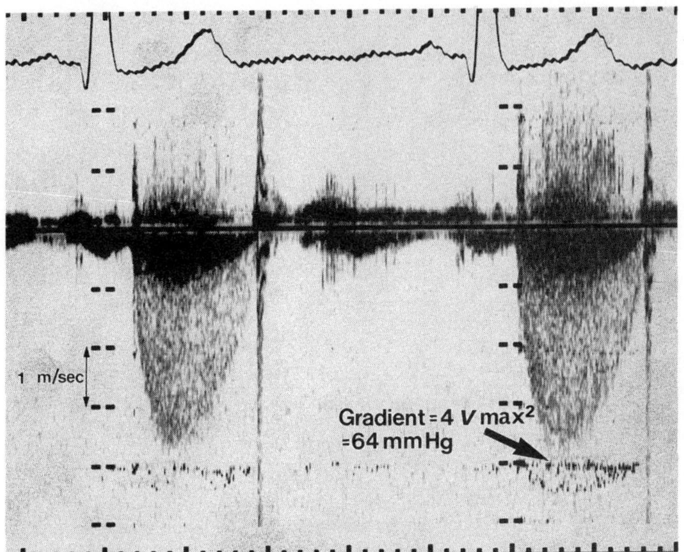

Fig. 10.24 Continuous wave Doppler signal in a patient with moderate aortic valve stenosis (apical view). Peak velocity = 4 m/sec (*V*max). Peak systolic gradient = 4 $V\text{max}^2$ = 64 mmHg.

Mitral valve area:

Measurement of pressure half time is needed to calculate mitral valve area.

$V_1 = 0.7 \times V\text{max}$, and occurs at the time (t) when the pressure gradient has fallen to half its maximum value. t = pressure half time.

Mitral valve area = $220/t$

= 759 /BT where BT is the base time of the extrapolated slope to zero.

($t = 0.29 \times \text{BT}$)

These formulae cannot be used for the tricuspid valve.

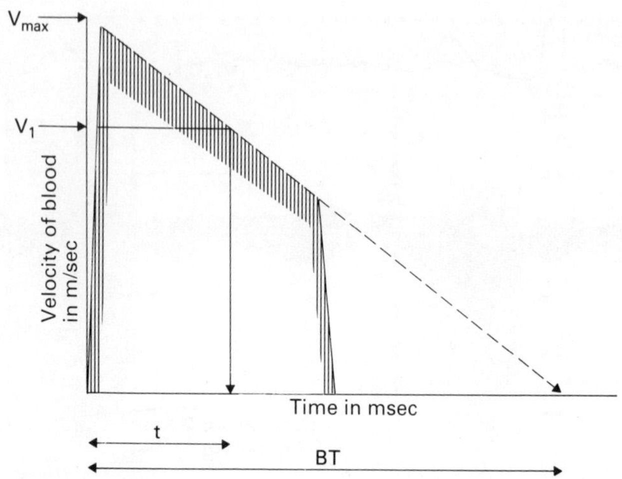

Fig. 10.25 Calculation of mitral valve gradient and valve area from a diagramatic apical continuous wave Doppler signal. Vmax = peak velocity in m/sec, V_1 = 0.7 × peak velocity in m/sec, t = pressure half time in msec (=0.29 × BT), BT = base time, Peak mitral gradient = 4 Vmax^2; mitral valve area = 220/t = 759/BT.

Fig. 10.26 Apical continuous wave Doppler echocardiography with sample volume in mitral valve orifice. ▶
1 = Normal laminar flow with minimal spectral broadening.
A = contribution of atrial systole; 2 = Normal laminar mitral flow but with high LVEDP. Early flow velocity 'E' is reduced, but late velocity is increased with the A wave; 3 = Mixed mitral valve disease with mitral stenosis and mild mitral regurgitation. Turbulent flow in both directions produces multiple velocities and marked spectral broadening. The turbulent signal above the base line is directed towards the transducer (stenotic jet), and the signal below the baseline is the regurgitant jet directed away from the transducer; 4 = Severe mitral regurgitation. Complete envelope of turbulent flow. Early peak velocity of severe regurgitation.

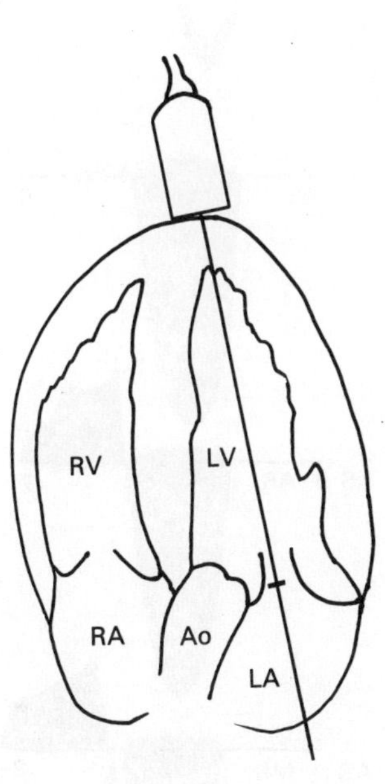
RV
LV
RA
Ao
LA

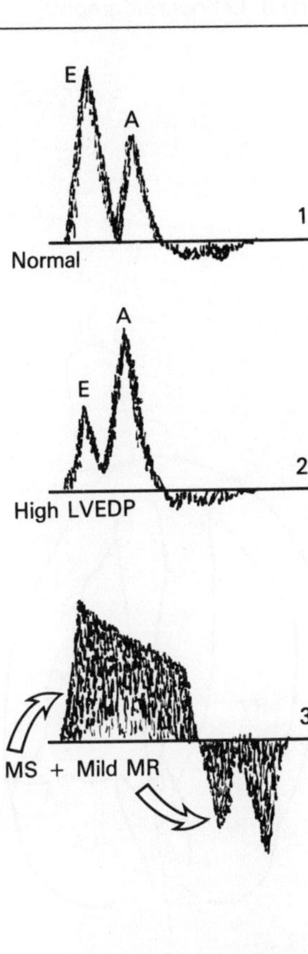
E
A
1
Normal
A
E
2
High LVEDP
3
MS + Mild MR

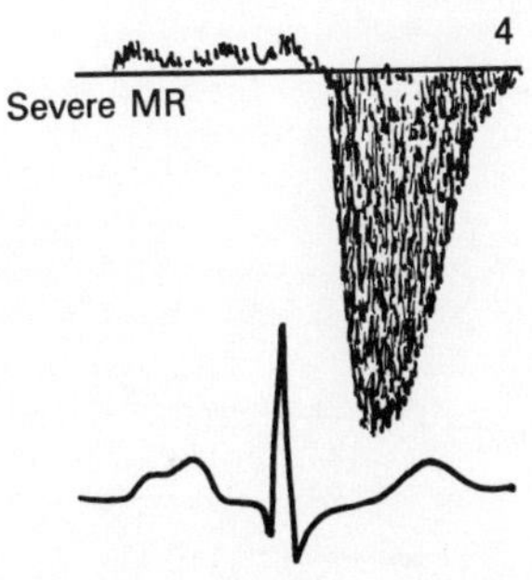
4
Severe MR

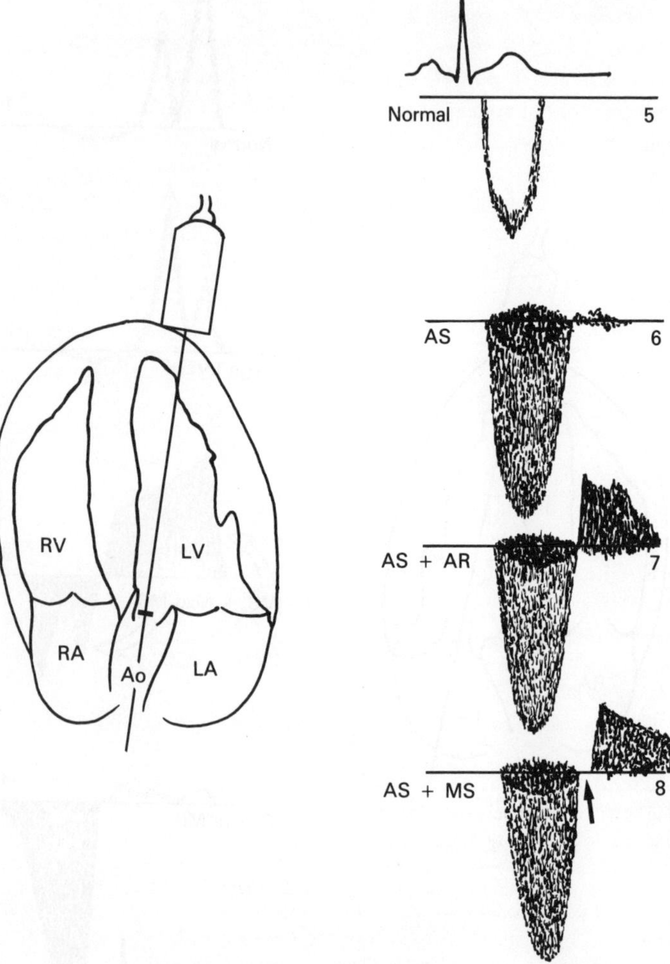
RV
LV
RA
Ao
LA
Normal
5
AS
6
AS + AR
7
AS + MS
8

10.4 Cardiac catheterisation

The advent of two dimensional and Doppler echocardiography has reduced the need for cardiac catheterisation in both congenital and adult heart disease. Newer forms of angiography such as digital subtraction angiography and radionuclide angiography together with magnetic resonance imaging may reduce the need still further. However it still plays a vital role in cardiac diagnosis. There is a rapid increase in the use of intervention techniques which avoid the need for cardiac surgical treatment, e.g.:

Congenital heart disease

• Rashkind balloon septostomy in TGA. Balloon dilatation of coarctation, mustard baffle, pulmonary venous obstruction, Blalock anastomosis, valve stenosis, etc.

Percutaneous transluminal coronary angioplasty (PTCA)

• Native coronary vessels, vein grafts, internal mammary grafts.

• Streptokinase infusion into main pulmonary artery in massive acute pulmonary embolism or into the coronary artery in acute myocardial infraction or during PTCA.

Valvuloplasty

• Balloon dilatation of all four valves is now a recognised procedure.

◀ **Fig. 10.27** Apical continuous wave Doppler echocardiography with sample volume in aortic valve orifice.
5 = Normal velocity profile with laminar flow; 6 = Aortic stenosis. Increased peak velocity with turbulent flow through the aortic valve; 7 = Mixed aortic valve disease. Turbulent flow in both directions, the stenotic component being away from the transducer with its signal below the baseline, and the regurgitant component above the baseline. Forward and reversed flow are continuous; 8 = Aortic and mitral stenosis with no aortic regurgitation. The two jet signals are not continuous with a small gap between (arrowed). This helps distinguish the signals of mitral stenosis from aortic regurgitation.

10.4 Cardiac catheterisation

Cardiac catheterisation is usually merely a diagnostic procedure with well defined mortality and morbidity risks. Since coronary arteriography was introduced by Mason Sones in 1962, great advances in catheterisation techniques and equipment have occurred.

Mortality and morbidity

Mortality in most centres is now approximately 0.1% in patients having coronary arteriography. The deaths occur in patients with the most severe coronary disease.

There is a definite morbidity relating to arterial entry site complications. The American Collaborative Study on Coronary Artery Surgery (CASS) published in 1979 suggested that the femoral entry site was safer. The brachial approach was only safe if the operator performed 80% or more of his procedures from the arm.

Most cardiologists are able to catheterise from either route with no morbidity.

What to tell the patient

The patient is told why the test is necessary and an explanation of what is involved and why local anaesthetic is preferred. The reasons that GA is usually unnecessary are as follows: it interferes with haemodynamics and oxygen saturations; patients cannot indicate if they develop angina or other symptoms; patients are usually required to perform respiratory manoeuvres, coughing, etc.; patients are sometimes required to perform exercise during the test.

The procedure should be painless, although the patient should be warned of the hot flush associated with angiography, and the very small risks should be explained.

Which route?

This is a matter of operator preference. Usually however the right brachial route is used for:

- patients on anticoagulants
- coarction of the aorta (or axillary cut down in babies)
- patients with intermittent claudication or those who have had aortic-iliac surgery
- aortic valve stenosis as a dominant lesion. (A few centres prefer the leg route using trans-septal puncture)
- hypertensive patients with high peak-systolic pressures, as femoral haemostasis may be difficult

The femoral route is usually preferred for patients with

- atrial septal defects and
- most congenital heart disease
- young women with atypical chest pain who may have small brachial arteries and a tendency to arterial spasm
- patients with Raynaud's phenomenon
- several (two or more) previous brachial catheterisations
- presence of a right subclavian bruit

Premedication

Some form of premedication is important as anxious patients may become vagal on arrival in the catheter laboratory or after withdrawal of the catheters. Anxiety may provoke angina before the procedure even starts in patients with ischaemic heart disease. The following is a suggested regime:

Adults:	Diazepam 10–20 mg orally 1–2 hours pre-catheter. A further dose may be given i.v. prior to the catheter if the patient is still anxious
Children: Up to 25 kg	Vallergan 4 mg/kg orally 2 hours pre-catheter
	Pethco 0.1 ml/kg im 1 hour pre-catheter
Children: 25–40 kg	Omnopon 10 mg } i.m.
	Scopolamine 0.2 mg } i.m.

Patients do not usually require GA if these doses are used, but an anaesthetist should be 'standing by' for paediatric cases.

Patients should be starved for >4 hours pre-catheter. Their cardiac medication should not be discontinued, except for diuretics which are best avoided on the morning of catheterisation.

Polycythaemic patients with cyanotic congenital heart disease are at risk (if the haemoglobin level is >18 g/100 ml) of both arterial and venous thrombosis. A few days prior to cardiac catheter the patients should be admitted for venesection, with concurrent plasma exchange if the haemoglobin exceeds this level (see **2.9**).

Coping with catheter complications occurring on the ward

1 *Haemorrhage*

Leg This is controlled by firm pressure. A Johns Hopkin's bandage is not effective and just obscures the puncture site. Firm pressure above the puncture site will help control the development of a haematoma. If the bleeding is not controlled after 30 min:

• check the clotting screen. If the patient is on warfarin fresh frozen plasma may help. Vitamin K is not recommended as it makes subsequent anticoagulation very difficult. If the patient has just had heparin then check the thrombin time as protamine reversal may help (dose = protamine 10 mg/1000 units heparin administered)

• is the patient hypertensive? High peak systolic pressure will exacerbate bleeding

• call for help. Very rarely femoral artery repair may be necessary for a false aneurysm. A hard tender pulsatile lump over the puncture site developing after cardiac catheterisation suggests a false aneurysm. The diagnosis can be confirmed by ultrasound imaging. Occasionally a small false aneurysm thromboses spontaneously, but most require surgical repair. The increasing use of PTCA and valvuloplasty require larger arterial sheaths and the use of additional streptokinase in the catheter laboratory during PTCA, all increase the risk of this complication.

Arm The same principles apply. However in this case the artery has been repaired by direct suture. Bleeding is often venous oozing only. Firm brachial pressure should not occlude the radial pulse. Protamine is not usually given following brachial artery catheterisation. Any haematoma development will require exploring and resuturing of the brachial artery.

2 *Infection*

Post catheter pyrexia is usually due to a dye reaction and settles within 24 hours. Persisting pyrexia should be investigated and treated on usual lines with blood cultures, urine cultures, etc. prior to antibiotics.

A tender pink area around the brachial cut down should be treated with complete rest (arm resting on a pillow), and oral amoxycillin 500 mg tds and flucloxacillin 500 mg qds for 5 days.

3 *Dye reaction*

This is commonly mild, causing: skin reaction, erythema, urticaria or even bullous eruption; nausea and vomiting, headache, hypotension, pyrexia, rigors. Very rarely it causes more severe reactions: fits, transient cortical disturbance, e.g. cortical blindness, anaphylactic shock

• urticaria and skin reaction is usually helped by intravenous antihistamines (e.g. chlorpheniramine 10 mg i.v.) and more severe cases by additional intravenous hydrocortisone 100 mg

• nausea, vomiting, i.v. metoclopramide 10 mg

• hypotension, i.v. fluids may be necessary, especially in patients who have been excessively diuresed or who have had a lot of dye (e.g. over 3 ml/kg)

• pyrexia and rigors are usually transient. Rest and sedation are all that is necessary

• anaphylactic shock. Occurs in the catheter laboratory rather than the ward, and should be treated by urgent volume replacement with i.v. plasma or N saline, hydrocortisone 200 mg i.v., adrenaline 1 in 1000, 1 ml slowly s.c.

• cortical disturbances are rare and again usually transient. They are not necessarily embolic, and may in part be due to vascular spasm, or an osmotic effect of the dye. Fits are controlled as in grand mal epilepsy with i.v. diazepam

4 *Cyanotic attacks*

These typically occur in the small child with Fallot's tetralogy and severe infundibular stenosis. The combination of metabolic acidosis, hypoxia and hypovolaemia predispose to infundibular shut down or spasm. Catecholamine release secondary to pain and/or fear will also exacerbate this. Treatment depends on reversing these factors:

- propranolol 0.025–0.1 mg/kg i.v., or
- morphine sulphate 0.1–0.2 mg/kg i.v. in severe cases
- check the arterial acid–base balance. If the base deficit is or exceeds −5 give i.v. $NaHCO_3$ 8.4% as:

$$\frac{\text{Body wt (kg)}}{6} \times \text{base deficit, then repeat the blood gases}$$

- exclude hypoglycaemia on above sample
- oxygen via a face mask
- placing the child in a knee-chest position acts in the same way as 'squatting' by cutting off acidotic venous return from the legs. As an initial manoeuvre it may help while drugs are being prepared

5 *The lost radial pulse*

This should be dealt with in the catheter laboratory at the time. If the patient is hypotensive volume replacement with intravenous heparisation may help. Nitrates are of little benefit. 50% of patients who do not regain the radial pulse will not develop claudication symptoms. A few patients will regain the radial pulse once they warm up and brachial spasm regresses. Overall a lost radial pulse occurs in less than 1% of brachial catheterisations.

A numb hand may occur in the presence of a good radial pulse. This is usually the effect of lignocaine on the median nerve at the catheter site and the sensation returns within 12 hours.

Residual median nerve damage is rare and probably due to unnecessary manipulation of the nerve during the catheter procedure.

A loss of the foot pulses following femoral artery catheterisation is also rare, but may be transient (24 hours) in children. In adults however loss of the foot pulses is usually irreversible and requires femoral thrombectomy.

6 *Angina*

May occur during or after coronary angiography, or as a result of paroxysmal tachycardia in the ischaemic patient. It usually responds to sublingual nitroglycerine and sedation. The ECG should be checked and if the angina recurs the patient should be monitored. Occasionally i.m. or i.v. diamorphine 2.5–5 mg is required.

In severe cases with recurrent pain intravenous nitrates should be started (p. 149).

If ST segment elevation occurs, the patient has probably occluded a major coronary artery due to thrombus or dissection following intubation or instrumentation of the coronary artery. Very occasionally it may be due to coronary spasm. In either case treatment with i.v. nitrates is started. The next stage depends on the findings at cardiac catheterisation. The patient may be suitable for an immediate angioplasty, or emergency coronary artery by-pass surgery may be necessary. If immediate surgery or PTCA are not possible then intra-aortic balloon pumping is considered. This will help maintain coronary flow and reduce infarct size until a more definitive treatment is available. In the elderly, or those who have had a difficult salvage angioplasty, it may be felt that supportive medical treatment is appropriate. (See **5.7**).

7 *Dysrhythmias*

These are usually transient and dealt with during catheterisation. They may occasionally recur on the ward, e.g. paroxysmal AF or SVT, more rarely paroxysmal ventricular dysrhythmias. Each dysrhythmia must be treated on its merits along the lines discussed in **6.12**.

8 *Pericardial tamponade*

This should be considered in any patient who becomes hypotensive and anuric following catheterisation. It is a very rare complication of routine cardiac catheterisation but is a recognised complication of the trans-septal puncture procedure or RV biopsy. Diagnosis is confirmed by M-mode and 2D echocardiography. Pericardial aspiration may be required.

Valve area calculation

Calculation of aortic or mitral valve area from cardiac catheter data is possible if the cardiac output is measured together with simultaneous pressures from either side of the aortic or mitral valve. Calculations of tricuspid and pulmonary valve area are perfectly possible but rarely needed.

The calculation of valve area thus depends on:

- the mean valve gradient
- the forward flow across the valve
- a constant

The constant used derives from the calculations of Gorlin and Gorlin (1951) which has been established by comparing calculated valve area and actual valve area measured at autopsy or at operation. Since the calculation depends on 'forward flow' the method is invalidated in the presence of regurgitation unless angiographic output is used.

The range of aortic and mitral valve area

Valve area in adult (cm^2)	Aortic	Mitral
Normal	2.5–3.5	4–6
Mild stenosis	1.0–1.5	1.5–2.0
Moderate stenosis	0.5–1.0	1.0–1.5
Severe stenosis	<0.5	<1

This table relates to native valves. The method can also be used for prosthetic valves.

The Gorlin formula tends to over estimate the true valve area at high cardiac outputs, and under estimate valve area at low cardiac outputs.

Aortic valve area (same formula for pulmonary valve) (Fig. 10.28)

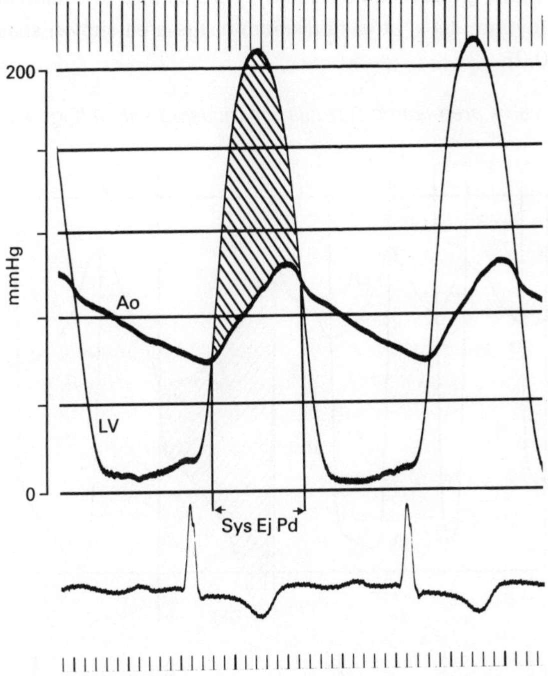

Fig. 10.28 Aortic valve area. Hatched area is that planimetred for calculation of mean aortic gradient. Sys Ej Pd = systolic ejection period in sec/min.

10.4 Cardiac catheterisation

$$\text{Aortic valve area} = \frac{\text{Aortic valve flow (ml/sec)}}{44.5\sqrt{\text{Mean aortic gradient (mmHg)}}}$$

$$\text{Aortic valve flow} = \frac{\text{Cardiac output (ml/min)}}{\text{Systolic ejection period (sec/min)}}$$

44.5 = The Gorlin constant for aortic (or pulmonary) valves.

Mean aortic gradient is calculated by planimetry (5 cycles in sinus rhythm, 10 in atrial fibrillation) of the area shown shaded in Fig. 10.28.

Mitral valve area (same formula for tricuspid valve) (Fig. 10.29)

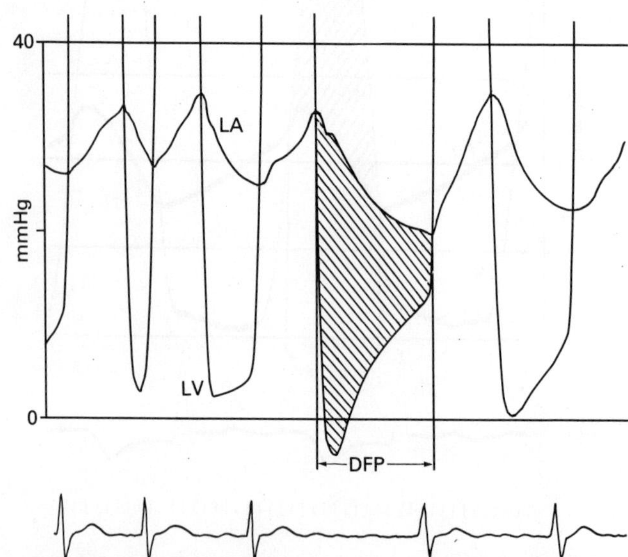

Fig. 10.29 Mitral valve area. Hatched area is that planimetred for calculation of mitral valve area. Ten consecutive cycles should be measured for patients in AF. DFP = diastolic filling period in sec/min.

$$\text{Mitral valve area} = \frac{\text{Mitral valve flow (ml/sec)}}{31\sqrt{\text{Mean mitral gradient (mmHg)}}}$$

$$\text{Mitral valve flow} = \frac{\text{Cardiac output (ml/min)}}{\text{Diastolic filling period (sec/min)}}$$

Mean mitral gradient is calculated by planimetry of the area shown in Fig. 10.29.

31 = The Gorlin constant for mitral (or tricuspid valves) (0.7 × 44.5) in the original calculation where LV mean diastolic pressure was assumed to be 5 mmHg.

With simultaneous measurement of LV and LA (or PAW) pressures the constants 38 or 40 are frequently used.

Angiographic estimation of LV volume

In spite of the facts that gross assumptions are made about the shape of the LV cavity, that magnification errors may arise, and that single plane cine is usually used, the angiographic assessment of LV volume correlates very closely with ventricular cast measurements or echocardiographic estimations of LV volume.

Although formulae for biplane cineangiography have been produced, most centres use a single plane 30° RAO projection for the LV cine. Most formulae assume the left ventricular cavity is an ellipsoid of revolution: thus assuming that the minor axes in two planes are identical.

$$V = \frac{4\pi}{3} \times \frac{D}{2} \times \frac{D}{2} \times \frac{L}{2} = \frac{\pi}{6} \times D^2 \times L \text{ (uncorrected for}$$

magnification)

The magnification factor (f) is calculated from filming a marked catheter or grid/ruler of known length (at central chest level). The corrected volume equation becomes:

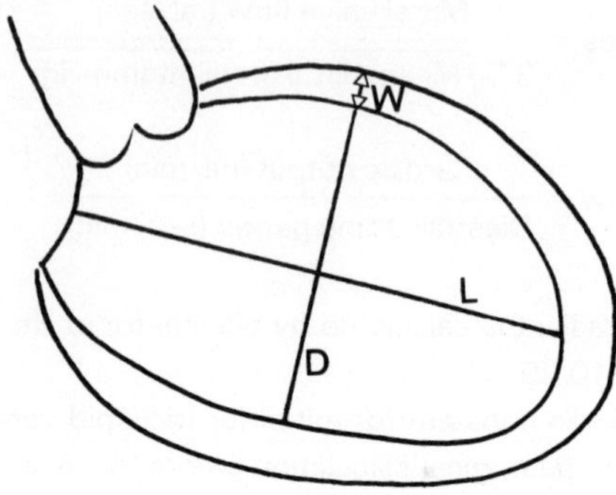

Fig. 10.30 Estimation of LV volume by single plane 30° RAO projection. L = major axis (cm), D = minor axis in two planes (cm), V = ventricular volume (ml), W = wall thickness (cm, see LV mass estimation).

$$V = \frac{\pi}{6} D^2.L.f^3 = 0.524.D^2.L.f^3 \text{ (Greene formula)}$$

The formula can be modified by calculation of the area (A cm^2) and length (L cm) only. The area is measured by planimetry or more usually by a light-pen computer system. Using this area length method the minor axis need not be measured as:

$$\frac{D}{2} = \frac{2A}{L} \text{ where A = area of LV in cm}^2$$

Substituting this in the original volume equation we can simplify the equation to:

$$V = \frac{0.849.A^2.f^3}{L} \text{ (Dodge formula)}$$

Programming this formula into a computer, rapid sequential LV volume analysis is possible.

10.4 Cardiac catheterisation

Formulae for the calculation of right ventricular volume have been derived but each make assumptions of RV cavity shape which are even more unfounded than the assumption of LV cavity shape.

Angiographic assessment of LV mass

The volume of the left ventricular cavity is subtracted from the volume of cavity and LV wall. Uniform wall thickness is assumed.

If W = wall thickness at midpoint of intersection of the minor axis, and specific gravity of heart muscle is 1.05 then:

$$\text{LV mass} = 1.05 \times \underbrace{\left[\frac{4}{3}\pi f^3 \left(\frac{D}{2} + W\right)^2 \left(\frac{L}{2} + W\right)\right]}_{\text{LV wall + cavity volume}} - \underbrace{\left[\frac{\pi}{6} f^3.D^2.L\right]}_{\text{Cavity volume}}$$

In spite of the obvious invalidity of the assumptions involved in the calculation this estimate of LV mass has been shown to correlate well with post mortem measurements.

Normal values for LV angiographic volumes (Kennedy)

LVEDVI	70 ± 20 (mean $\pm$ SD) ml/m^2
LVESVI	24 ± 10ml/m^2
Ejection fraction	0.67 ± 0.08
LV mass	92 ± 16 g
Wall thickness	10.9 ± 2.0 mm

Cardiac output calculations

Direct Fick method

The main difficulty with this method is an accurate measurement of oxygen consumption.

$$\text{Cardiac output} = \frac{\text{Oxygen consumption}}{\text{Arteriovenous oxygen content difference}}$$

10.4 Cardiac catheterisation

$$\text{or CO (l/min)} = \frac{O_2 \text{ consumption ml/min}}{(A_0 - PA)\ O_2 \text{ content ml/100 ml} \times 10}$$

Oxygen content calculation

The haemoglobin and oxygen saturation must be known.

$$\text{Oxygen content} = (\text{Hb} \times 1.34 \times \%\ \text{saturation}) + \text{Plasma } O_2 \text{ content}$$

Where Hb = haemoglobin; 1.34 is derived from the fact that 1 g Hb when 100% saturated combines with 1.34 ml O_2.

$$\text{Plasma } O_2 \text{ content in 100 ml plasma } \frac{100 \times 0.0258 \times PO_2}{760}$$

Thus with Hb of 15 g/100 ml and 97% saturation the arterial oxygen content is = (15 × 1.34 × 0.97) + 0.3 = 19.65 ml/100 ml where 0.3 is the plasma correction factor.

Plasma correction factors

Saturation %	Correction	Saturation %	Correction
97	0.3	75	0.12
96	0.27	70	0.11
94	0.24	60	0.10
92	0.21	50	0.08
90	0.19	40	0.07
85	0.17	30	0.05
80	0.14	20	0.04

It does not matter from which systemic artery the O_2 content is calculated. Only the pulmonary artery should be used for mixed venous oxygen content calculation.

Oxygen content can also be measured by specific equipment

containing a galvanic fuel cell which releases electrons on absorbing oxygen (Lexington instruments) or by a manometric method (Van Slyke).

Oxygen consumption calculation

Expired air is collected for 3–10 min of steady state respiration. The method is only really possible or accurate in the basal state. Three methods are available:

- closed circuit spirometer—containing 100% oxygen and expired CO_2 is absorbed by soda-lime canister
- open circuit: with expired air collected in a Douglas bag
- fuel cell technique—with a sample of expired air measured for oxygen concentration using purpose built equipment

$$\dot{V}O_2 = \dot{V}_E \, STP \, (F_{IO_2} - F_{EO_2}) \times 10 \text{ ml/min}$$

where $\dot{V}O_2$ = Oxygen consumption in ml/min

$\dot{V}_E$ STP = expired volume of air corrected for standard temperature and pressure

F_{IO_2} = concentration of inspired oxygen. In room air this is 20.93% and need not be measured

F_{EO_2} = concentration of expired oxygen

The correction of $\dot{V}_E$ for standard temperature and pressure is:

$$\dot{V}_E \, STP = \dot{V}_E \, ATP \times \frac{273}{273 + T} \times \frac{P - W}{P} \times \frac{P}{760}$$

Where $\dot{V}_E$ ATP = measured expired volume at atmospheric temperature and pressure

T = room temperature in °C

P = barometric pressure in the room (mmHg)

W = water vapour pressure (mmHg)

Table of water vapour pressure (W) at various room temperatures

Temp °C	W mmHg	Temp °C	W mmHg	Temp °C	W mmHg
15	12.79	21	18.65	27	26.74
16	13.63	22	19.83	28	28.35
17	14.53	23	21.07	29	30.04
18	15.48	24	22.38	30	31.82
19	16.48	25	23.76	31	33.70
20	17.54	26	25.21	32	35.60

Indirect Fick method

Using the table of estimated oxygen consumption the direct Fick measurement or an indicator dilution method can be checked. The table is a guide and cannot be comprehensive for all ages at any heart rate.

Mean oxygen consumption in the basal state per body surface area in ml/min/m^2. (See body surface area nomogram on p. 473.)

Basal state: Adults approx 70 bpm, Children approx 120 bpm

Age	Male	Female	Age	Male	Female
3	185	178	23	129	118
4	180	173	24	129	117
5	177	170	25	127	117
6	174	167	27	127	117
7	169	163	28	127	117
8	166	155	30	125	117
9	162	151	32	125	116
10	158	146	33	124	115
11	153	143	35	124	114
12	150	137	36	123	113
13	147	133	38	123	112
14	143	127	40	122	112
15	140	124	42	119	112
16	137	122	45	118	111
17	135	121	50	117	110
18	134	120	55	115	109
19	132	119	60	114	108
20	131	118	65	113	107
21	130	118	70	112	106
22	130	118	75	110	105

Cardiac output by indicator dilution

Indocyanine green (peak absorption at 800 nm) is injected into the right heart or main pulmonary artery. Downstream sampling is from the aorta, brachial or femoral artery through a densitometer. The Gilford densitometer is often used. It is insensitive to changes in O_2 saturation. Background dye causes a baseline shift.

The disadvantage of the technique is that two catheters are involved and that recirculation occurs. Also a calibration factor (K) must be calculated from known concentrations of green dye in fresh heparinised non-smokers blood.

$$\text{Then } K = \frac{\text{Indicator concentration in mg/l}}{\text{Deflection through densitometer (mm)}}$$

Several concentrations of dye in blood must first be prepared (e.g 1–10 mg/l).

From the Hamilton equation:

$$CO = \frac{I \times 60}{C \times t}$$

Where I = amount of green dye injected (mg)

C = mean concentration of dye (mg/l)

t = duration of curve (sec)

The product ($C \times t$) is the area under the curve excluding the recirculation component, the primary curve. There are two chief methods for calculation of the area. The most accurate is to reconstruct the primary curve by plotting the time-concentration curve on semi-logarithmic paper with the indicator concentration on the semi-log axis. The straight line on the descending limb is extrapolated and the primary curve reconstructed from the semi-log plot: it is assumed that the decay of the primary curve is exponential (Fig. 10.31).

The second type of calculation employs short cuts which ignore the recirculation component and do not involve reconstruction of the primary curve.

1 *Reconstruction of the primary curve* (Fig. 10.31)
Once the primary curve is constructed there are several methods for calculation of the area, some of which are discussed below

- By planimetry (Fig. 10.32)
- Summation of one second interval concentration values

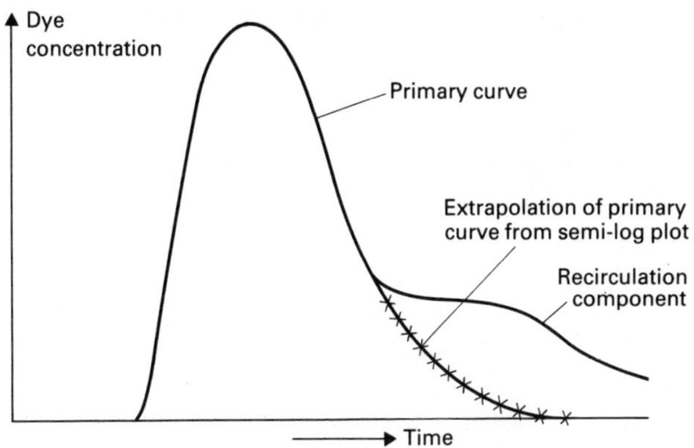

Fig. 10.31 Reconstruction of the primary curve.

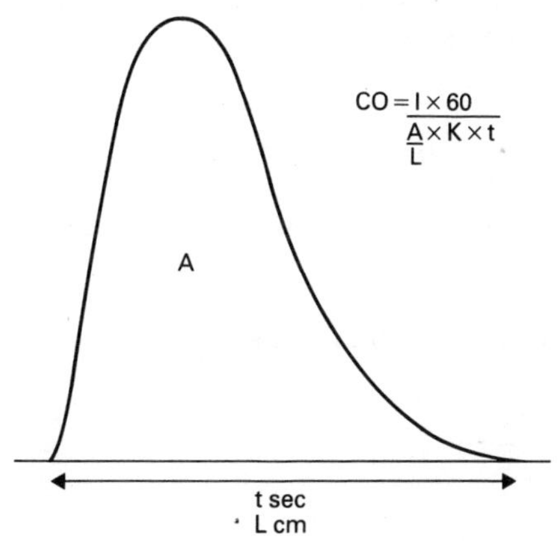

Fig. 10.32 Calculation of the area by planimetry. A = planimetred area of curve in cm^2. L = length of base line in cm. K = calibration factor. t = time of curve in sec. 1 = quantity of dye injected in mg.

(ordinates). This is easier if the curve is traced on to graph paper (Fig. 10.33).

2 *Short cuts not requiring primary curve reconstruction*
These methods are quicker and reconstruction of the primary curve from the dye curve is unnecessary. Several other measurements are required depending on the method used. (Fig. 10.34)

Where AT = appearance time of dye in sec

BT = build up time in sec from onset of curve

T_{50} = time at half peak concentration

C_p = peak concentration in mg/l

PCT = time to peak concentration from dye injection

Dow's formula:

$$\text{Area} = \frac{\text{PC} \times \text{PCT}}{3 - 0.9\ (\text{PCT}/\text{AT})}\ \text{mm sec}$$

Hetzel *et al.* formula (forward triangle method)

$$\text{CO} = \frac{\text{I} \times 60 \times \text{K}}{\text{BT} \times C_p/2}$$

K in this case is an empirical constant (0.37 for central injection, 0.35 for peripheral injection)

Bradley and Barr formula (fore-'n-aft triangle method)
Area = $C_p \times T_{50}$ mm sec

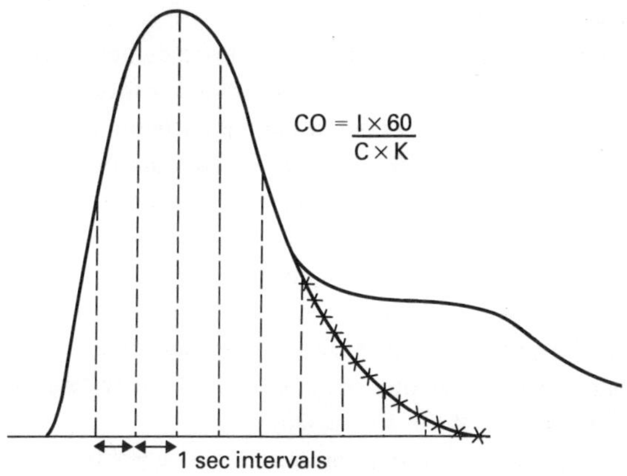

Fig. 10.33 Summation of 1 sec intervals. C = sum of ordinate values (mm sec) at one second intervals.

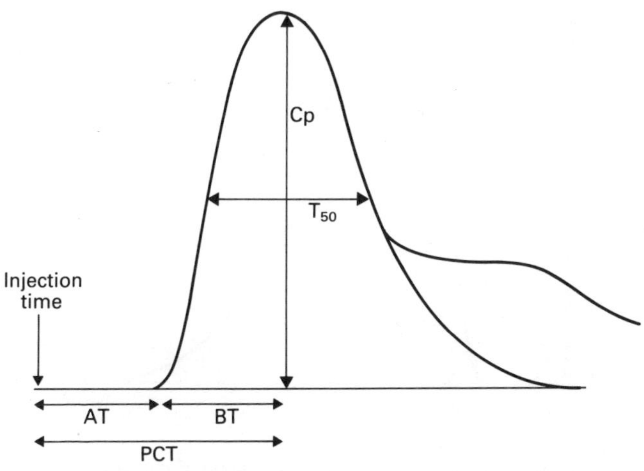

Fig. 10.34 Calculation of area under the curve without planimetry.

Thermodilution method

This is usually performed using a Swan–Ganz catheter in the right heart. 5 or 10 ml of 5% dextrose (at either room temperature or 4°C) are injected in the right atrium, and the thermister at the catheter tip in the pulmonary artery senses the transient fall in temperature as a rise in resistance.

Advantages over green-dye measurements are:

- the recirculation curve can be ignored
- only one catheter is needed
- the method can be repeated rapidly following drug intervention and the catheter may be left in the right heart for further assessment of the sick patient

A variety of cardiac output computers are available which integrate electronically the area under the curve. Several methods are used, all of which assume the downslope of the curve is exponential (Fig. 10.35).

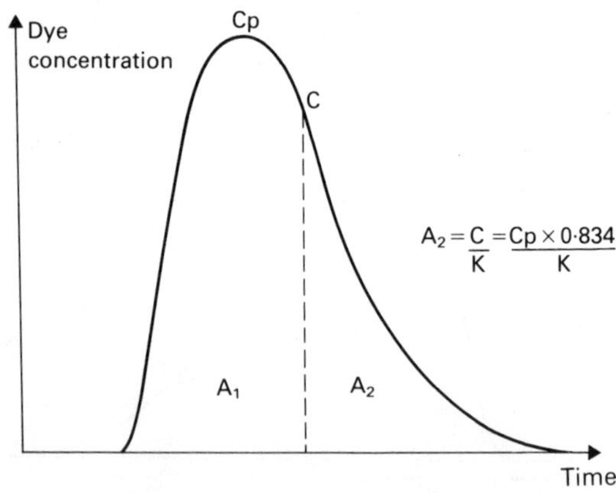

Fig. 10.35 Measuring area, where the downslope of the curve is exponential. K is the decay constant of the downslope. The exponential decay is assumed to start at 83.4% of peak concentration.

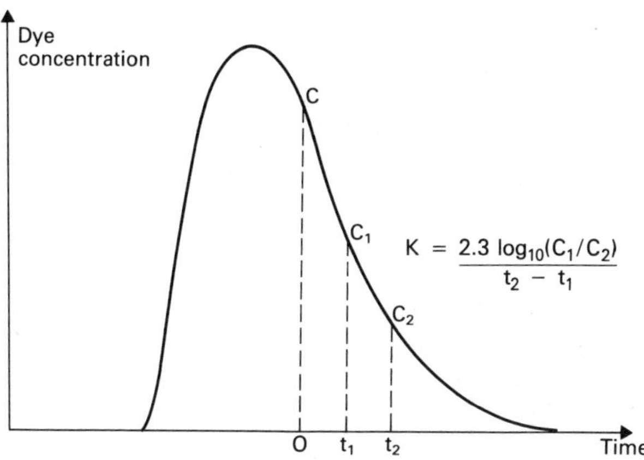

Fig. 10.36 Calculation of the decay constant (K).

Shunt quantitation by dye dilution

Shunt quantitation is possible by either dye-dilution or oximetry. Dye dilution is more sensitive but more complex. Two types of curve may be produced. The normal curve is superimposed in each case. In both cases peak concentration is less. Early appearance of dye occurs in the right-to-left shunt and the curve has a double hump, with the unshunted dye forming the second peak (Fig. 10.37)

1 *Left-to-right shunt*

The dye must be injected in main pulmonary artery and sampled in descending aorta or more peripherally. If the dye is injected in the left heart distal to the shunt site the curve will have a normal appearance.

Using the method of Carter *et al.* for the left → right shunts (Fig. 10.38)

The ratio of $\frac{C_{(p+BT)}}{C_p}$ and $\frac{C_{(p+2BT)}}{C_p}$ is calculated

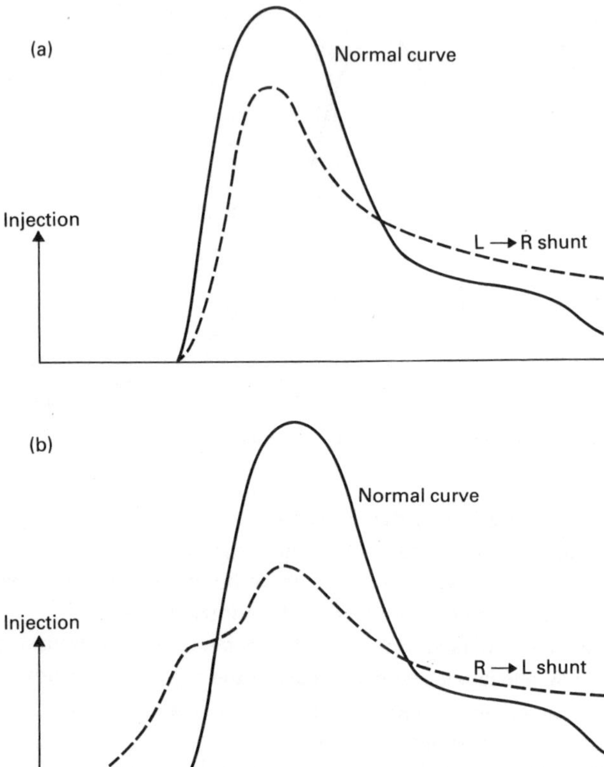

Fig 10.37 Shunt qualification by dye dilution. (a) Left-to-right shunt (b) Right-to-left shunt.

$$\text{Then: } \frac{\text{left-to-right shunt}}{\text{pulmonary flow}} \times 100 = 141 \times \frac{C_{(p+BT)}}{C_p} - 42 \text{ (A)}$$

$$\text{and} = 135 \times \frac{C_{(p+2BT)}}{C_p} - 14 \text{ (B)}$$

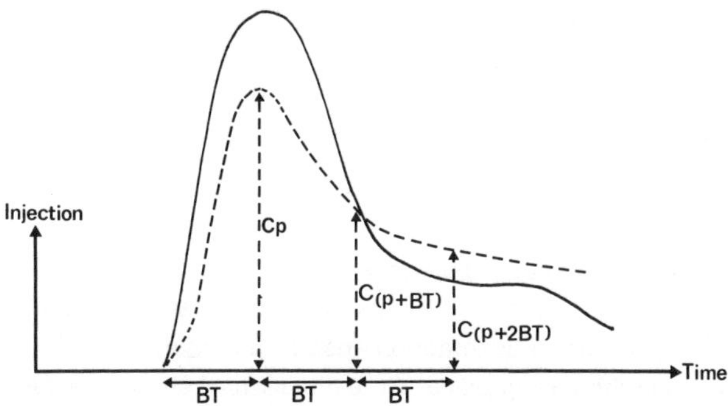

Fig 10.38 Calculation of left-to-right shunt. Where C_p = peak concentration, BT = build-up time, $C_{(p+BT)}$ concentration one build-up time after peak, $C_{(p+2BT)}$ = concentration two build-up times after peak.

A and B are averaged to produce the ratio of shunt to pulmonary flow. (The equations are derived from regression lines of studies by Carter *et al.*)

2 *Right-to-left shunt*

The forward triangle method compares areas under the early and late hump of the curve. The early hump is assumed to be due

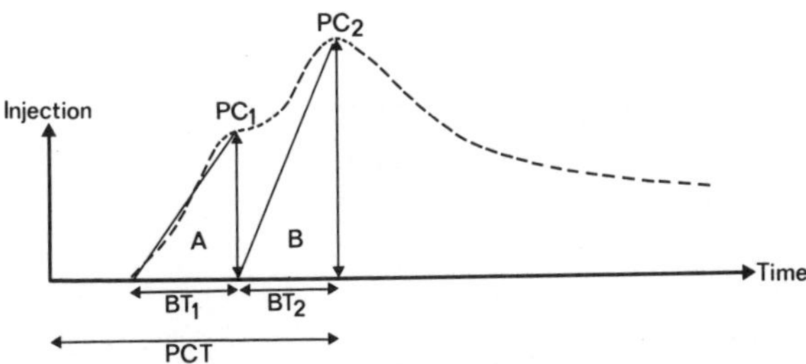

Fig. 10.39 Calculation of the right-to-left shunt. A = shunt triangle, B = systemic flow triangle, PC_1 = peak concentration of initial hump (shunt) (mg/l), PC_2 = peak concentration of second hump (systemic) (mg/l), BT_1 build-up time of initial hump (sec), BT_2 build-up time of second hump (sec) ($= 0.46 \times$ PCT), PCT = time to peak concentration PC_2.

to the right-to-left shunt only. The later hump is assumed to be due to systemic flow (Fig. 10.39).

$$\text{Then } \frac{\text{Right-to-left shunt}}{\text{Systemic flow}} = \frac{BT_1 \times PC_1}{(BT_1 \times PC_1) + (BT_2 \times PC_2)}$$

Shunt quantitation by oximetry

Oximetry is used to detect shunts rather than quantitate them accurately. Errors in quantitation arise from streaming and sampling in the wrong place. An estimation of shunt size can be made from saturation measurements during catheterisation.

From the Fick equation:

$$\text{Pulmonary flow} = \frac{O_2 \text{ consumption}}{(\text{PV}-\text{PA } O_2 \text{ content})}$$

Pulmonary vein sampling is not possible unless there is an ASD or trans-septal catheterisation is performed. PV saturation is assumed to be 98%.

The equation becomes:

1 Pulmonary flow =

$$\frac{O_2 \text{ consumption}}{\frac{(98 - \text{PA saturation})}{100} \times \text{Hb} \times 1.34 \times 10} \text{ l/min}$$

Similarly:

2 Systemic flow =

$$\frac{O_2 \text{ consumption}}{\frac{(A_0 \text{ saturation} - \text{mixed venous saturation})}{100} \times \text{Hb} \times 1.34 \times 10}$$

Mixed venous saturation is calculated as:

$$\frac{(3 \times \text{SVC saturation}) + (1 \times \text{IVC saturation})}{4}$$

SVC saturation is usually lower than IVC saturation.

Rather than measure O_2 consumption the ratio of pulmonary to systemic flow can be estimated by dividing **1 by 2** i.e.

$$\frac{\text{Pulmonary}}{\text{Systemic flow}} = \frac{A_0 \text{ saturation} - \text{mixed venous saturation \%}}{98 - \text{PA saturation \%}}$$

True pulmonary vein saturation is substituted for 98% if it is obtained. Small left-to-right shunts may be missed by oximetry and green dye or ascorbate techniques are more sensitive. Oximetry will not usually detect a PDA or small VSD. A primum ASD may be mistaken on oximetry as a VSD with the oxygenated stream being missed in low right atrial sampling.

Nevertheless it provides a useful check during catheterisation and an estimate of shunt size. A routine saturation run during catheterisation usually involves sampling from:

High SVC	RV inflow
Low SVC	RV body
R_A/SVC junction	RV outflow
High RA	Main PA (RPA + LPA)
Mid RA	LA and PV if possible
Low RA	LV
IVC	A_0

Sampling through the right atrium is performed down the lateral RA wall to detect anomalous venous drainage. Bidirectional shunting can be detected but not accurately quantitated using oximetry.

Assessment of left ventricular function

The importance of the assessment of LV function to the cardiologist is in the prognosis following cardiac surgery. To the clinical pharmacologist the importance lies in the measurement of the effects of drugs and to the physiologist the understanding of the heart as a pump.

The problem remains that there is no single index of LV function which can be used to diagnose early myocardial damage.

Compensatory mechanisms for volume or pressure overload result in many of the indices mentioned below remaining normal even in the presence of some myocardial damage or disease.

Myocardial mechanics is a complex subject which cannot be covered here. The indices discussed briefly below are those which are most commonly used. None of the contractility indices are entirely independent of preload or afterload.

Compensatory autoregulation mechanisms

1 Frank–Starling effect (heterometric autoregulation). Increasing fibre length results in increased velocity of contraction. Thus an increase in end-diastolic volume results in an increased stroke volume. The descending limb of the curve does not exist in man.

2 Anrep effect (homeometric autoregulation). Increasing afterload resulting in increased contractility. Possibly due to noradrenaline release from the myocardium.

3 Bowditch effect (in ochronic autoregulation). Increasing heart rate resulting in increased contractility. Mediated via calcium flux.

These three mechanisms are independent of the sympathetic or parasympathetic system influences on the heart. During exercise the increase in cardiac output is primarily due to an increase in heart rate (and not stroke volume) mediated via the sympathetic nervous system.

Parameters of ventricular function

1 Angiographic (p. 442)

LVEDV	LV mass
LVESV	LV ejection rate
Ejection fraction	

2 Radionuclide

Ejection fraction

3 Haemodynamic

Cardiac index	Minute work index
LVEDP	LV power
Stroke work index	Myocardial O_2 consumption and efficiency

4 Pre-ejection/isovolumic phase indices

Systolic time intervals

Max dP/dt Min dP/dt

Derivatives of max dP/dt correcting for preload, e.g.

$$\frac{\text{max dP/dt}}{\text{LVEDP}}$$

V_{pm} maximum measured rate of contractile element shortening from force-velocity loop

V_{max} maximum rate of contractile element shortening at zero pressure (extrapolated from force-velocity loop)

5 Ejection phase indices (derived from echo- or angiogram), e.g. Peak V_{cf}

6 Diastolic indices

dP/dV (diastolic stiffness) or dV/dP (compliance)

Left ventricular work

Left ventricular work is commonly calculated as the LV stroke work index (LVSWI)

$$\text{LVSWI} = \text{LV} \times \text{SVI} \times 0.0136 \text{ g m/m}^2$$

where LV = mean LV pressure in mmHg during ejection (as in calculation of TTI – see Fig. 10.41)

SVI = Stroke volume index ml/m^2/beat (calculated from angiogram or from thermodilution cardiac output)

Common indices of cardiac function

Index	How derived	Normal range
Cardiac index	Cardiac output/body surface area	2.5–4.0 $l/min/m^2$
Stroke volume index (SVI)	Stroke volume/body surface area	40–70 ml/m^2
LV Stroke work index (LVSWI)	Stroke volume index × 0.0136 × Mean arterial − mean wedge pressure	40–80 g m/m^2
LV Minute work index (LVMWI)	Stroke work index × heart rate/1000	4.5–5.5 kg m/m^2/min
Systemic vascular resistance (SVR)	(a) $\frac{80\,(\overline{A_0} - \overline{RA})}{CO}$ or (b) $\frac{(\overline{PA} - \overline{PAW})}{CO}$	(a) 770–1500 dynes sec cm^{-5} (b) 10–20 units
Pulmonary vascular resistance (PVR)	(a) $\frac{80\,(\overline{PA} - \overline{PAW})}{CO}$ or (b) $\frac{(\overline{PA} - \overline{PAW})}{CO}$	(a) <200 dynes sec cm^{-5} (b) <2.5 units
Tension time index (TTI)	LV pressure during ejection × HR × systolic ejection period (mmHg.sec/min)	DPTI/TTI ratio > 0.7 (applies to TTI and DPTI)
Diastolic pressure time index (DPTI)	LV pressure during diastole ×HR × Diastolic filling period. mmHg.sec/min.	
LV dP/dt max	Differentiated LV pressure from micromanometer	Approx 1000 − 2400 mmHg/sec
V_{max}	$\frac{dP/dt}{K.P.}$	Developed pressure V_{max} Approx 2.0 − 3.3. sec^{-1}

Since planimetering the LV pressure during ejection to derive LV is time consuming, provided there is no aortic valve gradient mean aortic pressure may be used. This calculates systolic work.

Net LV work is calculated as:

$$\text{LVSWI} = (\text{LV} - \text{LVED}) \times \text{SVI} \times 0.0136$$

or

$$(A_0 - \text{PAW}) \times \text{SVI} \times 0.0136$$

Where A_0 = mean aortic pressure
PAW = mean pulmonary artery wedge pressure
LVED = mean LV end-diastolic pressure

LV minute work index

LVMWI is calculated as LVSWI $\times \dfrac{\text{HR}}{1000}$ in kg $\text{m/m}^2\text{/min}$

This allows consideration of heart rate in work calculation as HR tends to have an inverse relation with SVI.

Pressure volume loops (Fig. 10.40)
Left ventricular work may be calculated by measuring the area within a pressure volume loop. Intra-ventricular pressure is measured during an LV angiogram. By recording ECG timing on cine film instantaneous LV pressure can be calculated at any LV volume (Fig. 10.40).

The pressure volume loop is used to study LV compliance $\left(\frac{dV}{dP}\right)$ and stiffness $\left(\frac{dP}{dV}\right)$. There are major problems in the study of LV compliance as in contractility. The slope of the diastolic pressure volume plot at any instant of volume is a measure of diastolic stiffness. Assumptions from the excised dog's heart that the diastolic pressure volume relation is an exponential are not necessarily valid in man.

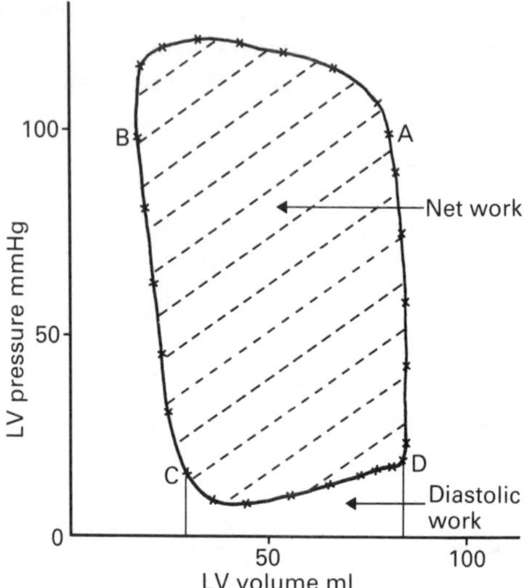

Fig. 10.40 Pressure-volume loop to show calculation of net left ventricular work. A = aortic valve opening, B = aortic valve closure, C = mitral valve opening, D = mitral valve closure.

Diastolic pressure time index/tension time index (Fig. 10.41)
The diastolic pressure time index (DPTI)/tension time index (TTI) ratio is established as a measure of subendocardial ischaemia. The DPTI gives a measurement of myocardial oxygen supply, and the TTI a measure of myocardial oxygen consumption. It is thus a supply/demand ratio (Buckberg and Hoffman).

DPTI = Mean LV pressure during diastole × diastolic filling period × heart rate

TTI = Mean LV pressure during ejection × systolic ejection period × heart rate

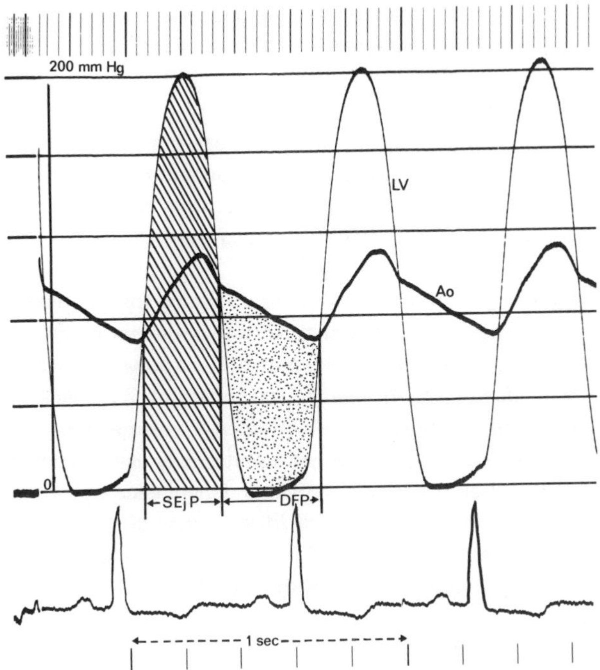

Fig. 10.41 Calculation of tension time index and diastolic pressure time index in aortic stenosis.

Figure 10.41 shows simultaneous pressure recordings of LV and aorta in a patient with aortic stenosis. The stippled area represents the area planimetred to calculate mean LV pressure in diastole and hence DPTI. The hatched area represents the area planimetred to calculate mean LV pressure in systole and hence TTI. Normal ratio = > 0.7, typical range in aortic stenosis 0.3–0.5. S Ej P = Systolic ejection period in sec/min. DFP = diastolic filling period in sec/min.

Inotropes will reduce the ratio by increasing TTI and decreasing DPTI (by shortening diastole with the inevitable chronotropic effect). Beta-blockade will increase the ratio by reducing TTI and by increasing DPTI (longer diastole).

Indices of ventricular contractility

The ideal index of contractility should be easily measurable in the contact heart, reproducible and independent of changes in preload or afterload. No ideal index exists. Only two pre-ejection phase indices will be briefly discussed.

1 Max dP/dt

The maximum rate of rise of LV pressure during the isovolumic phase is recorded via a catheter tip micromanometer in the left ventricle and the pressure differentiated. It is known that max dP/dt depends not only on the inotropic state of the muscle, but also on preload, afterload and left ventricular volume (end-diastolic fibre length). It is thus not a particularly useful index of contractility. Attempts to avoid preload dependence by deriving other indices from max dP/dt (e.g. max dP/dt ÷ LVEDP) do not solve the problem. Min dP/dt (Peak negative dP/dt) depends on the inotropic state of the muscle, and on end-systolic volume.

2 V_{max} (Fig. 10.42)

This index is defined as the maximum velocity of contractile element shortening at zero load. As with max dP/dt it is derived from hi-fidelity catheter tip manometer recordings of LV pressure. The LV pressure is differentiated and divided by the instantaneous LV pressure. This is plotted on the vertical axis with LV pressure on the horizontal axis. Using numerous assumptions about the left ventricle it can be shown that:

$$VCE = \frac{dP/dt}{KP}$$

The force-velocity loop appears as shown in Fig. 10.42.

Conversion of the vertical axis to a log scale allows for a straight line extrapolation. The extrapolation distance is shorter if 'developed pressure' is used (i.e. LVEDP).

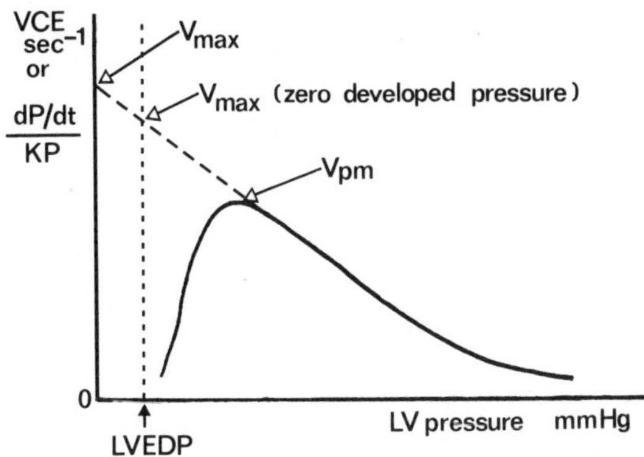

Fig. 10.42 Force-velocity loop to show extrapolation of curve to zero developed pressure (LVEDP) to calculate V_{max}. VCE = velocity of contractile element shortening (sec^{-1}). dP/dt = rate of rise of LV pressure (mmHg/sec). K = coefficient of series elasticity (calculated in dogs as = 28, but unknown in man). P = instantaneous LV pressure − LVEDP, i.e. this is developed LV pressure.

Some workers prefer to express results as KV_{max} since K, the coefficient of series elasticity, has not been calculated in man. Many of the assumptions used to generate V_{max} are generally agreed to be invalid. It is probably dependent on preload.

Systolic time intervals

This non-invasive assessment of LV function is mainly used in the study of drugs on LV performance and in the follow up of cardiac disease in a single patient. However it should not really be used in inter-patient comparisons.

Intervals measured (see Fig. 10.43)

$Q - S_2$: Onset of Q wave to onset of aortic valve closure. This is total electromechanical systole

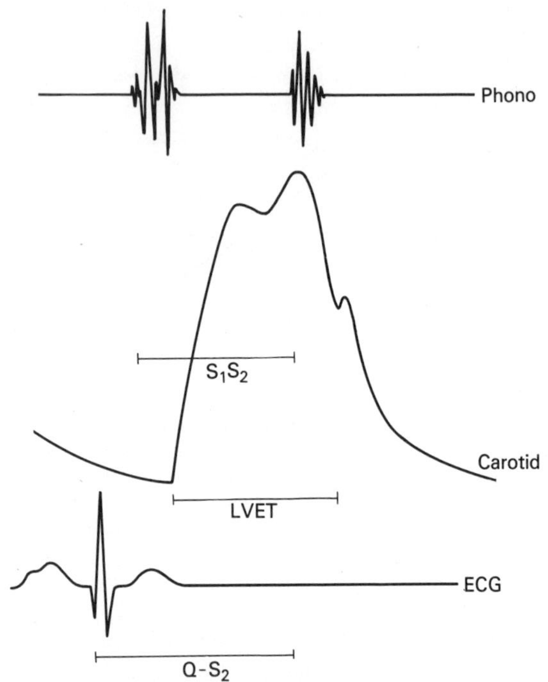

Fig. 10.43 Systolic time intervals. $Q - S_2$ = electromechanical systole. LVET = left ventricular ejection time.

LVET: LV ejection time. Onset of carotid upstroke to dicrotic notch. This interval has been shown to equal ejection time measured from the same interval in the aortic root.

PEP: Pre-ejection period. This is taken from onset of Q wave to aortic valve opening. However unless taken at cardiac catheterisation with LV and A_0 pressures recorded the non-invasive measurement is:

$$PEP = QS_2 - LVET$$

There are two components to the PEP:
(a) The electromechanical interval (Q wave to onset of systolic rise of LV pressure)
(b) The isovolumic contraction time (IVCT). Onset of rise of LV pressure to aortic valve opening

IVCT: Isovolumic contraction time = $S_1 - S_2$ interval − LVET. The exact definition of the onset of mitral valve closure from the beginning of S_1 may be difficult. It is not usually measured non-invasively. The indices QS_2, PEP, and LVET are dependent on heart rate. The ratio $\frac{PEP}{LVET}$ has been widely used to avoid this dependence.

Predicted normals (intervals in msec)

	Male	**Female**
QS_2	546 − 2.1 × HR	549 − 2.0 × HR
LVET	413 − 1.7 × HR	418 − 1.6 × HR
PEP	131 − 0.4 × HR	133 − 0.4 × HR
$\frac{PEP}{LVET}$	0.35 ± 0.04 (1SD)	

Range of abnormality of PEP/LVET in LV dysfunction:

Mild	Moderate	Severe
(0.44 − 0.52)	(0.53 − 0.6)	(>0.6)

The ratio increases with a combination of prolonged PEP and shortened LVET. The ratio may also be increased by:
- LBBB (lengthens PEP)
- beta-blockade
- reduction in LV volume, diuretics, haemorrhage

The ratio decreases (shortening of PEP) if inotropes are given (digoxin or catecholamines). Moderate aortic valve disease also reduces the ratio by lengthening the LVET. As LV function in aortic valve disease deteriorates the ratio returns towards normal. It is thus not a useful index in aortic valve disease. It has been found useful however in assessing prognosis following myocardial infarction.

Coronary artery nomenclature

Key to coronary artery anatomy Figs. 10.44 and 10.45, as seen at coronary angiography.

A	Atrial branch
AM	Acute marginal artery
AVC_x	Atrioventricular groove branch of circumflex
AVN	Atrioventricular node artery
CB	Conus branch
D	Diagonal branch of LAD
LAC	Left atrial circumflex
LAD	Left anterior descending
LAO	30° left anterior oblique projection
LAT	Left lateral projection
LMS	Left main stem
LV	Left ventricular branches
MC_x	Main circumflex
PD	Posterior descending
PLC_x	Posterolateral circumflex branch (obtuse marginal)
RA	Right atrial branch
RAO	30° right anterior oblique projection
RV	Right ventricular branch
1^{st}S	First septal perforator
S	Septal perforating arteries
SN	Sinus node artery

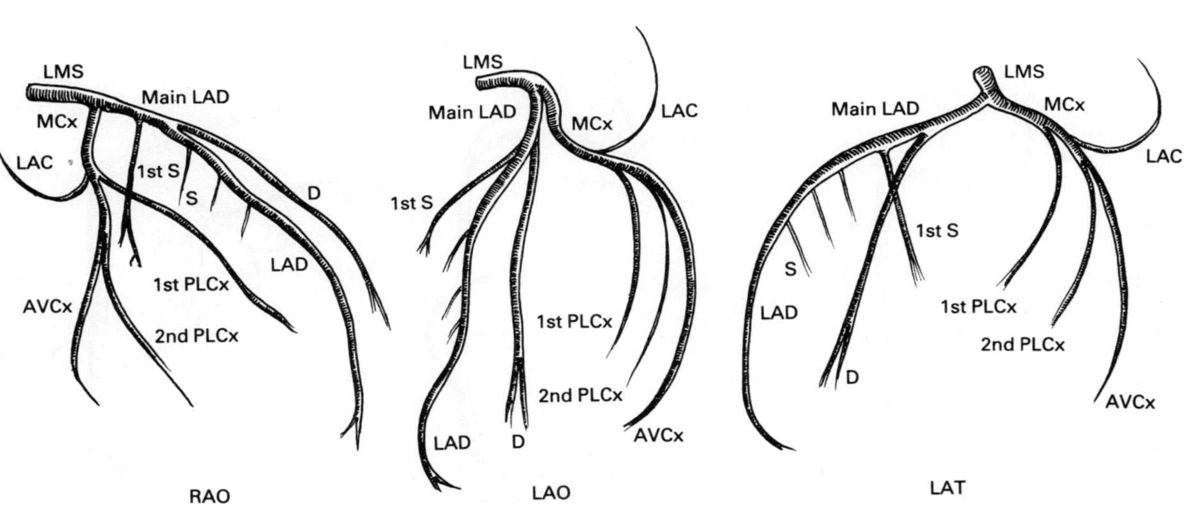

Fig. 10.44 Left coronary artery.

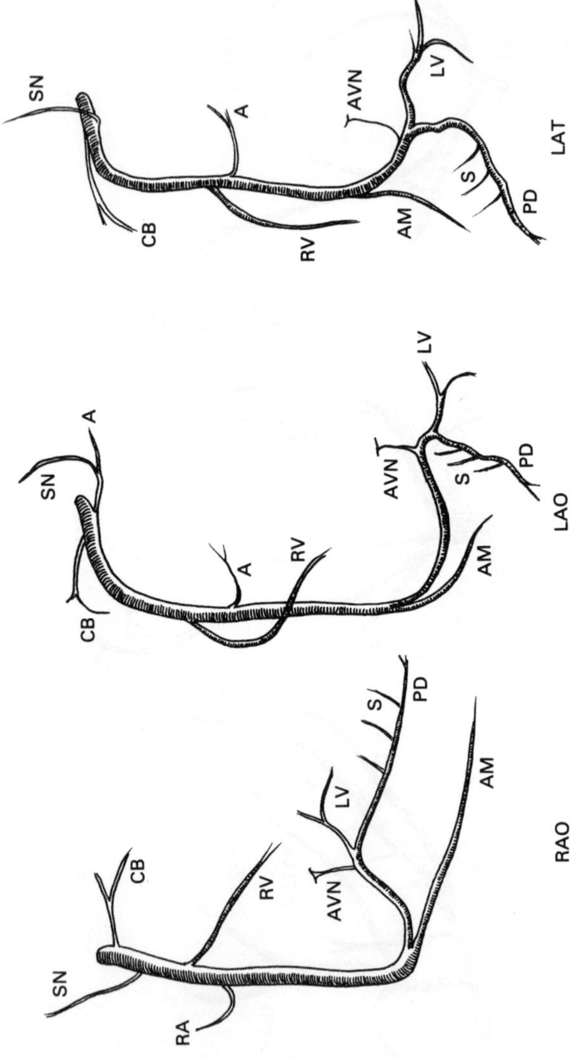

Fig. 10.45 Right coronary artery.

Appendices

Appendices

1 Nomogram for body size

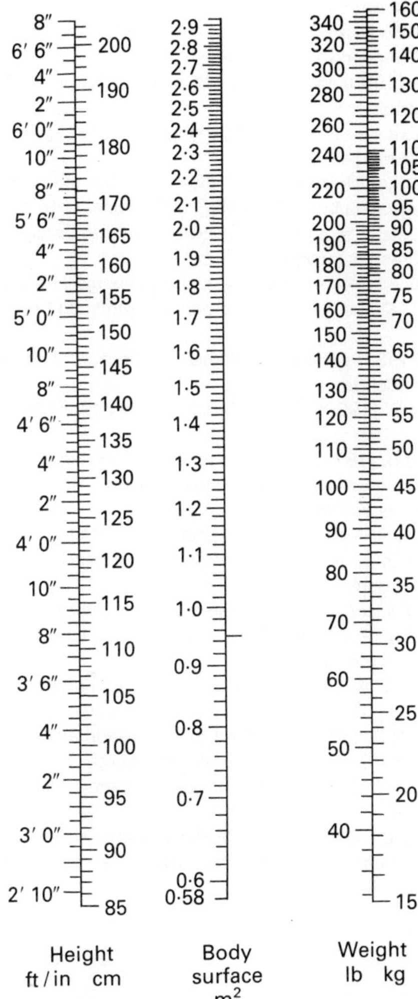

2 Further reading

Anderson R.H. & Shinebourne E.A. (eds)(1978 and 1981) *Paediatric Cardiology*. Churchill Livingstone, Edinburgh.

Bennett D.H. (1985) *Cardiac Arrhythmias*. Wright, Guildford.

Braunwald E. (ed) 1988 *Heart Disease. A Text-Book of Cardiovascular Medicine*. W.B. Saunders, Philadelphia.

Camm J. & Ward D. (1983) *Pacing for Tachycardia Control*. Telectronics, London.

Chung E.K. (1983) *Exercise Electrocardiography. Practical Approach*. Williams and Wilkins, Baltimore.

Cleland W., Goodwin J., McDonald L. & Ross D. (1969) *Medical and Surgical Cardiology*. Blackwell Scientific Publications, Oxford.

Dickinson C.J. & Marks J. (eds) (1978) *Developments in Cardiovascular Medicine*. MTP Press, Lancaster.

Feigenbaum H. (1986) *Echocardiography*. Lea and Febiger, Philadelphia.

Hamer J. (ed) (1987) *Drugs for Heart Disease*. Chapman and Hall, London.

Harrison D.C. (ed.) (1981) *Cardiac Arrythmias. A Decade of Progress*. G.K. Hall and Co, Boston.

Jefferson K. & Rees S. (1980) *Clinical Cardiac Radiology*. Butterworths, London.

Kleid J.J. & Arvan S.B. (1978) *Echocardiography. Interpretation and Diagnosis*. Appleton-Century-Crofts, New York.

Opie L.H. (1987) *Drugs and the Heart*. The Lancet.

Oram S. (1981) *Clinical Heart Disease*. Heinemann, London.

Perloff J.K. (1987) *Clinical Recognition of Congenital Heart Disease*. W.B. Saunders, Philadelphia.

Schrire V. (1971) *Clinical Cardiology*. Staples Press, London.

Sokolow M. & McIlroy M.B. (1986) *Clinical Cardiology*. Lange Medical Publications, Los Altos, California.

Varriale P. & Naclerio E.A. (1979) *Cardiac Pacing*. Lea and Febiger, Philadelphia.

Verel D. & Grainger R.G. (1978) *Cardiac Catheterisation and Angiocardiography*. Churchill Livingstone, Edinburgh.

Weyman A.E. (1982) *Cross-Sectional Echocardiography*. Lea and Febiger, New York.

Yang S.S., Bentivoglio L.G., Maranhao V. & Goldberg H. (1978) *From Cardiac Catheterisation Data to Haemodynamic Parameters*. F.A. Davis Company, Philadelphia.

3 Useful addresses

British Heart Foundation, 102 Gloucester Place, London W1H 4DH. *Tel:* 01-935-0185

British Cardiac Society, 7 St Andrews Places, Regents Park, London NW1 4LB. *Tel:* 01-486-6430

British Heart Journal or Cardiovascular Research, BMA House, Tavistock Square, London WC1H 9JR. *Tel:* 01-387-4499

British Pacing Group, 47 Wimpole Street, London W1. *Tel:* 01-953-3259

European Heart Journal (Journal of the European Society of Cardiology), Academic Press (London), 24–28 Oval Road, London NW1 7DX
or
Academic Press Inc, 111 Fifth Avenue, New York 10003

American College of Cardiology, Heart House, 9111 Old Georgetown Road, Bethesda, Maryland, MD 20814

American Heart Association or Circulation, 7320 Greenville Avenue, Dallas, Texas 75231

America Heart Journal, C.V. Mosby Co, 11830 Westline Industrial Drive, St Louis MO 63141

American Journal of Cardiology, 875 Third Avenue, New York NY 10022

Journal of the American College of Cardiology, Elsevier Science Publishing Co Inc, 52 Vanderbilt Avenue, New York, NY 10017.

NASPE, North American Society of Pacing and Electrophysiology, 13 Eaton Court, Wellesley Hills, MA 02181. *Tel:* (617) 237-1866

4 List of abbreviations

ACE	Angiotensin converting enzyme
AF	Atrial fibrillation
AML	Anterior mitral leaflet
ANF	Antinuclear factor
AP	Aortopulmonary
APD	Action potential duration
APSAC	Anisoylated plasminogen streptokinase activator complex
AS	Aortic stenosis
ASD	Atrial septal defect
AV	Atrioventricular
AVD	Aortic valve disease
AVR	Aortic valve replacement
BCR	British corrected ratio
CAD	Coronary artery disease
CCF	Congestive cardiac failure
CFT	Complement fixation test
COCM	Congestive cardiomyopathy
CVS	Cardiovascular system
CW	Continuous wave Doppler
CxR	Chest x-ray
Dd	Diastolic dimension
DFP	Diastolic filling period
DOLV	Double outlet left ventricle
DORV	Double outlet right ventricle
DPTI	Diastolic pressure time index
ERP	Effective refractory period
ESR	Erythrocyte sedimentation rate
FDPs	Fibrin degradation products
HRAE	High right atrial electrogram
HOCM	Hypertrophic obstructive cardiomyopathy
HV	His-ventricular
IABP	Intra-aortic balloon pumping
ISA	Intrinsic sympathomimetic activity
IVS	Interventricular septum
JVP	Jugular venous pulse

4 List of abbreviations

LA	Left atrium
LAD	Left axis deviation. Left anterior descending
LAHB	Left anterior hemiblock
LAID	Left atrial internal dimension
LAO	Left anterior oblique projection
LAT	Lateral projection
LBBB	Left bundle branch block
LPHB	Left posterior hemiblock
LSE	Left sternal edge
LV	Left ventricle
LVEDP	Left ventricular end-diastolic pressure
LVEDV	Left ventricle end-diastolic volume
LVESV	Left ventricle end-systolic volume
LVET	Left ventricular ejection time
LVF	Left ventricular failure
LVFP	Left ventricular filling pressure
LVIDd	Left ventricular internal dimension at end-diastole
LVIDs	Left ventricular internal dimension at end-systole
LVMWI	Left ventricular minute work index
LVOT	Left ventricular outflow tract obstruction
LVSWI	Left ventricular stroke work index
MAOIs	Monoamine oxidase inhibitors
MB	Creatine phosphokinase isoenzyme of cardiac muscle
MIC	Minimum inhibitory concentration
MR	Mitral regurgitation
MS	Mitral stenosis
MV	Mitral valve
MVR	Mitral valve replacement
NYHA	New York Heart Association
PA	Pulmonary artery
PAEDP	Pulmonary artery end-diastolic pressure
PATB	Paroxysmal atrial tachycardia with varying block
PAW	Pulmonary artery wedge
PDA	Patent ductus arteriosus
PE	Pulmonary embolism
PEP	Pre-ejection period
PFO	Patent foramen ovale
PGE_2	Prostaglandin E_2
PGI_2	Prostaglandin I_2
PHT	Pulmonary hypertension
PLVW	Posterior left ventricular wall

4 List of abbreviations

PND	Paroxysmal nocturnal dyspnoea
PR	Pulmonary regurgitation
PS	Pulmonary stenosis
PTCA	Percutaneous transluminal coronary angioplasty
PVR	Pulmonary vascular resistance
PW	Pulsed wave Doppler
PXE	Pseudoxanthoma elasticum
RA	Right atrium
RAD	Right axis deviation
RAO	Right anterior oblique projection
RBBB	Right bundle branch block
REM	Rapid eye movement
rt-PA	Recombinant tissue plasminogen activator
RV	Right ventricle
RVEDP	Right ventricular end-diastolic pressure
RVID	Right ventricular internal dimension
RVOT	Right ventricular outflow tract
SAM	Systolic anterior movement of the mitral valve
SACT	Sino-atrial conduction time
S Ej P	Systolic ejection period
SLE	Systemic lupus erythematosus
SNRT	Sinus node recovery time
SSS	Sick sinus syndrome
SV	Stroke volume
SVC	Superior vena cava
SVT	Supra-ventricular tachycardia
TAPVD	Total anomalous pulmonary venous drainage
TGA	Transposition of the great arteries
TS	Tricuspid stenosis
TSH	Thyroid stimulating hormone
TR	Tricuspid regurgitation
TS	Tricuspid stenosis
TTI	Tension time index
TV	Tricuspid valve
TXA_2	Thromboxane A_2
VCE	Velocity of contractile element shortening
VCF	Velocity of circumferential fibre shortening
VPB	Ventricular premature beats
VSD	Ventricular septal defect
VT	Ventricular tachycardia

4 List of abbreviations

WPW	Wolff–Parkinson–White.
WT	Wall thickness

Index

Index

Index

Index